ALLE ZEIT WACH
SJ
1842

Investigative Urology 3

Edited by
H. Rübben · D. Jocham · G. H. Jacobi

With 180 Figures and 42 Tables

Springer-Verlag Berlin Heidelberg New York
London Paris Tokyo Hong Kong

Volume 1 of the series "Investigative Urology" is "Experimentelle Urologie" edited by R. Harzmann, G. H. Jacobi, L. Weißbach, 1985

Professor Dr. HERBERT RÜBBEN
Knappschaftskrankenhaus Bardenberg
Abteilung Urologie
Dr.-Hans-Böckler-Platz 1, D-5102 Würselen 1

Professor Dr. DIETER JOCHAM
Urologische Klinik und Poliklinik
Klinikum Großhadern
Ludwig-Maximilian-Universität München
Marchioninistr. 15, D-8000 München 80

Professor Dr. GÜNTHER H. JACOBI
Urologische Fachpraxis
Friedrich-Ebert-Str. 176, D-4100 Duisburg 18

ISBN-13:978-3-642-74440-2 e-ISBN-13:978-3-642-74438-9
DOI: 10.1007/978-3-642-74438-9

Product Liability: The publisher can give no guarantee for information about drug dosage and application thereof contained in this book. In every individual case the respective user must check its accuracy by consulting other pharmaceutical literature.

2122/3130-543210 – Printed on acid-free paper

List of Contributors

The addresses are given at the beginning of each contribution

Preface

The first symposium of the working group on experimental urology of the German Society of Urology was held in Cologne in 1972. It was meant to be a platform to present and, in particular, to discuss experimental studies developing new diagnostic and therapeutic approaches, and to promote innovation in urology in Germany. This plan was well received, and during the last 16 years both the number of participants from other European and overseas countries and the number and quality of presentations have been continuously increasing. At the most recent meeting, held in Aachen in 1988, new data were presented on renal cell cancer, andrology, prostatic cancer and adenoma, bladder cancer, urinary diversion, urodynamics, renal pathophysiology, transplantation and the pathogenesis and treatment of urolithiasis.

The present book contains 44 of the 109 papers given at the Aachen meeting, covering both basic and clinical research. It will be of eminent interest to all scientifically minded urologists, oncologists, neurophysiologists, endocrinologists, and pathologists because it is a synopsis of all the major scientific research currently being conducted in urology in Europe. There are no other books available which offer as comprehensive a coverage of recent experimental issues in urology. The aim of the series *Investigative Urology* is to demonstrate the continuous development of research in urology and to encourage all colleagues interested in experimental urology to continue their important activities and create new international cooperation.

Aachen — H. Rübben
Munich — D. Jocham
Duisburg — G. H. Jacobi

Preface

Contents

III. BPH-Prostate Cancer

IV. Bladder Cancer

V. Urodynamics

VI. Kidney Trauma, Pathophysiology, Urolithiasis

Contents

I. Renal Cancer

Biological Markers in the Evaluation of Prognosis in Patients with Renal Cell Carcinoma*

B. J. Schmitz-Dräger[1], D. Rohde[1], H. Frenzel[2], and R. Ackermann[1]

Introduction

Successful treatment of malignant disease is based on extensive knowledge of the biology of a given tumor and, as a consequence, the prognosis of the disease. At the moment, only a few parameters are known which correlate with the prognosis of renal cell carcinoma (RCC). Several investigators could demonstrate a close correlation between tumor stage and patient survival (Böttiger 1970; Golimbu et al. 1986; Giuliani et al. 1983; Klöppel et al. 1986; Robson et al. 1969). The impact of the tumor grade on the prognosis of the disease is a matter of discussion. While some authors report a good correlation between tumor grade and the course of the disease, this could not be confirmed by others (Donhuijsen 1986; Fuhrman et al. 1982; Klöppel et al. 1986; Kofler et al. 1975; Syrjänen and Hjelt 1978). Recently, the value of biological markers, e.g., DNA content, the expression of differentiation or proliferation antigens and of antigens belonging to the cytoskeleton, has been investigated (Bohle et al. 1986; Fleming and Symes 1987; Fleming and Brown 1987; Ljungberg et al. 1986; Loy et al. 1986).

The monoclonal antibody Due ABC 3 recognizes an antigen which is present on the membrane of urothelial tumor cells but not on normal urothelium. The specificity analysis demonstrates cross reactions with proximal tubular epithelium and some renal cell carcinoma specimens (Schmitz-Dräger et al. 1988). The aim of this retrospective analysis is to investigate whether the expression of the ABC 3 antigen is correlated with the course of disease in patients with RCC.

Materials and Methods

A total of 64 patients who underwent nephrectomy between 1979 and 1983 were investigated. In 59 patients retrospective tumor staging was performed according to the recommendations of the UICC from 1987 (Hermanek 1986). Of these, 21 patients had a RCC stage 2, 16 stage 3, and 22 patients with lymph node or distant metastases were classified as stage 4. The determination of the tumor grade was performed according to the criteria proposed by Hermanek and coworkers (Hermanek et al. 1976). Follow-up data could be obtained from 49 patients, who were either alive at

* Supported by the Bundesminister für Forschung und Technologie and the Minister für Wissenschaft und Forschung des Landes Nordrhein-Westfalen, FRG

[1] Department of Urology, University of Düsseldorf, Medical School, Moorenstr. 5, 4000 Düsseldorf, FRG

[2] Institute of Pathology, University of Düsseldorf, FRG

Investigative Urology 3
Edited by H. Rübben et al.

the time of the investigation or had died from their tumor. The follow-up interval ranged from 5 to 9.5 years.

The production of monoclonal antibody Due ABC 3 was performed using a modification of the hybridoma technique as described by Köhler and Milstein (1975). Details have been reported recently (Schmitz-Dräger et al. 1988). Briefly, bladder tumor cell line SW 1710, which was established from a moderately differentiated bladder tumor, was used as immunogen (Wright et al. 1981). Spleen cells of an immunized BALB/c mouse and the nonimmunoglobulin-secreting myeloma cell line X63-Ag8.563 were fused using polyethylene glycol 1500 as fusing agent (Kearny et al. 1979). Hybridoma cells were cultured, expanded, and cloned by limiting dilution. Specificity analysis was performed on shock frozen sections derived from tissues of various origin.

The immunohistochemical investigation was performed on deparaffined 5–6 µm sections. Endogenous peroxidases were blocked with 3% H_2O_2 in methanol at 4°C for 30 min. After washing in phosphate buffered saline (PBS) 0.1 ml tissue culture supernatant containing monoclonal antibody (mAb) Due ABC 3 was given on the sections and incubated for 12–20 h at room temperature. After removal of free mAb by washing in PBS the sections were incubated subsequently with peroxidase-labeled rabbit anti-mouse immunoglobulin and goat anti-rabbit immunoglobulin antisera (JRL, West Grove, PA, USA; 1:100 in PBS) for 30 min at room temperature. The enzyme reaction was started adding 0.05% diaminobenzidine and 0.01% H_2O_2 in PBS. After 10 min in complete darkness the reaction was terminated by washing the slides with PBS. Counterstaining was performed with hemalum for 10 s. The slides were mounted and examined. The percentage of positive tumor cells was analysed by two independent investigators. At least 200 cells were examined. The results were attributed to three different grades: grade 1 (61%–100%), grade 2 (31%–60%), grade 3 (0%–30%), based on the number of positive tumor cells.

Results

Table 1 demonstrates the distribution of tumor stage and tumor grade. The tumor grade was found to be equally distributed in all tumor stages. Grade 2 tumors were predominantly represented (33/56). The distribution of tumor stage and the percent-

Table 1. Distribution of tumor stage and tumor grade in patients with renal cell carcinoma

Tumor grade	Tumor stage: 2	3	4
1	1	2	0
2	12	10	11
3	8	3	9

Table 2. Distribution of tumor stage and amount of ABC 3 antigen-positive cells in renal cell carcinoma

ABC 3 antigen-positive cells (%)	Tumor stage: 2	3	4
61–100	17	6	3
31– 60	1	4	2
0– 30	3	6	17

Table 3. Correlation between prognosis and tumor stage in patients with renal cell carcinoma

Tumor stage	Prognosis: (within the follow-up interval)	
	Death from disease	Survival
2	3	8
3	5	6
4	11	2

Table 4. Correlation between prognosis and tumor grade in renal cell carcinoma

Tumor grade	Prognosis: (within the follow-up interval)	
	Death from disease	Survival
1	1	1
2	14	18
3	7	7

Table 5. Correlation between prognosis and percentage of ABC 3 antigen-positive cells in renal cell carcinoma

ABC 3 antigen-positive cells (%)	Prognosis: (within the follow-up interval)	
	Death from disease	Survival
61–100	6	17
31– 60	4	2
0– 30	13	7

Table 6. The development of local recurrence or distant metastases in patients with renal cell carcinoma stages 2 and 3 in correlation with the amount of ABC 3 antigen-positive tumor cells

ABC 3 antigen-positive cells (%)	Local recurrence/distant metastases after nephrectomy (within the follow-up interval)	
	+	–
61–100	2	15
31– 60	0	1
0– 30	5	5

age of ABC 3 positive cells are listed in Table 2. A negative correlation between tumor stage and expression of the ABC 3 antigen was observed. While 17 out of 21 tumor specimens (81%) from patients with RCC stage 2 had a high amount of antigen-positive cells, 17 out of 22 specimens (77%) derived from patients with RCC stage 4 were either antigen-negative or had less than 30% ABC 3-positive tumor cells.

The correlation between tumor stage and prognosis of disease is demonstrated in Table 3. While 8 out of 11 patients (73%) with RCC stage 2 were still alive after at least 5 years of follow-up this was only true for 2 out of 13 patients (15%) suffering from metastasized RCC. No correlation was observed between survival and tumor grade (Table 4). In all tumor grades approximately 50% of the patients were alive after more than 5 years. In contrast, a good correlation was found comparing patient survival and the loss of ABC 3 antigen expression (Table 5): 74% of patients with a high amount and 35% of those with a low percentage of ABC 3 antigen-positive cells survived during the follow-up interval.

Some 27 patients with RCC stages 2 and 3, who were nephrectomized with curative intention, were evaluated for the appearance of late metastases or local tumor recurrence (Table 6). Out of 17 patients with a high percentage of ABC 3 antigen-positive tumor cells (12%) developed tumor recurrence within the follow-up interval. However, in 5 out of 10 patients (50%) with a loss of the ABC 3 antigen, metastases or local tumor recurrence occurred.

Discussion

The most common tumor-related parameter is the determination of the tumor grade. However, the morphological diversity of the RCC led to the proposal of different grading classifications. Besides those based on histological and/or cytological criteria, others have been reported relying exclusively on the nuclear morphology (Donhuijsen 1986; Hermanek et al. 1976; Syrjänen and Hjelt 1978; Thoenes et al. 1985). A poor correlation between histological classifications and the course of the disease has been reported by other investigators (Donhuijsen 1986; Klöppel et al. 1986; Syrjänen and Hjelt 1978). This observation was confirmed here.

The immunohistochemical investigation of RCC for different antigens, e.g., differentiation antigens, tumor or proliferation antigens, and antigens belonging to the cytoskeleton, has been reported (Bohle et al. 1986; Fleming and Symes 1987; Fleming and Brown 1987; Loy et al. 1986). Fleming and Symes investigated the expression of different cytokeratins in RCC (Fleming and Symes 1987). No significant difference of the binding pattern between normal renal tissue and tumor tissue was observed. In contrast, another component of the cytoskeleton, vimentin, was found to be preferably expressed in tumor tissue as compared with normal kidney (Fleming and Brown 1987).

Loy and coworkers reported on the expression of the S-phase antigen Ki-67 in RCC specimens (Loy et al. 1986). The amount of Ki-67-positive tumor cells ranged between 0.4% and 25%. No correlation was observed between the tumor grade and the percentage of Ki-67-positive cells. Bohle and coworkers investigated 27 RCC specimens for the presence of various antigens (Bohle et al. 1986). Using monoclonal antibody 28 C 1, directed against an antigen present on proximal tubular epithelium, they found a negative correlation between tumor grade and expression of the corresponding antigen (Falkenberg et al. 1981). A positive correlation was observed between tumor grade and the expression of vimentin and the proliferation antigen TPA (Bohle et al. 1986). However, until now the expression of these markers was only correlated with tumor stage or grade. A confirmation of the predictive value of these markers for the patient's survival is still lacking. A major handicap is the sensitivity of most markers against fixatives, e.g., formaldehyde or acetone, thus not allowing a retrospective analysis of fixed tumor specimens.

The present study demonstrates that the loss of the expression of the ABC 3 antigen is indicative of an unfavourable prognosis. This is also suggested by the negative correlation between tumor stage and the expression of the ABC 3 antigen. The poor correlation between tumor grade and other parameters related to patient survival confirms the observations of other authors who concluded that a tumor grading based exclusively on histological criteria does not reflect the prognosis of patients with RCC (Böttiger 1970; Skinner et al. 1971; Lieber et al. 1981). The combination of several parameters related to the course of the disease might be helpful to identify those patients with an increased risk of tumor recurrence, who require follow-up investigations within short intervals in order to recognize a tumor recurrence as early as possible.

References

Bohle B, Waldherr R, Schwechheimer K, Moldenhauer G, Momburg F (1986) Immunhistochemische Charakterisierung von Nierenzellkarzinomen. Verh Dtsch Ges Pathol 70:274–278

Böttiger LE (1970) Prognosis in renal carcinoma. Cancer 26:780–787

Donhuijsen K (1986) Nierenzellkarzinome: Prognostische Bedeutung der Zellkerngröße. Verh Dtsch Ges Pathol 70:634

Falkenberg FW, Ruffelmann HB, Müller E, Gutenberg W, Behrendt B, Waks T (1981) Monoclonal antibodies against antigens in the human kidney. In: Hämmerling GJ, Hämmerling U, Kearney JF (eds) Monoclonal antibodies and T-cell hybridomas. Elsevier/North-Holland, Amsterdam, pp 148–155

Fleming S, Brown G (1987) The expression of 3-fucosylated-*N*-acetyl lactosamine carbohydrate determinants in renal tumours. Histopathol 11:171–182

Fleming S, Symes CE (1987) The distribution of cytokeratin antigens in the kidney and in renal tumours. Histopathol 11:157–170

Fuhrman SA, Lasky LC, Limas C (1982) Prognostic significance of morphologic parameters in renal cell carcinoma. Am J Surg Pathol 6:655–663

Giuliani L, Martorana G, Giberti C, Pescatore D, Magnani C (1983) Results of radical nephrectomy with extensive lymphadenectomy for renal cell carcinoma. J Urol 130:664–668

Golimbu M, Joshi P, Sperber A, Tessler A, Al-Askari S, Morales P (1986) Renal cell carcinoma: survival and prognostic factors. Urology 27:291–301

Hermanek P (1986) Neue TNM/pTNM-Klassifikation und Stadieneinteilung urologischer Tumoren ab 1987. Urologe (B) 26:193–197

Hermanek P, Sigel A, Chlepas S (1976) Histological grading of renal cell carcinoma. Eur Urol 2: 189–292

Kearny JF, Radbruch A, Liesegang B, Rajewsky K (1979) A new mouse myeloma cell line that has lost immunoglobulin expression but permits the construction of antibody-secreting hybrid cell lines. J Immunol 123:1548–1550

Klöppel G, Knöfel WT, Baisch H, Otto U (1986) Prognosis of renal cell carcinoma related to nuclear grade, DNA content and Robson stage. Eur Urol 12:426–431

Kofler K, Reichl ER, Zischka-Konorsa W (1975) Statistische Untersuchungen zur Frage der Beziehungen zwischen Morphologie und Prognose bei Nierenparenchymcarcinomen. Virchows Arch [A] 368:347–359

Köhler G, Milstein C (1975) Continuous culture of fused cells secreting antibody of predefined specificity. Nature 256:495–497

Lieber MM, Tomera FM, Taylor WF, Farrow GM (1981) Renal adenocarcinoma in young adults: survival and variables affecting prognosis. J Urol 125:164–168

Ljungberg B, Forsslund G, Stenling R, Zetterberg A (1986) The prognostic significance of nuclear DNA content in renal cell carcinoma. J Urol 135:422–426

Loy V, Krech R, Gerdes J, Kramer W, Stein H (1986) Malignitätsgrad und Wachstumsfraktion beim Nierenzellkarzinom. Verh Dtsch Ges Pathol 70:633

Robson CJ, Churchill BM, Anderson W (1969) The results of radical nephrectomy for renal cell carcinoma. J Urol 101:297–301

Schmitz-Dräger BJ, Rohde D, Peschkes C, Ebert T, Ackermann R (1988) Monoklonale Antikörper gegen Harnblasenkarzinome – ein Beitrag zur Verbesserung der Diagnostik? Akt Urol 19: 217–223

Skinner DG, Colvin RB, Vermillion CD, Pfister RC, Leadbetter WF (1971) The diagnosis and management of renal cell carcinoma: a clinical and pathologic study of 309 cases. Cancer 28: 1165–1177

Syrjänen K, Hjelt L (1978) Grading of human renal adenocarcinoma. Scand J Urol Nephrol 12: 49–55

Thoenes W, Störkel St, Rumpelt HJ (1985) Pathomorphologische Systematik und Nomenklatur der Nierenzelltumoren (insbesondere Nierenzellkarzinome) der Erwachsenen. Verh Dtsch Ges Pathol 69:429

Wright WC, Daniels WP, Fogh J (1981) Distinction of seventy-one cultured human tumor cell lines by polymorphic enzyme analysis. J Natl Cancer Inst 66:239–247

Comparison of Human Normal Renal Cells and Malignant Renal Cells In Vivo and In Vitro Using Cytological, Cytochemical, and Immunocytochemical Methods

W. DE RIESE[1], E. P. ALLHOFF[1], U. POHL[1], G. LENIS[1], S. LIEDKE[1], Z. ATAY[2], U. JONAS[1], and S. O. WARNAAR[3]

Introduction

In vitro culturing of subprimary cells obtained from solid tumors often leaves differentiation of dignity equivocal. Employing conventional cytological, cytochemical, and immunocytochemical measures we tried to characterize benign and malignant renal cells (RCC) in vivo and in vitro. The preparation of solid tumor tissue itself does not necessarily result in unadulterated tumor cell cultures. Our intention, therefore, was to develop a fast as well as practicable method to determine the percentage of tumor cells within the primary cultures. Up to now there has been a lot of experience as far as cytological diagnosis in vivo is concerned but limited information regarding in vitro preparations (Morasca 1976; Thoenes 1986).

Material and Methods

Tumor tissue and normal kidney tissue of 10 patients were prepared and analyzed. According to the method recently described (Kovacs et al. 1987), the procedure of

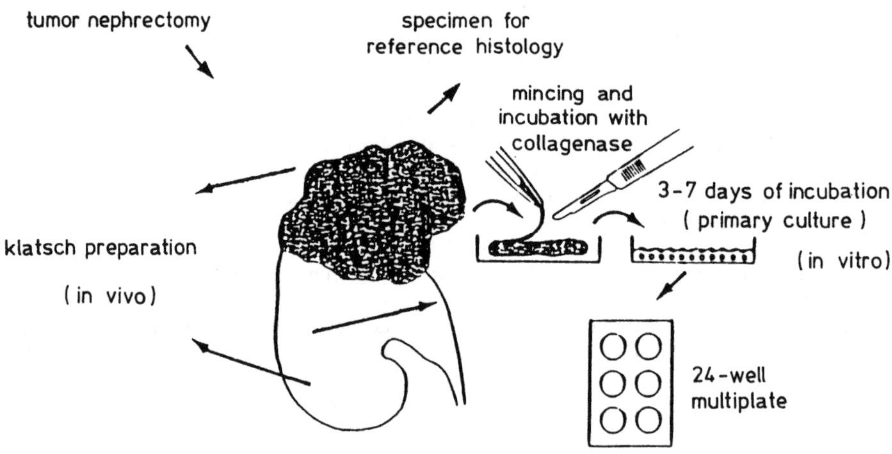

Fig. 1. In vivo and in vitro preparation of normal and malignant renal cells

[1] Dept. of Urology, Medical School Hannover, Konstanty-Gutschow-Str. 8, 3000 Hannover 61, FRG
[2] Fachpraxis für Zytologie, Siegesstr. 8, 3000 Hannover 1, FRG
[3] Centocor Comp., Leiden, The Netherlands

Investigative Urology 3
Edited by H. Rübben et al.

cell preparation was chosen as follows: tumors from previously untreated patients were obtained by conventional tumor nephrectomy and a macroscopically homogeneous area lacking fibrosis, necrosis, or hemorrhage was excised for preparation. Figure 1 exhibits schematically the tumor cell preparation. One sample of the excised tumor tissue was taken for conventional klatsch preparation and another one for in vitro cell preparation. A third one was taken for histological examination as a "reference slide."

Preparation of Primary Cell Cultures

Samples of tumor tissue were cut into pieces of approximately 2–3 mm^3 and minced with a surgical scalpel under sterile conditions in a petri dish containing RPMI 1640 medium. Subsequently, the minced tissue was washed twice in PBS. The small fragments, thus freed from cell debris, were incubated for 2–3 h in 0.1% collagenase (Worthlington CLS III) and then dissolved in culture medium (RPMI 1640 supplemented with 15% fetal calf serum and 1% penicillin) for 30–60 min at 37°C. The tissue fragments were centrifuged and washed twice in medium. Finally, the samples were resuspended in a centrifuge tube containing 2–4 ml culture medium and dispersed vigorously with a pasteur pipette.

The suspension was sedimented for 1 min and the supernatant, containing over 90% of single cells with low viability and the cell debris, was decanted. The pellet, consisting of over 90% of small cell clusters with approximately 10–15 cells, was resuspended and seeded in culture. The cell clusters were incubated at 37°C in a humidified atmosphere with 5% CO_2 in 25 cm^3 Falcon flasks (Biochrom, Berlin) containing 5 ml culture medium each. During in vitro growth the cells were observed with an inverted phase-contrast microscope. The small cell clusters attached to the flasks within 24 h and grew out to a near confluent monolayer, in most cases within 3–7 days after seeding.

Preparation of In Vitro Slides

After decanting the medium of the primary cultures, the cells were washed twice with warm (37°C) trypsin to remove cell debris and remaining blood cells. Half of the cell clusters were transferred to another 25 cm^2 flask for further subculturing processes, the other half was equally pipetted into a 24-well multiplate containing 3 ml culture medium (without any antibiotics) per well. Each well was equipped with one plastic "Thermanox" platelet (NUNC, Wiesbaden, FRG). This approved technique was developed at our institution to increase the amount of cells on the slides, thus diminishing the loss of material, because cells grow much better on the rougher surface of plastic than on glass. About 3–7 days later the cells had grown out to a confluent monolayer. The platelets were air dried and then attached to conventional glass slides by using a special adhesive (Loctite, FRG). Subsequently, the slides were stained for further diagnosis.

Staining Methods

Pappenheim and Papanicolaou staining were used for cytomorphological judgement; for cytochemical diagnosis periodic acid-Schiff reaction (PAS), and staining for alka-

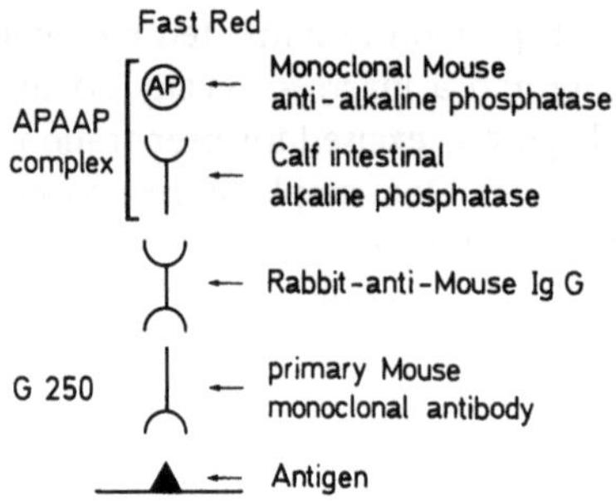

Fig. 2. Immunocytochemical labeling using the monoclonal antibody G 250 and the alkaline phosphatase anti-alkaline phosphatase *(APAAP)* complex

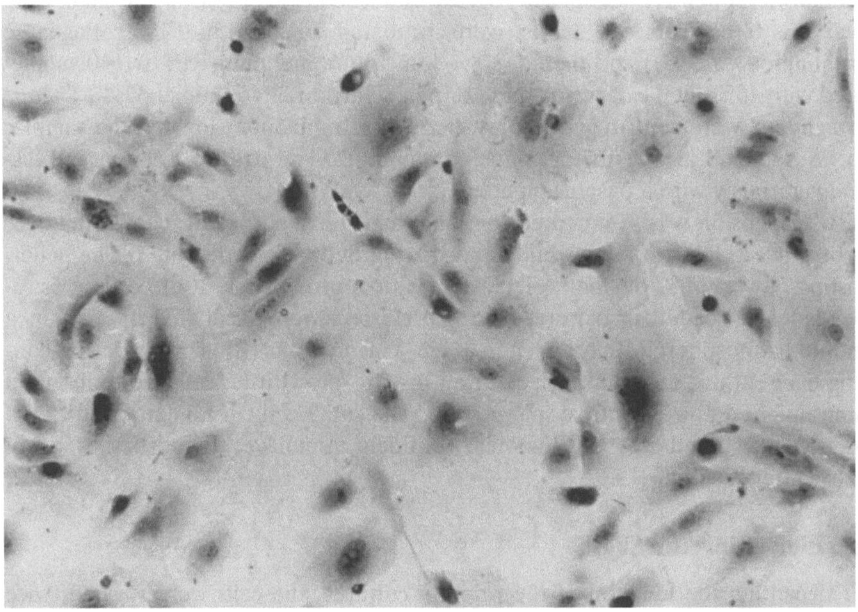

Fig. 3. In vitro normal renal cells stained with the G 250 technique; original magnification × 140

line and acid phosphatase as well as for the unspecific esterase were employed. Two monoclonal antibodies against tumor-associated antigens (CEA and G 250) were chosen for immunocytochemical examination.

CEA is a well-known antigen, whereas G 250 was first isolated and described in 1986 by Oosterwijk et al. The antibody against G 250 – a subclass of IgG – recognizes a specific antigen, which is only expressed on the surface of RCC cells but not on cells of normal proximal tubular epithelium (Oosterwijk et al. 1986b). It's staining pattern differs from that of other RCC-related antibodies (Oosterwijk et al. 1986b; Bander et al. 1983; Bander 1984).

The staining technique detecting G 250 corresponds with that used for Ki-67 described earlier in detail by Gerdes (1985) and delineated schematically in Fig. 2. The acetone and cloroform fixed cells are exposed for approximately 30 min to the mono-

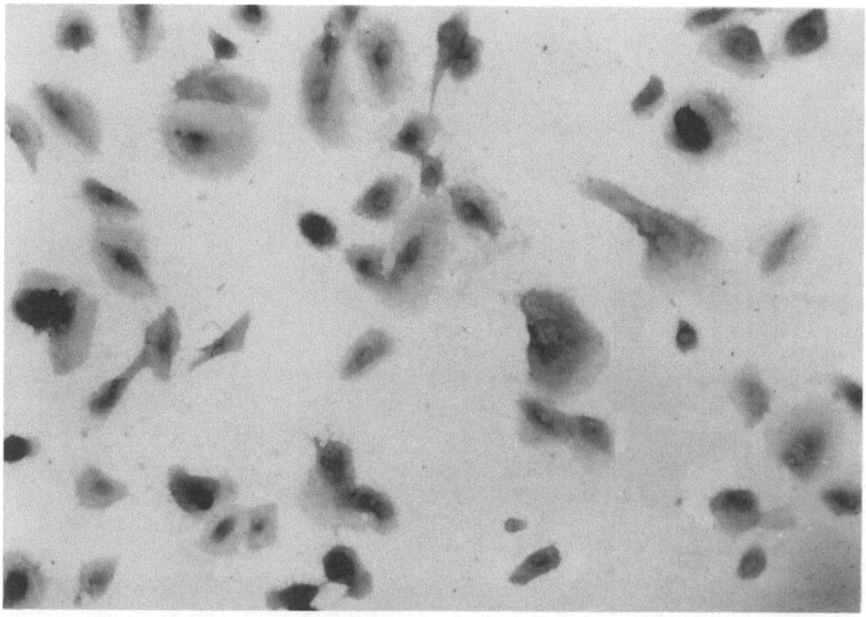

Fig. 4. In vitro malignant renal cells (RCC) stained with the G 250 technique original magnification ×140

clonal antibody diluted in RPMI 1640 medium. After washing in Tris-buffered solution (pH 7.4–7.6), the cells are incubated with rabbit mouse-specific IgG and after another washing with the alkaline phosphatase anti-alkaline phosphatase (APAAP) complex (Cordell et al. 1984). Subsequently, the slides are stained with fast red and counterstained with hemalum. Presence of the specific antigen is indicated by a red color reaction instead of the blue counterstaining (Figs. 3 and 4).

Results

Cytomorphological Examination

Since Papanicolaou stain exhibits a less precise pattern of cytological characteristics, such as granula and delicate shades of color of the cytoplasm, than the Pappenheim stain, we preferred the latter for examination. The air-dried and Pappenheim-stained in vivo and in vitro slides were examined by an experienced cytologist. He compared the cultured benign as well as malignant cells with the corresponding in vivo klatsch slides, trying to characterize normal renal and RCC cells in vitro by conventional cytology. Figures 5–8 are the in vivo and in vitro slides of normal and malignant renal cells.

Comparing the in vivo klatsch preparations (Figs. 5, 6) different patterns could be observed: Cells of normal kidney were isomorphic with round and smooth-faced nuclei and homogeneous chromatin. In contrast to this, the malignant cells were pleomorphic, with different sized and sometimes with hyperchromatic nuclei. Fur-

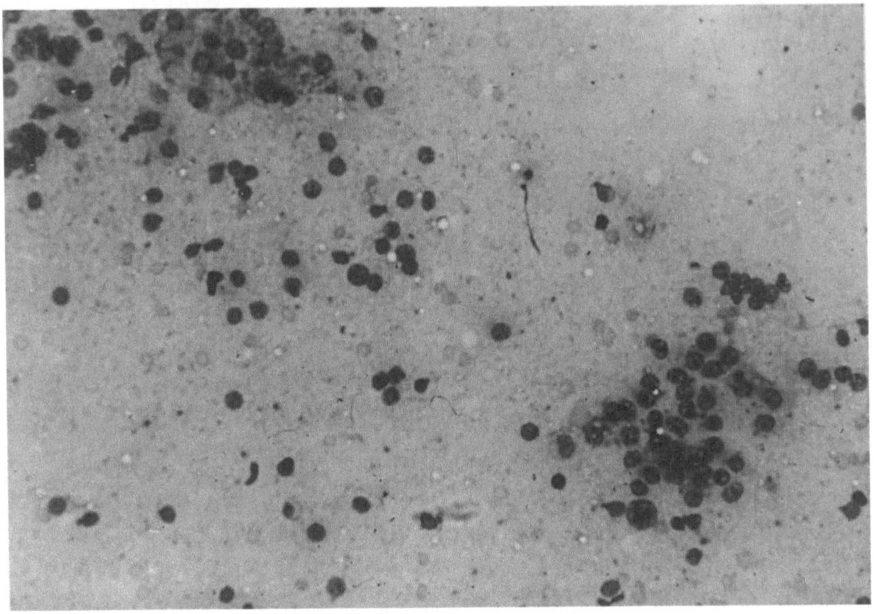

Fig. 5. In vivo Pappenheim-stained normal renal cells, klatsch preparation; original magnification ×140

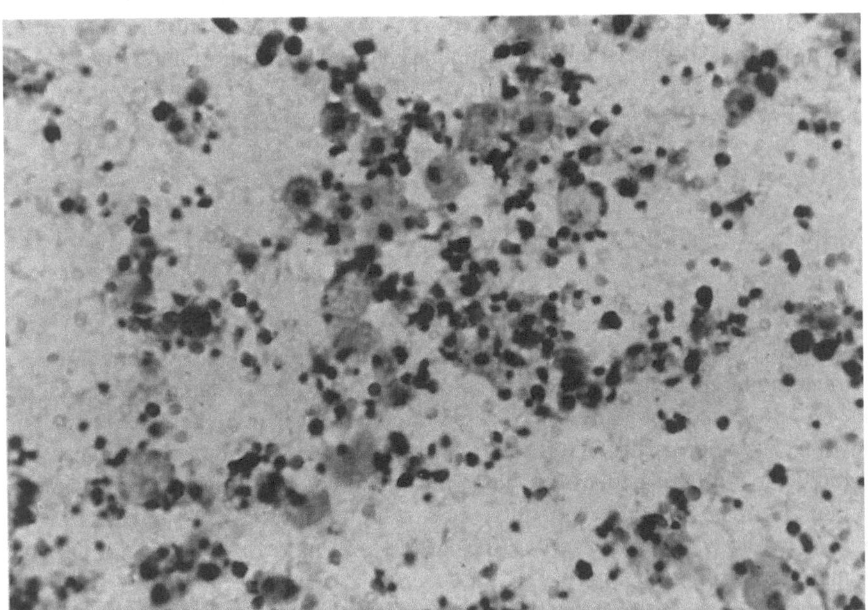

Fig. 6. In vivo Pappenheim-stained malignant renal cells, klatsch preparation; original magnification ×140

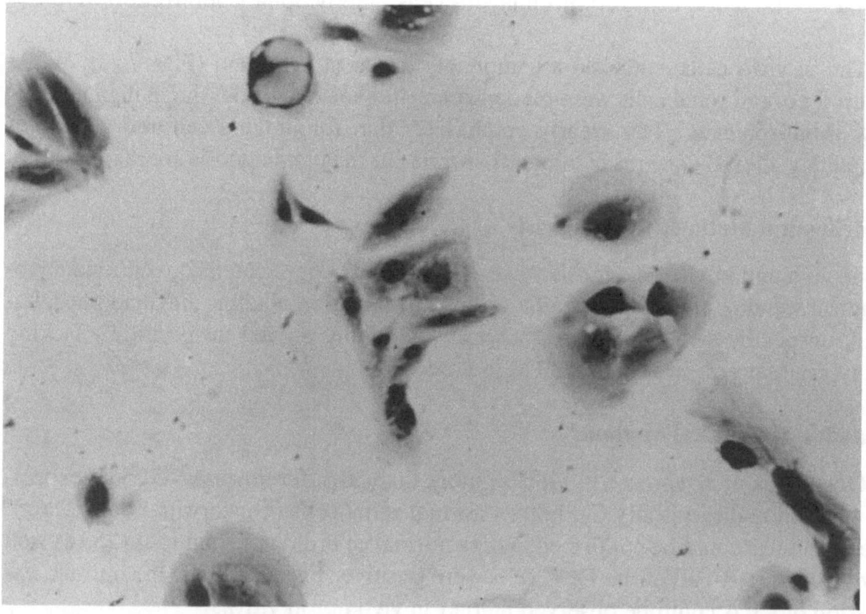

Fig. 7. In vitro Pappenheim-stained normal renal cells; original magnification ×140

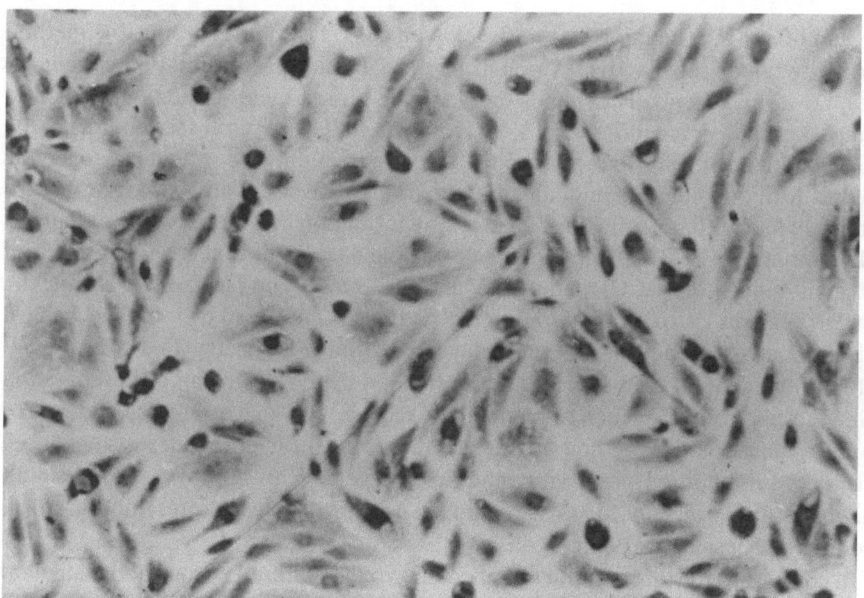

Fig. 8. In vitro Pappenheim-stained malignant renal cells; original magnification ×140

thermore, red blood cells, erythrophagous cells, and lymphatic infiltration were observed.

The in vitro cells exhibited a completely different cytogram (Figs. 7, 8): While cultured normal renal cells were pleomorphic and anisokaryotic, the malignant cells grew isomorphically. This clearly emphasizes that for judging cultured cells with completely altered patterns cytological criteria for in vivo diagnosis are inapplicable.

Cytochemical Methods for Diagnosis

For in vivo and in vitro diagnosis we used commonly appreciated conventional cytochemical staining methods (periodic acid-Schiff reaction, alkaline and acid phosphatases, unspecific esterase); these, however, generally proved unspecific by lacking any typical pattern, in vivo as well as in vitro.

Immunocytochemical Methods

As Oosterwijk et al. showed in 1986 for more than 50 different cases, G 250 is expressed only on malignant (RCC), not on normal renal cells (Oosterwijk et al. 1986a). These findings could be confirmed: While normal cells did not stain for G 250 as well in vivo as in vitro, all of the RCC cells were positive (Figs. 3 and 4). In contrast, expression of CEA could be observed neither in vivo nor in vitro.

Discussion

The aim of our investigation was to develop an easy, fast, and reproducible method to identify tumor cells in vivo as well as in vitro. Reliable interpretation of cell cultures, however, essentially depends on the precise assessment of the tumor cell rate (Hanauske and Von Hoff 1985; Von Hoff 1987). Up to now this could not be achieved unequivocally except through time- and money-consuming cytogenetic analyses with only limited amounts of karyograms (Kovacs et al. 1987). For in vitro culturing of solid tumors the "soft agar colony formation assay" according to Salmon and Hamburger (1978) is recommended, but the success rate of in vitro growth of malignant renal cells (RCC) amounts to just 50%–60% (Von Hoff 1987). During the past few years in vitro cell preparation methods were improved by using mechanical and enzymatic techniques. The monolayer procedure according to Kovacs et al. (1987) provides an in vitro success rate for RCC of nearly 90%. This cell preparation technique underwent further refinement to achieve cytological in vitro slides. For routine application this method proved advantageous, providing slides with high cell density and in addition preserving material and cells. This approach allows simultaneous assays especially for in vitro drug sensitivity studies as presented in detail recently (de Riese et al. 1987).

In contrast to the information obtained in vivo the cultured normal and malignant cells in our study completely differed with regard to their morphological and cytochemical phenotype; thus, conventional cytology and cytochemistry (PAS, staining for alkaline and acid phosphatase and unspecific esterase) are reliable only for the in vivo diagnosis of malignant renal tumor cells. According to these observations the in vitro diagnosis currently remains troublesome even for experienced cytologists.

More recently several studies on the expression of different antigens on the surface of normal and malignant renal cells were presented (Bander et al. 1983; Bander 1984; Oosterwijk et al. 1984; Oosterwijk et al. 1986a, b). However, with regard to histogenetic considerations the renal cell associated antigens like RC 8 and RC 38 appear promising (Oosterwijk et al. 1986b). Nevertheless, immunocytochemical identification of the renal origin itself does not allow any judgement concerning dignity. Furthermore, staining for CEA does not provide any indication of pathologic changes including malignant transformation.

This, however, can be effectively achieved by using a new monoclonal antibody designated G 250, subclass IgG, which preferentially recognizes an antigen expressed on the membranes of RCC but not on benign renal cells. In 1986, Oosterwijk et al. first isolated and characterized this glycoprotein, which was present on 46 of 47 primary RCCs, on 7 of 8 RCC metastases, and only on a few other nonrenal tumors (8% of colonic carcinomas, 5% of sarcomas, 5% of ovarian carcinomas) (Oosterwijk et al. 1986a). To our knowledge this study represents the first investigation of the G 250 in vitro expression in renal cancer. The combination of tissue culture methods and immunocytochemical techniques outlined above offers a novel approach of considerable promise for in vitro studies on RCC.

G 250 is the first immunocytochemical marker to distinguish unequivocally between normal and malignant renal cells in vitro.

Summary

Tumor tissue (RCC) as well as normal renal tissue of 10 patients were processed for conventional cytology and for subprimary cell culturing. Employing different cytologic, cytochemical and immunocytochemical measures the in vitro cells exhibited completely altered staining patterns compared to normal and malignant cells in vivo. Thus cytologic criteria valuable for in vivo diagnosis cannot be reliably applied under in vitro conditions. Furthermore expression of two cell-surface antigens was evaluated using monoclonal antibodies (CEA, G 250). While expression of CEA neither in-vivo nor in-vitro was observed, staining for G 250 proved a reliable immunocytochemical technique to identify the tumor-cell rate in-vitro.

Acknowledgements. We thank Mrs. M. Akkermann and Mrs. C. Pütz for their expert technical assistance.

References

Bander NH (1984) Comparison of antigen expression of human renal cancers in vivo and in vitro. Cancer 53:1235–1239

Bander NH, Cordon-Cardo CC, Finstad CL, Houghton AN, Whitmore WF, Melamed MR (1983) Monoclonal antibody defined antigens of normal and neoplastic human kidney cells. Proc ASCO C:49

Cordell JL, Falini B, Erber WN, Ghosh AK, Abdulaziz Z, Macdonald S, Pulford KAF, Stein H, Mason DY (1984) Immunoenzymatic labeling of monoclonal antibodies and monoclonal antialkaline phosphatase (APAAP complexes). J Histochem Cytochem 32(2):219–229

de Riese W, Szücs S, Hoene E, Lenis G, Kovacs G (1987) Short term in-vitro sensitivity testing of human renal cell carinoma. Invest Urology 2:81–86

Gerdes J (1985) An immunohistological method for estimating cell growth fractions in rapid histopathological diagnosis during surgery. Int J Cancer 35: 169–171

Gerdes J, Schwab U, Lemke H, Stein H (1983) Production of a mouse monoclonal antibody reactive with a human nuclear antigen associated with cell proliferation. Int J Cancer 31: 13–20

Hanauske AR, Von Hoff DD (1985) Clinical correlations with the human tumor cloning assay. Cancer Investigation 3(6): 541–551

Kovacs G, Szücs S, de Riese W, Baumgärtel H (1987) Specific chromosome aberration in human renal cell carcinoma. Int J Cancer 40: 171–178

Morasca L (1976) Advances in morphological identification of cell types in primary culture. In: Dendy PP (ed) Human tumours in short term culture. Academic, London, pp 78–84

Oosterwijk E, Fleuren GJ, Jonas U, Zwartendijk J, Te Velde J, Warnaar SO (1984) The expression of renal antigens in renal cell carcinoma. World J Urol 2: 156–158

Oosterwijk E, Ruiter DJ, Hoedemaeker PJ, Pauwels EKJ, Jonas U, Zwartendijk J, Warnaar SO (1986a) Monoclonal antibody G250 recognizes a determinant present in renal cell carcinoma and absent from normal kidney. Int J Cancer 38: 489––494

Oosterwijk E, Ruiter DJ, Wakka JC, Huiskens v d Meij JW, Jonas U, Fleuren GJ, Zwartendijk J, Hoedemaeker P, Warnaar SO (1986b) Immunohistochemical analysis of monoclonal antibodies to renal antigens. Am J Pathol 123: 301–309

Salmon SE, Hamburger AW (1978) Quantitation of differential sensitivity of human tumor stem cells to anti-cancer agents. N Engl J Med 298: 1321–1327

Thoenes W (1986) Histopathology and classification of renal-cell tumors (adenomas, oncocytomas, carcinomas). Path Res Pract 181: 125–143

Von Hoff DD (1987) In-vitro predictive testing. Int J of Cell Cloning 5: 179–190

Growth and Cell Proliferation of Human Renal Cell Carcinomas Xenografted into BALB/c *nu/nu* Mice

M. Harasim[1], E. Loer[1], M. Wirth[2], and B. Maurer-Schultze[1]

Introduction

Since the first report of a human malignant tumor growing in a mouse mutant by Rygaard and Povlsen in 1969, the nude mouse model has been frequently used in studies of growth (Katsuoka et al. 1976; Shimosato et al. 1976; Giovanella et al. 1978; Auerbach et al. 1978; Kyriazis et al. 1978) and therapy (Otto et al. 1984a, b; Bubenik et al. 1987; Taetle et al. 1987; Byers et al. 1987) of human tumors. Although this model is much closer to the human tumor than experimental animal tumors, the question is how far the nude mouse model actually represents the conditions in human beings. Furthermore, investigations in this field are mainly based on measurements of the tumor size (Giovanella et al. 1978; Auerbach et al. 1978; Höehn and Schroeder 1978; Naito et al. 1987) as well as of the DNA content of the tumor cells and its distribution by flow cytometry (Otto et al. 1984a, b; Baisch et al. 1986) There are almost no studies on cell proliferation of human tumors in nude mice apart from occasional determinations of the labeling and the mitotic index (Heller et al. 1987). The aim of the present study was a quantitative analysis of the growth and proliferation of human renal cell carcinomas growing in the nude mouse.

Materials and Methods

Animals. Male and female BALB/c *nu/nu* mice (own breeding facilities), 20–25 g, 4–8 weeks old, were kept under constant conditions: temperature-controlled laminar flow hoods, 27°C, 12-h light-dark regimen, Nohrlin diet (12 ZH 10, Bad Salzuflen, FRG) and water (pH 2.5, vitamins and antibiotics added) ad libitum.

Labeled Thymidine (TdR). [^{3}H]methyl-thymidine (6700 mCi/mmol) and 2[^{14}C]-thymidine (52 mCi/mmol) from New England Nuclear (Boston, MA, USA) were used.

Xenografting. Tumor tissue of 50 human renal cell carcinomas was obtained directly at the time of radical nephrectomy. Specimens were transported in warm RPMI 1640 culture medium (37°C; Grand Island Biological, NY, USA) supplemented with 10% fetal calf serum. Tissue specimens of about 2 × 2 × 2 mm were implanted subcutaneously into each side of the anterior-lateral thoracic wall of BALB/c *nu/nu* mice (Kyriazis and Kyriazis 1980) within 30–60 min after removal of the tumor. After

[1] Institut für Medizinische Strahlenkunde der Universität Würzburg, Versbacher Str. 5, 8700 Würzburg, FRG
[2] Urologische Klinik und Poliklinik der Universität Würzburg, Josef-Schneider-Str. 2, 8700 Würzburg, FRG

Investigative Urology 3
Edited by H. Rübben et al.

growing up to a sufficient tumor size, pieces of $2 \times 2 \times 2$ mm were serially transplanted in the same way.

Tumor Size Measurements. Tumor size was determined weekly by external caliper measurements of two perpendicular tumor diameters. The largest dimension has been chosen as one diameter. Results were expressed as length times width (cm^2).

Flow Cytometry. Single cell suspensions of tumor samples were obtained by mincing the tumor tissue and filtering it through a 50-µm mesh. The cells were washed in lymphocyte buffer and stained with DAPI (4,6-diamidino-2-phenylindole dihydrochloride; Serva, Heidelberg, FRG). Flow measurements of DAPI-fluorescence intensity were carried out with an EPICS V system (Coulter Electronics Inc, Hialeah, FL, USA).

Histology and Autoradiography. Immediately after killing the animals by cervical luxation the solid tumors were removed, fixed in 4% formalin, and embedded in paraplast. Half of the 4-µm serial cross sections was Feulgen stained, the other half was stained with hematoxylin and eosin. For single labeling experiments slides were covered with a thin emulsion layer by dipping them into diluted Ilford K2 emulsion (emulsion : distilled water, 3:2), exposed, and developed with Amidol. In case of double labeling experiments two emulsion layer autoradiographs were prepared according to the method of Schultze et al. (1976).

Evaluation of the Autoradiographs. For determining the mitotic index (MI) and the labeling index (LI) at least 1000 tumor cells/animal were counted. Mitoses were registered from late prophase to early telophase. In the double labeling experiments the percentages of each category of labeled cells (purely ^3H-labeled, double labeled, and purely ^{14}C-labeled) and of unlabeled cells were determined according to the method of Schultze et al. (1976). At least 100 cells of the smallest category per animal, i.e., up to 3500 tumor cells per animal, were evaluated.

Results

The overall *take rate* of the tumors was 34% (Table 1). According to *nuclear grading* the majority (68%) of human tumor specimens belonged to grade II tumors. Take

Table 1. Take rate, nuclear grading, and ploidy of 50 human renal cell carcinomas

Nuclear grading			Take rate
		Overall	34%
I	22%		0%
II	68%		35%
III	10%		100%
Ploidy			
Diploid	70%		27%
Nondiploid	30%		53%

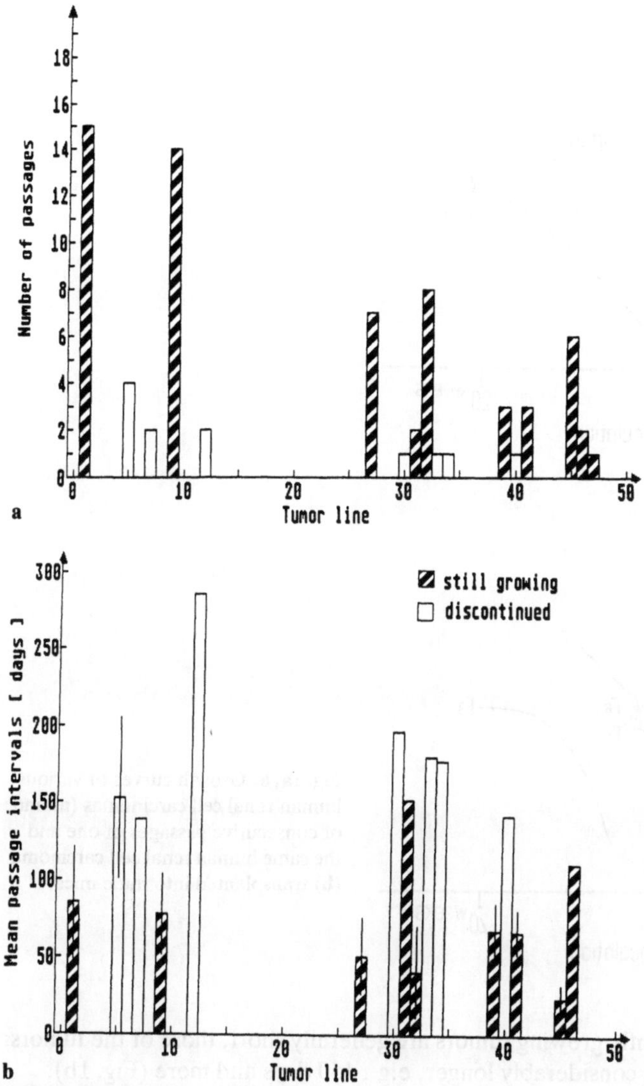

Fig. 1a, b. Take rate, number of passages (**a**), and time intervals between passages (**b**) of human renal cell carcinomas transplanted into nude mice. The *hatched columns* represent the permanently growing tumors, the *white columns* those that stopped growing after a few transplantations. *Bars* indicate SD

rate of grade I tumors (22%) was zero in contrast to the 100% take rate of grade III tumors (10%). *Ploidy* of the tumors was examined by flow cytometry: 70% of the tumors were diploid and 30% were tetraploid or aneuploid. Take rate of diploid tumors was 27%, of nondiploid tumors, 53%.

From the 17 tumors that were growing in nude mice 10 are still growing and are serially passaged (1 to 15 generations), while 7 tumors stopped growing after 1 to 3 transplantations (Fig. 1a). Correspondingly, the mean time intervals between the

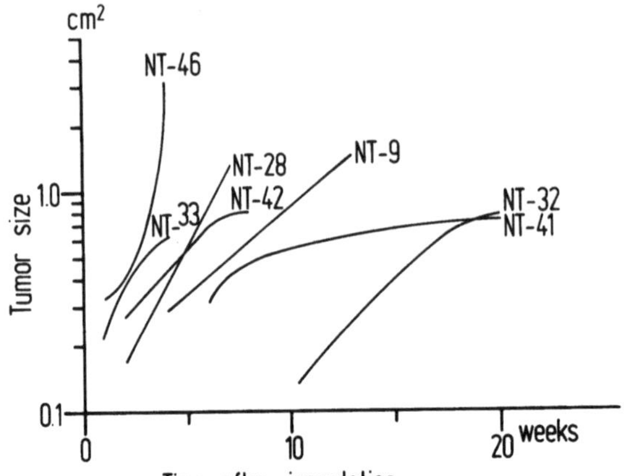

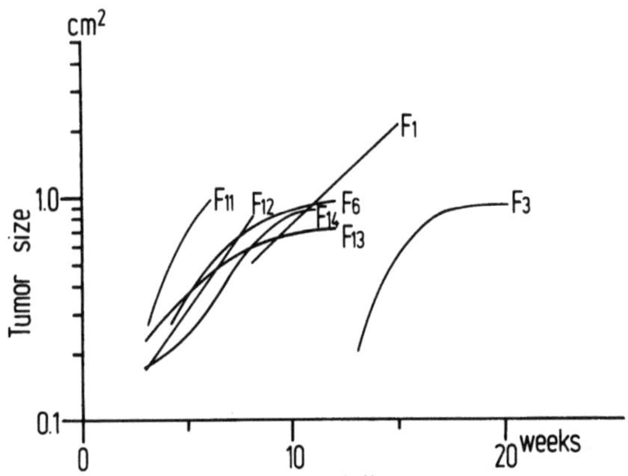

Fig. 2a, b. Growth curves of various human renal cell carcinomas (**a**) and of consecutive passages of one and the same human renal cell carcinoma (**b**) transplanted into nude mice

passages of the permanently growing tumors are generally short, those of the tumors that stopped growing are considerably longer, e.g., 150 days and more (Fig. 1b).

Figure 2 contains a selection of the numerous *growth curves* of the human renal cell carcinomas in nude mice presently studied. Figure 2a depicts growth curves of various human renal cell carcinomas. They show that tumor growth in the nude mouse differs considerably between the different tumors. It ranges from Gompertzian growth with an early delay (NT-41) or initial exponential growth with late and considerable delay (NT-42) to complete exponential growth with different slopes (NT-9, NT-28). The size of one tumor (NT-46) increases even faster than exponentially, most probably due to fluid retention in the tumor. Figure 2b demonstrates growth curves of different generations of the same human renal cell carcinoma (NT-1). They show that tumor growth also differs between the successive generations of one and the same tumor but not as much as between different tumors.

Table 2 contains the *cell kinetic parameters* of two human renal cell carcinomas, a primary tumor and a metastasis, growing in the nude mouse. For the purpose of

Table 2. Cell kinetic parameters of human renal cell carcinomas (one primary tumor, one metastasis) growing in nude mice as well as of a transplantable adenocarcinoma growing in C57b1/6j mice and after transplantation into nude mice. The methods used are listed at the bottom

Tumor	Animal	Tumor size (g)	T_{pot} (h)	T_C (h)	T_S (h)	L.I. (%)	M.I. (%)	GF	
AdCa (7 days old)	C_{57}	0.9	36	$17^{\square}$	$8.0^{\square}$	47.4	3.1	1.0	
EO 771 (7 days old)	BALB/c-nu/nu	1.0	32	$13^{\square}$	$8.0^{\square}$	48.6	3.1	0.75	
Human renal cell carcinoma	BALB/c-nu/nu	0.17	119°		6.3°	5.3			F_6
			150^{+}	112^{+}	9.4^{+}	8.4		0.7	
Human renal cell carcinoma Metastasis	BALB/c-nu/nu	0.23	69^{+}	53^{+}					
			68°		8.5°	7.8	0.8	0.7	F_3
			$75^{\bullet}$						
		0.42			$13.0^{\square}$				
			130^{+}	120^{+}	10.0^{+}	12.0	0.8	0.9	F_{10}
			76°		10.5°	1.40			

$^{+}$ Modified grain count halving method
$^{\circ}$ Double labeling with $[^3H]$- and $[^{14}C]$TdR
$^{\bullet}$ Stathmokinetic method with VCR
$^{\square}$ FLM method

comparison the cell kinetic parameters of a transplantable mouse tumor, the adenocarcinoma EO 771 in the C57 mouse and after transplantation into nude mice, are also listed in the table. For these cell kinetic studies different methods were used: a modified grain count halving method with $[^3H]$TdR (Bassukas and Maurer-Schultze 1988), double labeling with $[^3H]$- and $[^{14}C]$TdR, the stathmokinetic method with vincristine as well as the fraction of labeled mitoses (FLM) method.

The potential doubling time (T_{pot}) of the tumor cells of the renal cell carcinoma (primary tumor and metastasis) ranges from 68 h to 150 h. The cell cycle time of the primary tumor is 112 h, that of the metastasis is shorter, namely 53 h; it increases to 120 h after a further 7 passages. The S phase duration (T_S) is rather similar for all tumors studied, between 6.3 h and 13.0 h. The mean labeling index is for both primary tumor and metastasis about 7%. It increases to double the value up to the 10th generation of the metastasis. This agrees well with the tendency of this tumor to greater malignancy with an increasing number of passages as shown by histological criteria.

Discussion

The take rate of human renal cell carcinomas in the present study (34%; Table 1) agrees well with that reported by other authors (Clayman et al. 1985; Katsuoka et al. 1976) but contradicts the surprisingly high take rate (100%) stated by Otto et al. (1984a, b). This difference may be due to pretransplantational selection or to different criteria for a positive take. Growth to a size of about 8 mm in diameter was the criterion for a positive take in this study. The prevalence of grade II tumors can be explained by the more difficult detection of the lower malignant renal cell carcinomas (grade I) and the earlier metastasizing of the higher malignant tumors (grade III), preventing surgical intervention. The take rate of nondiploid tumors, which is twice as high as that of diploid tumors, stresses the importance of ploidy representing the aggressiveness of the corresponding tumor.

Apparently there is a correlation between the successful serial transplantation and the mean passage intervals with short passage intervals, i.e., faster growth and higher malignancy, resulting in permanently growing tumor lines (Fig. 1). These results together with the zero take rate of grade I tumors and the high take rate of grade III tumors demonstrate that the faster growing, more malignant tumors are selected by xenografting human renal cell carcinomas into nude mice.

The few examples from about 80 growth curves in Fig. 2 clearly demonstrate the great variation of tumor growth. This agrees well with numerous growth curves of human renal cell carcinomas published by other authors. This great variation can easily be explained by the well-known heterogeneity of renal cell carcinomas as such as well as by the arbitrary choice of the excised tumor material for xenografting. Variation of the growth curves of the successive generations of one and the same tumor (Fig. 2b) is less but still exists and demonstrates that growth in the nude mouse not only depends on the heterogeneity of the particular tumor but also on the arbitrarily transplanted amount of viable tumor cells or connective tissue. With respect to these results, i.e., to the different growth characteristics of human renal cell carcinomas, the question arises how far these differences in tumor growth without treatment influence the screening of cytotoxic drugs. In these studies of the drug effect the measured parameter is also tumor size, i.e., tumor growth, that differs greatly even without treatment.

There are only a few studies on cell proliferation of human tumors growing in nude mice. Similar values of T_{pot} as for the primary renal cell carcinoma (Table 2) were obtained for gastric, colon, and breast carcinomas by Kubato et al. (1986). Cell cycle times of these carcinomas and of the squamous cell carcinomas examined by Meck et al. (1981) are shorter (30 h to 47 h) than those of the renal cell carcinoma and the metastasis presently studied. The reliability of the methods used in the present work is demonstrated by the fact that the same potential doubling time (T_{pot}) of the tumor cells of the metastasis of a renal cell carcinoma, namely about 70 h, was obtained by applying three different methods (Table 2). T_{pot} as well as the cycle time (T_C) are somewhat longer in the case of the primary tumor.

The most striking result is that the S phase duration is rather short, namely 6–13 h. Similar values were obtained for human gastric, colonic, breast, and squamous cell carcinomas growing in nude mice (Meck et al. 1981; Kubato et al. 1986). This is considerably shorter than an S phase duration of about 20 h known from the few studies in human beings (see Steel 1977). On the other hand this S phase duration is quite similar to that measured for the transplantable mouse tumor in C57 and in nude mice (upper two lines in Table 2). Thus, the question arises whether S phase duration, and that means DNA synthesis, is controlled by the host. The S phase duration of the mouse cells is about 8 h. The same might be true for other cell kinetic parameters. The potential doubling and the cycle times of the renal cell carcinoma in the nude mouse are longer than those of the experimental mouse tumor but shorter than those known from tumors in human beings. This is also supported by the finding that the LI of the excised human renal cell carcinoma is lower than after transplantation into nude mice (Heller et al. 1987). Another explanation might be that clones of rapidly proliferating tumor cells are selected early after xenotransplantation into nude mice.

These results altogether suggest that we should be very cautious with respect to conclusions from the nude mouse model on the conditions in human beings.

Acknowledgements. We thank Miss T. Manger for her skillful technical assistance. This work was supported by the Deutsche Forschungsgemeinschaft.

References

Auerbach R, Morissey LW, Sidky YA (1978) Regional differences in the incidence and growth of mouse tumors following intradermal or subcutaneous inoculation. Cancer Res 38:1739–1744

Baisch H, Otto U, Klöppel G (1986) Long-term serial transplantation of 30 different human renal cell carcinomas into NMRI (nu/nu) mice: flow cytometric, histologic, and growth studies. JNCI 76:269–276

Bassukas ID, Maurer-Schultze B (1987) A modification of the grain count halving method for detailed analysis of cell kinetic parameters. Cell Tissue Kinet 20:527–537

Bubenik J, Kieler J, Tromholt V, Indrova M, Lotzova E (1987) Recombinant interleukin-2 inhibits growth of human tumor xenografts in congenitally athymic mice. Immunol Lett 14:325–330

Byers VS, Pimm MV, Scannon PJ, Pawluczyk I, Baldwin RW (1987) Inhibition of growth of human tumor xenografts in athymic mice treated with ricin toxin a chain-monoclonal antibody 791T/36 conjugates. Cancer Res 47:5042–5046

Clayman RV, Figenshau RS, Bear A, Limas C (1985) Transplantation of human renal cell carcinoma into athymic mice. Cancer Res 45:2650–2653

Giovanella BC, Stehlin JS, Williams LJ, Lee SS, Shepard RC (1978) Heterotransplantation of human cancers into nude mice. Cancer 42:2269–2281

Heller V, Bassukas ID, Grups JW, Wirth MP (1987) Growth of human renal cell carcinoma in nude mice. In: Jacobi GH, Rübben H, Harzmann R (eds) Investigative urology 2. Springer, Berlin Heidelberg New York, pp 75–80

Höehn W, Schroeder FH (1978) Renal cell carcinoma: two new cell lines and a serially transplantable nude mouse tumor (NC 65). Invest Urol 16:106–112

Katsuoka Y, Baba S, Hata M, Tazaki H (1976) Transplantation of human renal cell carcinoma to the nude mice as an intermediate of in vivo and in vitro studies. J Urol 115:373–376

Kubato T, Nakada M, Tsuyuki K, Inada T, Asanuma F, Ishibiki K, Abe O (1986) Cell kinetics and chemosensitivity of human carcinomas serially transplanted into nude mice. Gann 77:502–507

Kyriazis AA, Kyriazis AP (1980) Preferential sites of growth of human tumors in nude mice following subcutaneous transplantation. Cancer Res 40:4509–4511

Kyriazis AP, DiPersio L, Michael GJ, Pesce AJ, Stinnett JD (1978) Growth patterns and metastatic behaviour of human tumors growing in athymic mice. Cancer Res 38:3186–3190

Meck RA, Ingram M, Meck JM, McCulluogh JM, Wu M-C, Yunis AA (1981) Establishment and cell cycle kinetics of a human squamous cell carcinoma in nude mice and in vitro. Cancer Res 41:1076–1085

Naito S, von Eschenbach AC, Fidler IJ (1987) Different growth pattern and biological behaviour of human renal cell carcinoma implanted into different organs of nude mice. JNCI 78:377–384

Otto U, Klöppel G, Baisch H (1984a) Transplantation of human renal cell carcinoma into NMRI nu/nu mice. I. Reliability of an experimental tumor model. J Urol 131:130–134

Otto U, Huland H, Baisch H, Klöppel G (1984b) Transplantation of human renal cell carcinoma into NMRI nu/nu mice. II. Evaluation of response to vinblastine sulfate mono therapy. J Urol 131:134–138

Rygaard J, Povlsen CO (1969) Heterotransplantation of a human malignant tumor to "nude" mice. Acta Pathol Microbiol Scand 77:758–760

Schultze B, Maurer W, Hagenbusch H (1976) A two emulsion autoradiographic technique and discrimination of three different types of labelling after double labelling with [^{3}H] and [^{14}C]thymidine. Cell Tissue Kinet 9:245

Shimosato Y, Kameya T, Nagai K, Hirohashi S, Koide T, Hayashi H, Nomura T (1976) Transplantation of human tumors in nude mice. JNCI 56:1251–1257

Steel GG (1977) The growth kinetics of tumours. Oxford University Press, Oxford

Taetle R, Rosen F, Abramson I, Venditti J, Howell S (1987) Use of nude mouse xenografts as preclinical drug screens: in vivo activity of established chemotherapeutic agents against melanoma and ovarian carcinoma xenografts. Cancer Treat Rep 71:297–304

Expression of Epidermal Growth Factor Receptors on Renal Cell Carcinomas

W. Heckl, K. Becker, U. Wacker, and B. Halliger[1]

Introduction

The epidermal growth factor (EGF), a low molecular weight polypeptide, originally isolated from mouse submandibular glands and from human urine stimulates the proliferation of a variety of cells in cultures of both epithelial and mesenchymal origin (Cohen and Carpenter 1975; Gregory 1975). The EGF binds as well as the transforming growth factor-α (TGF-α) to the EGF-receptor located on the cell membranes of normal and transformed cells. This EGF-receptor is a 170000-dalton protein with an extracellular and an intracellular domain. The intracellular region of the EGF-receptor possesses tyrosine kinase activity, and there is autophosphorylation of tyrosine residues located near the carboxy terminus (Carpenter 1983; Downward et al. 1984b).

The finding that the v-*erb* B oncogene (from avian erythroblastosis virus) codes for the internal and membrane part of the EGF-receptor strengthens the link between oncogenic stimulation of a cell and its normal growth regulatory mechanism (Downward et al. 1984a). EGF-receptors are expressed on cells of various tumors including cancer of the breast, bladder, and lungs, gastric carcinomas, and nonneuronal brain tumors.

Because of the detection of TGF-α in kidney tumors, the aim of our study was to examine the distribution of EGF-receptors on human kidney carcinomas and to correlate these findings with the tumor stage and grade.

Material and Methods

Specimens from 37 patients with renal cell carcinomas nephrectomized at the Department of Urology, University of Würzburg, were immediately frozen and stored in liquid nitrogen. Out of the 20 men and 17 women there were 4 patients with pT1, 21 with pT2, 11 with pT3, and one with pT4 tumors. Two of the pT3 patients had a thrombus in the vena renalis. The patient with the pT4 tumor had a solitary metastasis in the pelvis.

Six patients from the pT2 group and three from the pT3/pT4 groups had paracaval and paraaortal lymph node metastases. A grade 1 tumor was found in 4 patients (4 pT2), grade 2 tumor in 23 (3 pT1, 12 pT2, 8 pT3), and a grade 3 tumor in 10 (1 pT1, 5 pT2, 3 pT3, 1 pT4). Four additional specimens of normal kidneys which

[1] Department of Urology, University of Würzburg Medical School, Josef-Schneider-Str. 2, 8700 Würzburg, FRG

Investigative Urology 3
Edited by H. Rübben et al.

have shown no evidence of a tumor under histological examination were taken as controls.

All specimens were snap frozen immediately after the nephrectomy, wrapped in metal foil to prevent dehydration, and stored in liquid nitrogen. The delay before freezing was no more than 30 min.

The EGF-receptors were identified by an indirect immunoperoxidase technique using a murine monoclonal antibody. This IgG1 antibody was raised against the extracellular domain of the EGF-receptor of A-431 cells (Schreiber et al. 1983), a epidermoid carcinoma cell line with high concentrations of EGF-receptors ($2–3 \times 10^6$ receptors/cell).

Air-dried, 20-µm cryostat sections were fixed in methanol: H_2O_2: acetone mixture at 4°C and washed twice for 5 min in saline. In order to reduce unspecific absorption, the sections were incubated with 100 µl of normal swine serum (1:5) for 10 min. The sections were incubated at room temperature with 100 µl of the primary antibody for 16 h (1:100). After washing with saline, the sections were incubated with 100 µl of biotinylated antimouse IgG (1:100) for 60 min followed by applying the VECTASTAIN ABC reagent. After two further washes with saline the peroxidase activity was developed by means of a solution of 3,3′-diamino-benzidine. The sections were again washed, counterstained with hematoxylin, dehydrated, and mounted.

As a positive control the A-431 cells which contain large numbers of EGF-receptors were used (Roberts et al. 1985). The EGF-receptors NR-6 cells served as negative controls (Pruss and Herschman 1977).

Staining by immunohistochemistry was graded semiquantitatively as follows: negative (−); weakly positive (+), if <25% of the cells were stained; positive (++), if 25%–50% of the cells were stained; strongly positive (+++), if >50% of the cells were stained.

Statistical analysis was done by calculating the P value <0.05. The correlation was estimated using the Kendall partial rank correlation coefficient.

Results

The tumor cell staining generally appeared to be cytoplasmic; staining was also found at the cell membranes (Fig. 1). Specimens from the normal kidneys did not stain positively for the EGF-receptors.

Out of the four pT1 tumors, two were graded as negative, one as positive, and one as strongly positive. In the pT2 group with 21 specimens, one specimen was not stained. Six patients showed a weak positive reaction, seven were graded as positive, and another seven as strongly positive. In the pT3 group with 11 patients all tumors were positive. One of them was weak positive, one positive, and the majority, namely 9 patients, had strongly positive staining. The only pT4 tumor was graded as strongly positive (Fig. 2).

Regarding the tumor grade in relation to the EGF-staining, all four G1 tumors were stained. Two of them stained only weakly, one strongly, and another very strongly. Out of the 23 patients with G2 tumors, all except three specimens were stained. Five stained weakly positive, 4 positively, and 11 strongly. Of the 10 G3 tumors, 4 stained positively and 6 strongly positive (Fig. 3).

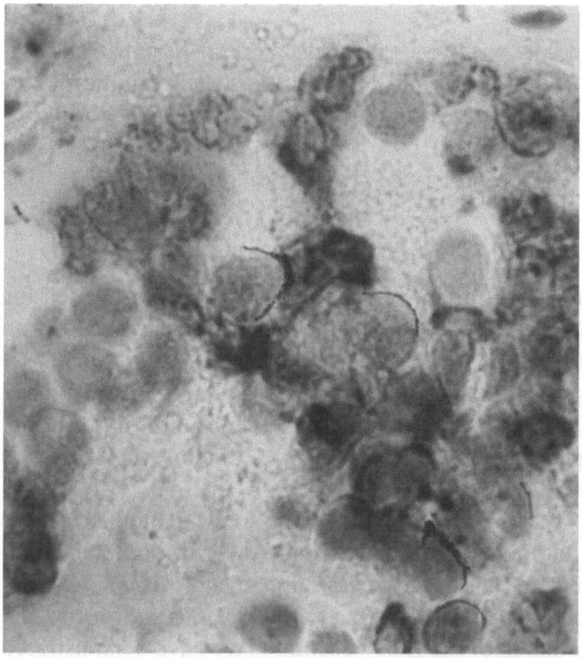

Fig. 1. Immunohistochemical localization of epidermal growth factor receptor in renal cell carcinoma. Staining is shown in the cytoplasm and at the cell membrane. × 960

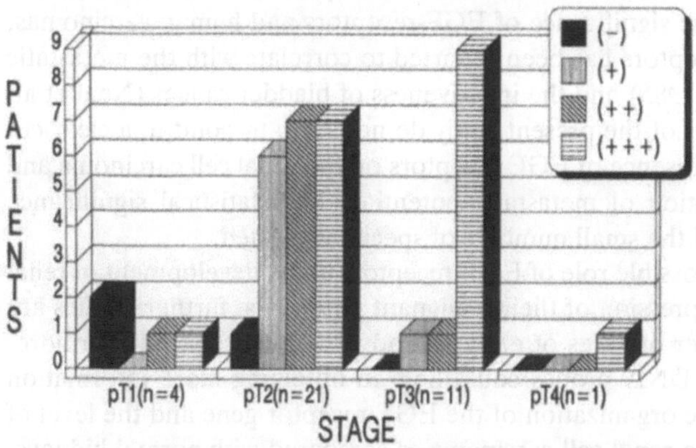

Fig. 2. Frequency of epidermal growth factor receptor positivity in primary renal cell carcinoma according to the tumor stage

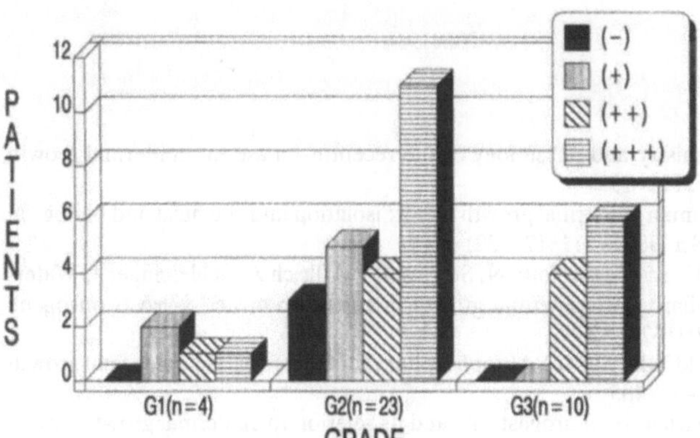

Fig. 3. Frequency of epidermal growth factor receptor positivity in primary renal cell carcinoma according to the tumor grade

Between the tumor stage and the positive stained cells there was a statistically significant correlation ($r = 0.33$, $P < 0.0075$). There was no statistically significant correlation between the tumor grade and the staining of the cells ($r = 0.23$, $P < 0.0613$).

Discussion

We have shown that human renal cell carcinoma contains EGF-receptors. Focusing only on the tumor stage the EGF-receptors were found immunohistochemically in all pT2, pT3, and pT4 tumors except in one pT2 tumor. Taking into account only those tumors with a positive staining of more than 50% of the cells, 33% (= 7) of the pT2 tumors, 82% (= 9) of the pT3 tumors, and the only pT4 tumor fulfill this criteria. The same quantitative staining was demonstrated in 25% G1 tumors, in 48% of the G2 tumors, and in 60% of the G3 tumors.

The identification of the EGF-receptors on human renal cell carcinoma cells has not been reported previously, although EGF can stimulate the growth of some kidney tumor cells. The monoclonal antibody, which was raised against the EGF-receptors of A-431 epidermoid carcinoma cells (Roberts et al. 1985) was shown to react with the extracellular binding domain of the EGF-receptors. We have demonstrated that normal kidney cells did not react with the EGF-receptor-specific antibody.

In regard to the biologic significance of EGF-receptors and human carcinomas, the expression of EGF-receptors has been reported to correlate with the metastatic potential (Sainsbury et al. 1985) and the invasiveness of bladder cancer (Neal et al. 1985). However, the results of the present study do not seem to point to a clear-cut relationship between the presence of EGF-receptors on the renal cell carcinoma and their histologic differentiation of metastatic potential. The statistical significance found is suspect because of the small numbers of specimens tested.

For elucidation of the possible role of EGF-receptors in the development of renal cell carcinomas and the expression of their malignant potentials, further studies are needed with a large number of cases of early and advanced cancers. Furthermore, the use of EGF-receptor cDNA probes could help in obtaining more information with respect to the genomic organization of the EGF-receptor gene and the level of expression of these genes in renal cell carcinoma as compared with normal kidneys.

References

Carpenter G (1983) The biochemistry and physiology of the receptor-kinase for epidermal growth factor. Mol Cell Endocrinol 31:1–19

Cohen S, Carpenter G (1975) Human epidermal growth factor: isolation and chemical and biological properties. Proc Natl Acad Sci USA 72:1317–1321

Downward J, Yarden Y, Mayes E, Scarce G, Totty N, Stockwell P, Ullrich A, Schlessinger J, Waterfield MD (1984a) Close similarity of epidermal growth factor receptor and v-*erb* B oncogene protein sequences. Nature 307:521–527

Downward J, Parker P, Waterfield MD (1984b) Autophosphorylation sites on the epidermal growth factor receptor. Nature 311:483–485

Gregory H (1975) Isolation and structure of urogastrone and its relation to epidermal growth factor. Nature 257:325–327

Neal DE, Bennett MK, Hall RR, Marsh C, Abel PD, Sainsbury JRC, Harris AL (1985) Epidermal-growth-factor receptors in human bladder cancer: comparison of invasive and superficial tumors. Lancet i: 366–368

Pruss RM, Herschman HR (1977) Variants of BT-3 cells lacking mitogenic response to epidermal growth factor. Proc Natl Acad Sci USA 74: 3918–3921

Roberts AB, Anzano MA, Wakefield LM, Roche NS, Stern DF, Sporn MB (1985) Type β transforming growth factor: a bifunctional regulator of cellular growth. Proc Natl Acad Sci USA 82: 119–123

Sainsbury JRC, Fardon JR, Sherbet GV, Harris AL (1985) Epidermal-growth-factor receptors and oestrogen receptors in human breast cancer. Lancet i: 364–366

Schreiber AB, Libermann TA, Lax I, Yarden Y, Schlessinger J (1983) Biological role of epidermal growth factor-receptor clustering. Investigation with monoclonal antireceptor antibodies. J Biol Chem 258: 846–853

In Vitro Sensitivity of Three Human Renal Tumor Xenografts Towards Tumor Necrosis Factor and Alpha and Gamma Interferon

A. J. M. C. Beniers[1], R. J. A. van Moorselaar[1], W. P. Peelen[1], B. T. Hendriks[1], U. Otto[2], J. A. Schalken[1], and F. M. J. Debruyne[1]

Introduction

Renal cell tumors rarely respond to conventional therapy with cytostatic drugs or hormones. Interest in biologic approaches to the treatment of this tumor has been fostered by the identification of unique antigens on the surface of some renal cell carcinomas (Ueda et al. 1981) and by well-documented observations of spontaneous regression of tumor metastases. The observations suggest that host factors may be capable of modifying the course of renal cell carcinoma (Krown 1985). Although the mechanisms of biological response modifiers (BRMs) are not well-defined, the possibility that interferons (IFNs) and tumor necrosis factor (TNF) might augment a host immune response against renal cell cancer provided a rationale for early clinical trials.

The IFNs comprise a complex family of several species and multiple subspecies of hormone-like cellular proteins. They can be produced by virtually all eukaryotic cells in response to a wide range of stimuli and are capable of acting on a range of homologous and heterologous cells with relative species specificity in these actions (Kirkwood and Ernstoff 1984). It is now accepted that IFN can be effective against a broad spectrum of tumors. Nevertheless, the mechanism by which IFN exerts its activity is still unknown. Presumably, it has a direct effect on host and tumor cells; there could also be IFN-induced, host-mediated components which are independent of the immune system (Nagy et al. 1988; Gresser 1986). IFN-α especially may act differently in the treatment of different malignancies (Porszolt et al. 1988).

Difficulties in evaluating IFN action arise from the fact that there is no good correlation between the in vivo and in vitro sensitivity of tumor cells, and particularly for renal cell carcinoma (RCC) there is no good correlation between in vivo results from multiple clinical trials with IFN-α and -γ (Bonnem and Spiegel 1984; Koiso 1987; Krown 1987; Muss 1987; Sarna et al. 1987).

Since TNF causes hemorrhagic necrosis of tumors in experimental tumor models 24–48 h after local or systemic injection (Brouckaert et al. 1986; Haranaka et al. 1984) and TNF induces IFN-γ production by T lymphocytes (Old 1985, 1987), much attention has been paid to this antitumor agent in combination with IFN-γ (Brouckaert et al. 1986; Fransen et al. 1986; Ruggiero et al. 1986; Wong and Goeddel 1986). Not only synergistic antitumor effects of TNF and IFN-γ were found but Williamson et al. (1983) also found a synergistic antitumor effect of IFN-α and TNF.

[1] Department of Urology, Radboud University Hospital, Nijmegen, The Netherlands
[2] Department of Urology, Eppendorf University Hospital, Hamburg, FRG

Investigative Urology 3
Edited by H. Rübben et al.

Because transplantation of human RCC into athymic nude mice provides experimental tumor models which make the development of new therapeutic approaches possible (Balkwill et al. 1985; Otto et al. 1984) and since IFN-α appears to be a potential active antitumor agent in patients with RCC (Buzaid et al. 1987; Muss et al. 1987) and TNF also shows in vitro cytostatic and cytolytic effects on human RCC cell lines (Heicappell et al. 1987), we decided to test the direct in vitro antiproliferative effects of human recombinant IFN-α and -γ as well as human recombinant TNF on three RCC tumor lines: NU-12, HAM-II, and HAM-III. In this study we show that they do have in vitro antiproliferative effects on RCC tumor cells.

Material and Methods

Renal Cell Carcinoma Xenografts. After original subcutaneous transplantation of small tumor pieces (2 mm^3) in both flanks of BALB-c *nu/nu* mice, the NU-12, HAM-II, and HAM-III xenografts were passaged every 4 weeks. Tumor material for testing was harvested after 4 weeks.

Biological Response Modifiers. Human IFN-α, IFN-γ and TNF-α, obtained from Boehringer, Ingelheim, were produced in *Escherischia coli* by recombinant DNA technology. The specific activity of IFN-α and IFN-γ was 3,2-10E8 units/mg protein and 2-10E7 units/mg protein, respectively. It was measured by inhibition of encephalomyocarditis (EMC) virus replication in A549 cells with reference to the National Institute of Health (NIH) leucocyte IFN-α standard Go 23-901-527 and the NIH IFN-γ standard Gg 23-901-530. The purity of both IFNs was > 98% as determined by SDS polyacrylamide gel electrophoresis and the amount of endotoxin was less than 1.0 ng/mg protein for IFN-α and less or equal to 0.5 ng/mg protein for IFN-γ, as based on the limulus amoebocyte lysate assay. The specific activity of TNF-α determined in the presence of actinomycin-D was 6E7 units/mg protein as determined in the L-929 cytotoxicity assay. The purity was > 99% as determined by SDS polyacrylamide gel electrophoresis, and it contained 1.0 ng or less endotoxin/mg protein based on the limulus amoebocyte lysate assay. The drugs were dissolved in the accessory solvent and diluted with double enriched (DE) CMRL 1066 medium (Gibco, Paisley, UK).

Preparation of Single Cell Suspensions. When tumors reached sizes of about 1.5 × 1.5 cm the mice were killed, and tumor material was suspended in McCoy's wash (Gibco, Paisley, UK). After careful removal of necrosis, tumors were cut into pieces of about 3–4 mm^3. The tumor pieces were then minced with scissors into a 300-μm metal sieve and continuously washed with McCoy's wash into a petri dish. The minced tumor tissue was passed twice through a 40–70 μm nylon filter (Ortho Diagnostics, Beerse, Belgium) to obtain a single cell suspension. The cells were centrifuged at room temperature at 400 *g* for 5 min after which the supernatant was discarded. Upon resuspension of the cell pellet in DE CMRL 1066, cell density and viability were determined by adding 15 μl trypan blue solution (25 mg in 5 ml 3% acetic acid) to 15 μl cell suspension and simultaneously counting colored and not colored cells using a Bürker Türk hemocytometer.

Human Tumor Colony Forming Assay. For detection of the growth potential of tumor cells in soft agar a modified, two-layer, soft agar culture method originally described by Hamburger and Salmon (1977) was used (Verheyen et al. 1985). Tumor cell suspensions were plated at a concentration of 1.10E5 tumor cells per dish in the upper layer of the two-layer agar culture system. The cells were cultured immediately after preparation of the single cell suspension, and growth potential was quantified using an Omnicon Fas II automated colony counter (Milton Roy, Rochester, New York, USA) (Herman et al. 1983). For dynamic colony growth development we used the temporal growth pattern method, giving an estimation of growth over a certain period of time (Feitz et al. 1986).

Drug Testing. Drug tests were performed by exposing the tumor cells to a single dose of the drug. The drugs were layered over the top agar in a volume of 200 µl DE CMRL 1066 medium. The dishes in the growth control were layered with 200 µl DE CMRL 1066 and as a cytotoxic growth control we used a 0.37 m*M* $HgCl_2$ solution.

Results

Effect of Single Doses of IFN-α, IFN-γ, and TNF on Colony Formation of the Human Tumor Xenografts NU-12, HAM-II, and HAM-III

Determination of optimal plating densities for analysis of colony formation according to the temporal growth curves revealed a tumor concentration of 1.10E5 cells per dish for all tumor lines (data not shown). Single drug tests were performed using 1500, 15000, and 150000 IU IFN/ml (10, 100, 1000 and 160, 1600, 16000 ng/dish

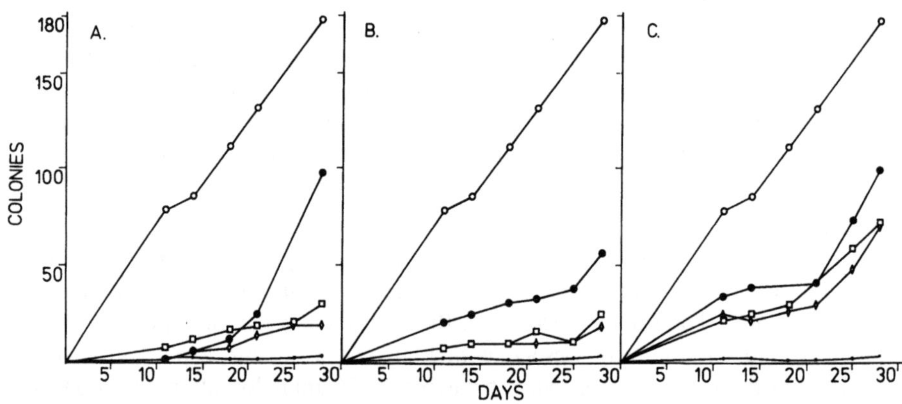

Fig. 1A–C. Effect of three different biological response modifiers on colony formation of NU-12 renal tumor xenograft in soft agar after application of a single dose of the drugs. **A** IFN-α. Specific activity: 3.2.10E8 IU/mg. ○—○, Growth control; •—•, cytotoxic control; ●—●, 10 ng/dish; □—□, 100 ng/dish; ◊—◊, 1000 ng/dish. **B** IFN-γ. Specific activity: 2.0.10E7 IU/mg. ○—○, Growth control; •—•, cytotoxic control; ●—●, 160 ng/dish; □—□, 1600 ng/dish; ◊—◊, 16000 ng/dish. **C** TNF. Specific activity: 6.0.10E7 IU/mg. ○—○, Growth control; •—•, cytotoxic control; ●—●, 10 ng/dish; □—□, 100 ng/dish; ◊—◊, 1000 ng/dish

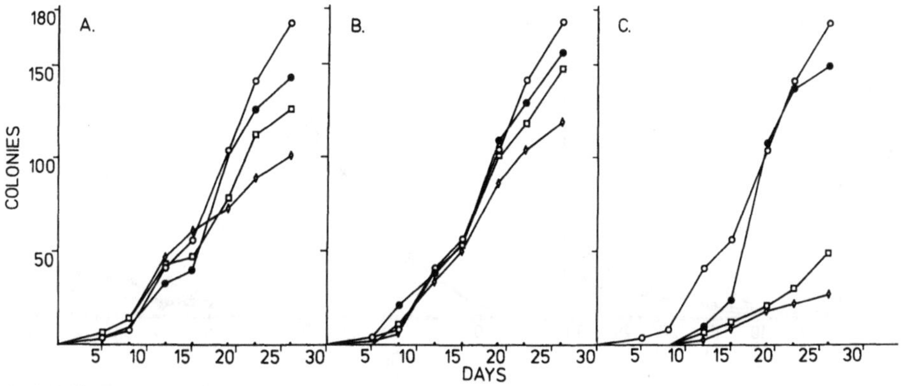

Fig. 2A–C. Effect of three different biological response modifiers on colony formation of HAM-II renal tumor xenograft in soft agar after application of a single dose of the drugs. **A** IFN-α. Specific activity: 3.2.10E8 IU/mg. ○—○, Growth control; •—•, cytotoxic control; ●—●, 10 ng/dish; □—□, 100 ng/dish; ◊—◊, 1000 ng/dish. **B** IFN-γ. Specific activity: 2.0.10E7 IU/mg. ○—○, Growth control; •—•, cytotoxic control; ●—●, 160 ng/dish; □—□, 1600 ng/dish; ◊—◊, 16000 ng/dish. **C** TNF. Specific activity: 6.0.10E7 IU/mg. ○—○, Growth control; •—•, cytotoxic control; ●—●, 10 ng/dish; □—□, 100 ng/dish; ◊—◊, 1000 ng/dish

(= ng/2 ml) for IFN-α and IFN-γ, respectively) and 600, 6000, and 60000 IU TNF/ml (10, 100, and 1000 ng/dish, respectively).

Figure 1 shows that sensitivity of the NU-12 xenograft is dose dependent for IFN-α, IFN-γ, and TNF. Sensitivity for the lowest tested doses of IFN-α and TNF was the same, resulting in a percentage survival fraction of about 60% as compared with the growth control. The higher doses of IFN-α resulted in a 15% survival fraction, but there was no or hardly any difference in the survival fraction between the intermediate and highest doses of IFN-α. TNF and IFN-γ both show the same pattern although the difference in activity between the lowest and intermediate concentrations of the BRMs is much less. Nu-12 is most sensitive for IFN-γ because a single dose of 160 IU/ml results in a percentage survival fraction of only 30% of growth control level.

Figure 2 shows the temporal growth curves of the HAM-II xenograft after application of single doses of the drugs. Although the sensitivity patterns are different, as with the NU-12 xenograft, inhibition of colony formation is dose dependent. This tumor line shows only very limited sensitivity for IFN-α, IFN-γ, and TNF. Only the intermediate (100 ng/dish) and high (1000 ng/dish) concentrations of TNF show percentage survival fractions which are 35% or less as compared with the growth control.

Figure 3 in which the temporal growth curves of the HAM-III tumor are shown, again gives different patterns of sensitivity towards the three tested BRMs. Sensitivity towards IFN-α and TNF is very high as compared with the other xenografts. A dose of 10 ng IFN-α and 10 ng TNF per dish resulted in a survival fraction of only 35% and 25%, respectively, as compared with the growth control. Remarkably, the effect of the intermediate concentration of 100 ng/dish is the same and a 10-fold rise of concentration to 1000 ng/dish diminishes the survival fraction by only 10%. Sensitivity of this line towards IFN-γ, however, appears to be very low. A concentration of 160 ng/dish results in a survival of 95% of growth control level, whereas the high-

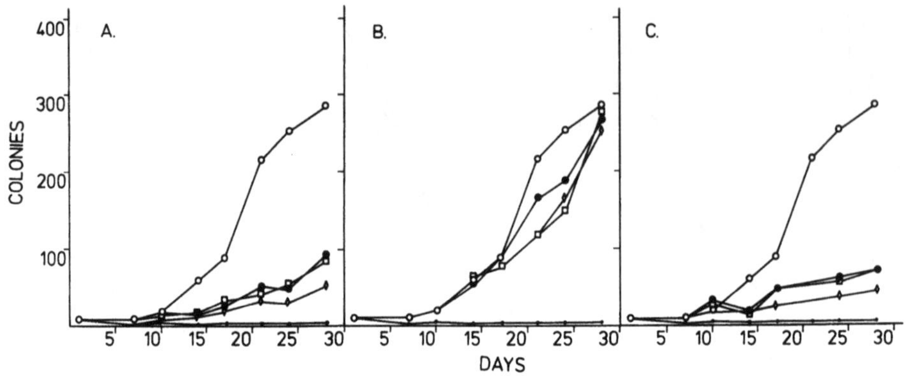

Fig. 3A–C. Effect of three different biological response modifiers on colony formation of HAM-III renal tumor xenograft in soft agar after application of a single dose of the drugs. **A** IFN-α. Specific activity: 3.2.10E8 IU/mg. ○—○, Growth control; •—•, cytotoxic control; ●—●, 10 ng/dish; □—□, 100 ng/dish; ◊—◊, 1000 ng/dish. **B** IFN-γ. Specific activity: 2.0.10E7 IU/mg. ○—○, Growth control; •—•, cytotoxic control; ●—●, 160 ng/dish; □—□, 1600 ng/dish; ◊—◊, 16000 ng/dish. **C** TNF. Specific activity: 6.0.10E7 IU/mg. ○—○, Growth control; •—•, cytotoxic control; ●—●, 10 ng/dish; □—□, 100 ng/dish; ◊—◊, 1000 ng/dish

est concentration of 16000 ng/dish still gives rise to about 85% of colonies as compared with the growth control.

Synergistic Antiproliferative Effects on Colony Formation of NU-12, HAM-II, and HAM-III Renal Tumor Cells After Application of a Single Dose of Combinations of IFN-α, IFN-γ, and/or TNF

Because IFNs and TNF can act synergistically (Hubbell et al. 1987; Salmon et al. 1987; Wong and Goeddel 1986), IFN concentrations of 10 and 160 ng/dish (1500 IU/ml) of IFN-α and IFN-γ, respectively, were used for the combination tests. The TNF concentration used was 100 ng/dish because preceding experiments with other RCC xenografts revealed a stimulation of colony formation in soft agar of one of the tested lines after application of 10 ng TNF/dish (Beniers et al. 1988).

The results of the combination tests are shown in Fig. 4 and are summarized in Table 1, which shows the percentage survival values for the combination tests as well as those for the single drug tests. Figure 4A shows the in vitro colony-forming capacity of NU-12 renal carcinoma cells when treated with different combinations of two of the above-mentioned BRMs. All combinations tested appear to have highly antiproliferative effects on the cells. Calculated according to Valeriote and Lin (1975), all combinations show highly synergistic antiproliferative effects on colony formation of this line. A 10% survival value is measured for the combination of 10 ng IFN-α/dish with 160 ng IFN-γ/dish. All other combinations, e.g., the combinations with TNF, coincide and give rise to only a 4% survival fraction as compared with the growth control.

Figure 4B, in which the in vitro colony-forming capacity of HAM-II renal carcinoma cells is shown after treatment with different combinations of the tested

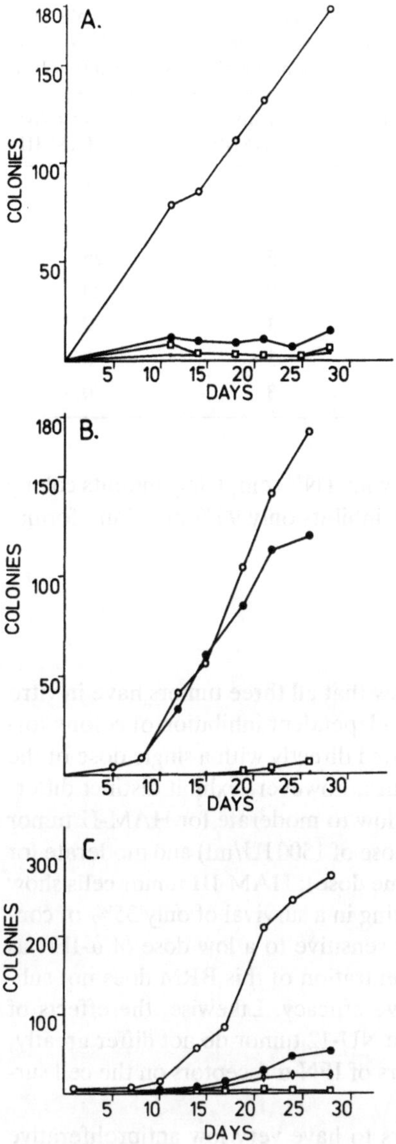

Fig. 4A–C. Effect of combinations of IFN-α (10 ng/dish), IFN-γ (160 ng/dish), and TFN (100 ng/dish) on colony formation of **A** NU-12, **B** HAM-II, and **C** HAM-III renal tumor xenograft cells in soft agar after application of a single dose of the drugs. The combinations of IFN-α/TNF, IFN-γ/TNF, and IFN-α/IFN-γ/TNF in **A** and **B** all coincide, as do the combinations of IFN-α/TNF and IFN-α/IFN-γ/TNF in **C**. ○—○, Growth control; •—•, cytotoxic control (200 µg $HgCl_2$/dish); ●—●, IFN-α/IFN-γ; □—□, IFN-α/TNF; ◊—◊, IFN-γ/TNF

BRMs, shows a rather high survival percentage with the drug combination IFN-α and IFN-γ. However, because of the low activities of the tested concentrations as shown in the single drug studies, this combination nevertheless results in a synergistic antiproliferative efficacy against the tumor cells, as do the other tested combinations which (as found for the NU-12 tumor cells) all give rise to the same antiproliferative effect on colony formation of the cells.

Figure 4C and Table 1 show that also for the HAM-III line all combinations tested act synergistically antiproliferatively on colony formation of these tumor cells. Least active again is the combination of IFN-α and IFN-γ which gives rise to a 20%

Table 1. Percentage survival of NU-12, HAM-II, and HAM-III renal tumor xenograft cells after growth in soft agar and application of a single dose of different combinations of IFN-α, IFN-γ, and TNF as compared with growth in the untreated control. Concentrations are given in ng/dish (ng/2 ml)

Drug combinations	% survival NU-12	% survival HAM-II	% survival HAM-III
α-IFN 10	55	85	35
γ-IFN 160	30	90	95
TNF 100	40	35	25
α-IFN 10, γ-IFN 160	10	70	20
α-IFN 10, TNF 100	3	3	0
γ-IFN 160, TNF 100	4	3	8
α-IFN 10, γ-IFN 160, TNF 100	4	3	0

survival rate, whereas the combination of IFN-α with TNF completely inhibits colony formation. The combination of IFN-γ with TNF inhibits only 90% of colony formation in the untreated growth control.

Discussion

Experimental results presented in this paper show that all three tumors have in vitro sensitivities for IFN-α, IFN-γ, and TNF. A dose-dependent inhibition of colony formation was evident for the three lines when treated directly with a single dose of the BRMs. Sensitivities of the three lines to the drugs, however, exhibit distinct differences. Sensitivity towards IFN-α appears to be low to moderate for HAM-II tumor cells (85% survival after application of a single dose of 1500 IU/ml) and moderate for NU-12 (55% survival after application of the same dose); HAM-III tumor cells show the highest sensitivity for this IFN-α dose, resulting in a survival of only 35% of control. Although the HAM-III tumor line is very sensitive to a low dose of α-IFN as compared with the other lines, raising the concentration of this BRM does not substantially contribute to a rise in antiproliferative efficacy. Likewise, the effects of intermediate and high IFN-α dose applied to the NU-12 tumor do not differ greatly, which may be an indication for different numbers of IFN-α receptors on the cell surface of the different tumors.

Except for the NU-12 tumor, IFN-γ appears to have very low antiproliferative efficacy against the tumors when applied as a single drug. Nevertheless, a dose-dependent inhibition is seen for all lines, and similar to the effect of the intermediate and high doses of IFN-α for the NU-12 tumor, there is no difference in antiproliferative efficacy between the intermediate and high doses of IFN-γ on colony formation of the NU-12 tumor line.

The same effect again was evident for the effect of TNF on this line. The HAM-II line shows only low sensitivity for the lowest TNF concentration of 300 IU/ml, resulting in only 30% inhibition of colony formation. Again, there is only little difference in antiproliferative efficacy between the intermediate and high doses of TNF for this line, and also the HAM-III line shows hardly any difference in sensitivity between the doses of 3000 and 30000 IU/ml.

The observed growth patterns in the combination tests showed that most combinations resulted in a high synergistic antiproliferative efficacy against the tumor cells. As found before (Beniers et al. 1988) the most effective drug combination for all tumor lines was the combination of IFN-α 10 ng/dish and TNF 100 ng/dish, resulting in a survival of 0% for the HAM-III line and of only 3% of the NU-12 and HAM-II lines, as compared with the growth control. As the mercury chloride cytotoxic growth control also gave rise to about 2% of growth control level of colony formation in the NU-12 experiments, we conclude that this combination completely inhibits colony formation of this line. The combination of IFN-α with IFN-γ acted synergistically but was the least active.

In conclusion, the three xenografts show distinct but different in vitro sensitivities towards IFN-α, IFN-γ, and TNF. Most sensitive was the NU-12 xenograft, which appeared sensitive for all three BRMs. Least sensitive was the HAM-II xenograft which was only moderately sensitive towards the three BRMs. The HAM-III xenograft appeared to be sensitive for IFN-α and TNF but showed no or hardly any sensitivity towards IFN-γ. All tested combinations of the three BRMs showed synergistic antiproliferative effects against colony formation of the three tumors. Most effective was the combination IFN-α 10 ng/dish plus TNF 100 ng/dish.

Acknowledgements. We want to thank Mr. J. Koedam and Mrs. M. Derks for their help in maintaining the tumors in nude mice. This work was supported by grants from the Netherlands Kidney Foundation (C85-563), the Maurits en Anna de Kock Foundation, the Nijbakker-Morra Foundation, and Boehringer, Ingelheim.

References

Balkwill FR, Goldstein L, Stebbing N (1985) Differential action of six human interferons against two human carcinomas growing in nude mice. Int J Cancer 35: 613–617

Beniers AJMC, Peelen WP, Hendriks BT, Schalken JA, Romijn JC, Debruyne FMJ (1988) In vitro antiproliferative efficacy of interferon-alpha, -gamma and tumor necrosis factor on two human renal tumor xenografts. Urol Res 16: 309–314

Bonnem EM, Spiegel RJ (1984) Interferon-alpha: current status and future promise. J Biol Resp Modif 3: 580–598

Brouckaert PGG, Leroux-Roels GG, Guisez Y, Tavernier J, Fiers W (1986) In vivo anti-tumour activity of recombinant human and murine TNF, alone and in combination with murine IFN-gamma, on a syngeneic murine melanoma. Int J Cancer 38: 763–769

Buzaid AC, Robertone A, Kisala C, Salmon SE (1987) Phase II study of interferon alfa-2a, recombinant (Roferon-A) in metastatic renal cell carcinoma. J Clin Oncol 5: 1083–1089

Feitz WFJ, Verheyen RHM, Kirkels WJ, Vooys GP, Debruyne FMJ, Herman CJ (1986) Dynamics of human renal tumor colony growth in vitro. Urol Res 14: 109–112

Fransen L, van der Heyden J, Ruysschaert R, Fiers W (1986) Recombinant tumor necrosis factor: its effect and its synergism with interferon-gamma on a variety of normal and transformed human cell lines. Eur J Cancer Clin Oncol 22: 419–426

Gresser I (1986) The antitumor effects of interferon. Med Oncol Tumor Pharmacother 3: 223–230

Hamburger AW, Salmon SE (1977) Primary bioassay of human tumor stem cells. Science 197: 461–463

Haranaka K, Satomi N, Sakurai A (1984) Antitumor activity of murine tumor necrosis factor (TNF) against transplanted murine tumors and heterotransplanted human tumors in nude mice. Int J Cancer 34: 263–267

Heicappell R, Naito S, Ichinose Y, Creasey AA, Lin LS, Fidler IJ (1987) Cytostatic and cytolytic effects of human recombinant tumor necrosis factor on human renal cell carcinoma cell lines derived from a single surgical specimen. J Immunol 138: 1634–1640

Herman CJ, Pelgrim OE, Kirkels WJ, Verheyen RHM, Debruyne FMJ, Kenemans P, Vooys GP (1983) In-use evaluation of the Omnicon automated tumor colony counter. Cytometry 3:439–442

Hubbel HR, Craft JA, Leibowitz PJ, Gillespie DH (1987) Synergistic antiproliferative effect of recombinant alpha-interferons with recombinant gamma-interferon. J Biol Resp Modif 6:141–153

Kirkwood JM, Ernstoff MS (1984) Interferons in the treatment of human cancer. J Clin Oncol 2: 336–352

Koiso K (1987) Phase II study of recombinant human interferon gamma (S-6810) on renal cell carcinoma. Cancer 60:929–933

Krown SE (1985) Therapeutic options in renal-cell carcinoma. Sem in Oncol [Suppl 5] 12:13–17

Krown SE (1987) Interferon treatment of renal cell carcinoma. Cancer 59:647–651

Muss HB (1987) Interferon therapy for renal cell carcinoma. Sem in Oncol [Suppl 2] 14:36–42

Muss HB, Costanzi JJ, Leavitt R, Williams RD, Kempf RA, Pollard R, Ozer H, Zekan PJ, Grunberg SM, Mitchell MS, Caponera M, Gavigan M, Ernest ML, Venturi C, Greiner J, Spiegel RJ (1987) Recombinant alfa interferon in renal cell carcinoma: a randomized trial of two routes of administration. J Clin Oncol 5:286–291

Nagy P, Kopper L, Gyapay G, Péterfy F, Lapis K (1988) Effect of interferon-alpha on various human tumor xenografts. Anticancer Res 8:467–470

Old LJ (1985) Tumor necrosis factor (TNF) Science 230:630–632

Old LJ (1987) Polypeptide mediator network. Nature 326:330–331

Otto U, Klöppel G, Baisch H (1984) Transplantation of human renal cell carcinoma into NMRI *nu/nu* mice. I. Reliability of an experimental tumor model. J Urol 131:130–133

Porzsolt F, Digel W, Jacobsen H, Mittnacht S, Kirchner H, Heimpel H (1988) Different antitumor mechanisms of interferon-alpha in the treatment of hairy cell leukemia and renal cell cancer. Cancer 61:288–293

Ruggiero V, Tavernier J, Fiers W, Baglioni C (1986) Induction of the synthesis of tumor necrosis factor receptors by interferon-gamma. J Immunol 136:2245–2450

Salmon SE, Yuong L, Scuderi P, Clark B (1987) Antineoplastic effects of tumor necrosis factor alone and in combination with gamma-interferon on tumor biopsies in clonogenic assay. J Clin Oncol 5:1816–1821

Sarna G, Figlin R, deKernion J (1987) Interferon in renal cell carcinoma. Cancer 59:610–612

Ueda R, Ogata S-I, Morrissay DM (1981) Cell surface antigens of human renal cancer defined by mouse monoclonal antibodies: identification of tissue-specific kidney glycoproteins. Proc Natl Acad Sci USA 78:5122–5126

Valeriote F, Lin H (1975) Synergistic interaction of anticancer agents: a cellular perspective. Cancer Chemother Rep 59:895–900

Verheyen RHM, Feitz WFJ, Beck JLM, Debruyne FMJ, Vooys GP, Kenemans P, Herman CJ (1985) Cell DNA content – correlation with clonogenicity in the human tumour cloning system (HTCS). Int J Cancer 35:653–657

Williamson BD, Carswell EA, Rubin BY, Prendergast JS, Old LJ (1983) Human tumor necrosis factor produced by human B-cell lines: synergistic cytotoxic interaction with human interferon. Proc Natl Acad Sci USA 80:5397–5401

Wong GHW, Goeddel DV (1986) Tumour necrosis factors alpha and beta inhibit virus replication and synergize with interferons. Nature 323:819–822

Water-Jet Cutting: A New Technique for Selective Parenchymal Surgery of the Kidney

J. Schüller[1], J. Pensel[2], A. J. A. Terzis[1], M. Florek[2], M. Steinmetz[2], S. Thomas[1], and P. Oehlert[1]

Introduction

One of the great difficulties in the development of surgery of parenchymal organs is the control of bleeding during dissection. This can be accomplished by cutting within intersegmental planes or by temporary occlusion of the vessels. Selective separation of tissue from vessels and fibrous structures is possible by focused ultrasonic energy (e.g., CUSA-System), which has found increasing application in liver and brain surgery. Another possibility of selective dissection is the method of water-jet cutting. This technique has been used in industry for a considerable time to separate soft and

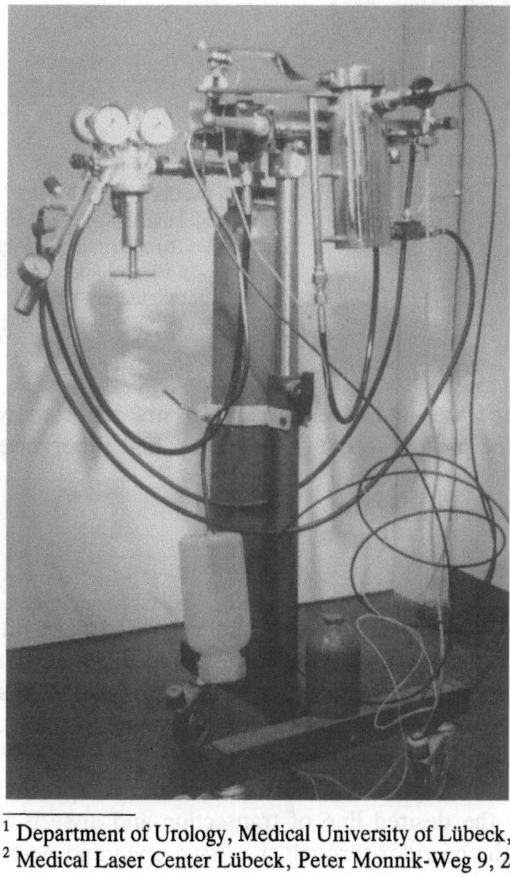

Fig. 1. Prototype of the water-jet system, pressure unit (BMTL, Lübeck)

[1] Department of Urology, Medical University of Lübeck, Ratzeburger Allee 160, 2400 Lübeck, FRG
[2] Medical Laser Center Lübeck, Peter Monnik-Weg 9, 2400 Lübeck, FRG

Investigative Urology 3
Edited by H. Rübben et al.

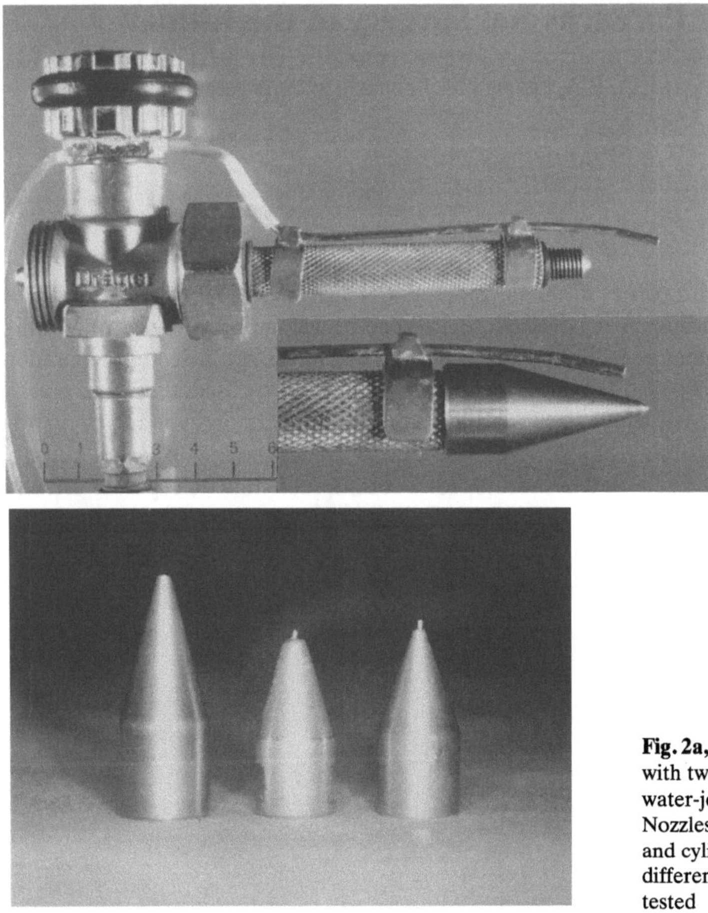

a

b

Fig. 2a, b. Handpiece (**a**) with two feed pipes for the water-jet and compressed air. Nozzles (**b**) with conical *(left)* and cylindrical shape and of different diameters were tested

hard materials. The application of the water-jet in liver surgery was first reported by Papachristou and Barters in 1982. The present report describes our first experience with the water-jet technique in the laboratory on cadaver organs.

Materials and Methods

In a cooperative venture between the Medical Laser Center Lübeck (MLL) and the company Biomedizinische Technik Lübeck (BMTL), a prototype of the water-jet system was developed. The system (Fig. 1) consists of three parts, a pressure unit, a connective unit, and a handpiece. The pressure obtained can be varied up to 50 bar. The system delivers normal saline solution.

The handpiece (Fig. 2) consists of feed pipes for the water-jet and compressed air. The water-jet hits the tissue at the desired line of transection and dissects it (Fig. 3). The compressed air keeps the corridor through the tissue open and pushes away the sprinkling water, which can obscure the view.

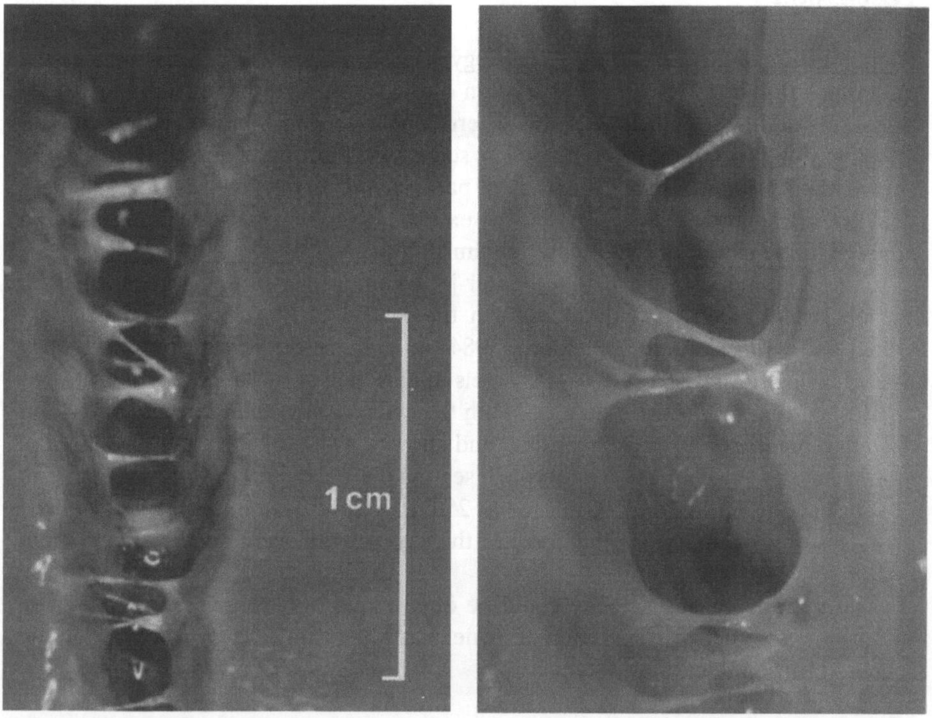

Fig. 3a, b. Dissection of the kidney using the water-jet scalpel (cylindrically shaped nozzle with inner diameter of 0.2 mm). The parenchyma is dissected, leaving fibrous structures intact (**a**). **b** Same cut magnified (× 4.4)

The aim of this pilot study was to find an optimal shape and diameter of nozzle. To this end, nozzles with cylindrical and conical shape and of three different diameters (0.1, 0.2, and 0.4 mm) were tested (Fig. 2b). Furthermore, the influence of the distance from the nozzle to the tissue, the cutting velocity, and the water-jet pressure on the quality of the cut had to be defined. Cadaver porcine kidneys were fixed on a specially designed cutting sled. The cuts were done with a nozzle perpendicular to the longitudinal axis of the organ.

Results

The best cutting results are obtained with cylindrically shaped nozzles with a diameter of 0.1 and 0.2 mm. The optimal distance between nozzle and tissue is between 0.5 and 1 cm. The optimal cutting velocity is between 3 and 5 mm/s.

The depths of the cuts increase linearly with the pressure in a range between 15 and 30 bar. A pressure between 20 and 25 bar produces ideal cuts with a depth of 0.7–1.0 cm.

The water consumption is dependent on the nozzle and the pressure. For a 0.2-mm nozzle and a pressure of 30 bar, it is 100 cc/min.

Discussion

High pressure fluid jet cutting technology has been used for cutting nonmetallic materials for about 30 years. By variation of the shape of the nozzle and the water pressure, biological structures with different solidity and consistency can be cut selectively and without thermic load. The selective dissection of vessels (Fig. 4) from surrounding tissue would allow cutting of parenchymal organs, which are not dependent on intersegmental lines. By this the extent of parenchymal resections could be adapted to the extent of the disease, minimizing damage of normal tissue.

Our preliminary studies with the water-jet technique for cutting parenchymal tissue on kidney, liver, and brain confirm the results of Papachristou and Barters (1982) and Nishisaka and Yonekawa (1984) in liver. Selective dissection of kidney tissue leaving fibrous structures and vessels undamaged seems to be possible.

Best cutting results were obtained with the cylindrically shaped nozzle of 0.1 and 0.2 mm diameter. The cut was precise and showed a fine delineation. The 0.4-mm nozzle gave a very deep cut with a rough sectional area and had a high consumption of saline solution (approx. 500 ml/min at 25 bar). The 0.1-mm nozzle often showed problems of obstruction, so that most of the experiments were done with a 0.2-mm nozzle.

The optimal cutting velocity could be determined between 3 and 5 mm/s. The water-jet system allows transection of tissue in a realistic time range in contrast to the focused ultrasound cutting system.

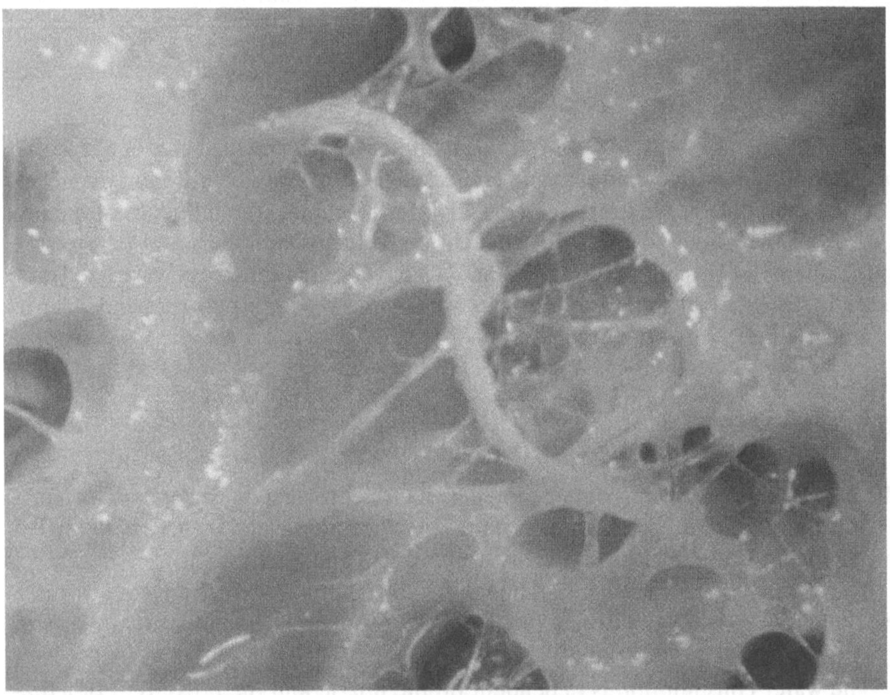

Fig. 4. Selective dissection of a vessel (1.5 mm outer diameter) from the surrounding liver tissue

The compressed air stream is an essential part of the new jet system, giving excellent viewing during dissection and obviating a plastic shield against spray as postulated by Papachristou.

The ideal distance between the nozzle and the tissue being transected is between 0.5 and 1 cm. Within this relatively wide range the management of the handpiece does not influence the cutting quality. Handheld application therefore seems possible.

The pressure of choice is between 20 and 25 bar, allowing cuts of approx. 1 cm in depth. With higher pressure the dissection is difficult to control. Application of a 40 bar water-jet will possibly completely transect the kidney in one cut.

The smallest diameter of vessels which will be left undamaged by the water stream is not exactly defined yet and will be determined in studies currently being performed on living perfused organs.

Summary

Water-jet cutting allows transection and dissection of biological structures independent of its solidity. Vessels of parenchymal organs as liver, kidney and brain show a higher solidity than the parenchyma and can therefore selectively by dissected from the surrounding tissue. Transection of parenchymal organs outside of the intersegmental planes can be performed with a water-jet without excessive blood loss. The extent of the resection can therefore be adapted to the extent of the disease, minimizing organs trauma.

References

Nishisaka T, Yonekawa M (1984) Development of the water jet scalpel. Proc Water Jet Technol Jpn, pp 55–61

Papachristou DN, Barters R (1982) Resection of the liver with a water jet. Br J Surg 69:93–94

II. Andrology and Testicular Cancer

Testicular Blood Supply with a View to Surgical Treatment

T. Strittmatter and G. Konrad[1]

Introduction

Andrology and research on fertility have offered many detailed aspects for surgical treatment in recent years. So, besides new surgical techniques and selection of a most beneficial time for intervention, for example, age of the patient (Hoechst and Hadziselimovic 1982), today's successful surgery of the testicles demands an intimate knowledge of their vascular anatomy. Harm to the testicles' blood supply should be avoided, but a surgeon has to think ahead as well about microsurgical possibilities in order to maintain suitable conditions in case of future repair. In the following, various indications for testicular surgery are discussed from the perspective of the vascular anatomy.

Vascular investigation of the human testicle and its epididymis by corrosion cast technique (Krienen et al. 1981; Steinmann and Frewein 1982; Wurzer 1987) presents detailed information about the distribution of even the smallest vessels. In spite of anatomic variations, corrosion casts of the human testis demonstrate three vessels, three main vascular supply areas, and three areas of anastomoses (Hundeiker 1970; Wurzer 1987).

Vessel Supply of the Testis

The spermatic artery (a. testicularis) supplies the testicular tissue itself.

The testicular artery enters the testicle at the mediastinum testis, lying immediately beneath the tunica albuginea, and courses from the extremitas caudalis along the margo liber to the extremitas cranialis. From this part of the spermatic artery (a. testicularis propria) the septal arteries descend, supplying as rami centripetales and rami centrifugales the germinative tissue.

The epididymic artery branches off from the spermatic artery 2–10 cm above the extremitas cranialis testis.

The a. ductus deferentis follows the course of the vas deferens and mainly supplies the cauda epididymis.

The a. cremasterica nurtures the tunica vaginalis.

Primarily the a. testicularis propria provides the blood circulation of the testicle itself. The epididymis receives approximately 84% of its blood supply via the a. epididymica in the region of the caput and 66% from the a. testicularis in the region of caput and corpus.

[1] Urologische Klinik – Franziskushaus, Viersenerstr. 450, 4050 Mönchengladbach 1, FRG

The region of the cauda epididymis is constantly supplied by the deferential artery. Participation of the cremasteric artery can be shown in 84%, and participation of the epididymis artery in 66% of patients. Blood supply from the testicular artery for the cauda epididymis can be shown in 84% of the testicles. To these anastomoses between the three vessel systems attention must be paid.

Vascular Supply by Anastomoses

Anastomoses between the testicular artery, cremasteric artery, and deferential artery can be found in three areas: (1) above the upper pole of the testis, (2) caput/corpus epididymis, and (3) cauda epididymis. While the anastomoses are subject to variation, only in the cauda epididymis region are anastomoses regularly to be found between all three vessel systems.

On the level of the upper testicular pole or up to 10 cm above it there are sporadically one or more thin-calibered anastomoses between a. spermatica and a. ductus deferentis. This anastomosis may be more or less strongly developed or not exist at all. To some extent (approximately 20%–30%) these anastomoses maintain a basic blood supply for the testicular tissue and for the caput epididymis if the spermatic

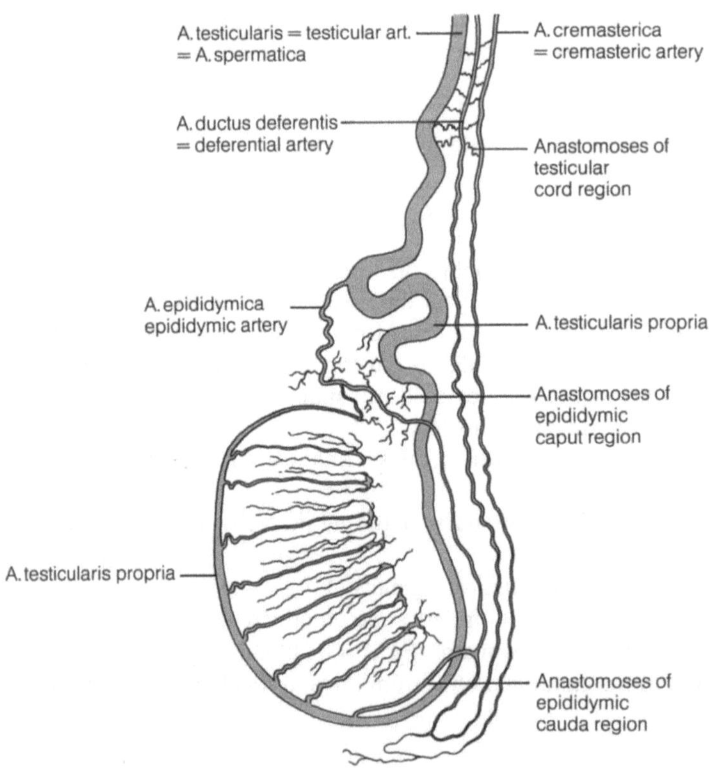

Fig. 1. Testicular blood supply

artery is cut off. A lack of nutrition endangers spermatogenesis in the tubules and maturation of the sperm in the caput epididymis. With respect to the caliber of a. spermatica, which we found regularly more than twice as wide in diameter compared with the a. ductus deferentis, the deficiency of blood perfusion is evident. The cremasteric artery is usually even smaller (Fig. 1).

Anastomoses on the level of the caput epididymis demonstrate a vast tributary variety but are weakly developed and, in general, follow the above-mentioned pattern.

As such the epididymic artery, as a branch of a. spermatica, provides the main nutrition for this tissue area.

In the area of the cauda epididymis and the lower pole of the testis, anastomoses between a. testicularis propria and a. ductus deferentis are constantly found. They are of extremely thin caliber. Infrequently, there are connections with a. cremasterica.

The investigations into the blood supply and the anastomotic connections of the vessels demonstrate clearly the main role of the spermatic artery for the vascularization of the testis, the caput, and corpus epididymis, as well as the importance of the three areas of anastomoses. So, after dissection of the testicular artery, the blood supply of the testis and epididymis depends on fine-calibered anastomoses. Even if the testicle is basically supplied by the cauda anastomoses and by the partly developed anastomoses of the spermatic cord region, the testis, and especially the caput, possibly as well the corpus epididymis are exposed to an enormous diminution of blood perfusion. This malperfusion distinctly harms the functional ability of the testis.

Surgical Methods and Vascular Supply

Some common surgical interventions to the male's genitals will be discussed in relation to blood supply. Awareness of prevalent anatomic vessel conditions should lead one to taking proper surgical steps so as to avoid a decline of spermatogenesis.

Orchidopexy. Cryptorchidism leads to the need for frequent surgical intervention. Relevant methods used for the repairing of maldescended testis are: conventional orchidopexy (Bevan 1899), two-stage orchidopexy (Persky and Albert 1971), long loop vas procedure (Fowler and Stephens 1959), and testicular autotransplantation (Silber 1981; Konrad et al. 1984, 1983; Konrad and Schwaiger 1984).

Conventional Orchidopexy. The majority of the undescended testicles can be placed successfully in the scrotum by conventional orchidopexy as proven by many basic surgical principles established as early as 1899 by Bevan. After mobilization of the testis and the spermatic cord, the dissection of the cremasteric fibers follows. After removing the peritoneal fold or hernia sac from the testicular cord, a sufficient length ought to be gained for scrotal fixation of the testis without undue tension. It is of course essential to protect the vessels of the spermatic cord and the possible high division of the epididymic artery and the anastomoses between a. spermatica and a. ductus deferentis. Special attention has to be given to the orchidopexy suture at the lower pole of the testis. The stitch should take only the connecting tissue between testis and epididymis – inferior epididymic ligament – thereby avoiding the tunica albuginea, because the a. testicularis propria courses immediately beneath it. An occlusion of this vessel by the thread severely disturbs the testicular blood supply and subsequently affects the reproductive system.

Two-Stage Orchidopexy. If conventional surgical maneuvers fail to gain enough length of the testicular cord, one method to bring the testicle into the scrotum is two-stage orchidopexy (Persky and Albert 1971). In the first stage, the testicle is fixed at the lowest possible inguinal position. A fixation suture is brought out through the skin and tied over a gauze sponge and must remain so for 4–5 days. A second stage follows from 6 months up to 2 years later. Most commonly, the two-stage orchidopexy is started with an attempt to gain length by extensive dissection of the cremasteric fibers along the vasal and testicular cord. If this is carried out too near to the testicle, then the risk of injuring the epididymic artery or the anastomoses of this region is very high. In the second stage, more preparation is required on the testicular cord, but it bears an additional danger for the vascular supply, especially for the secondary neovascular collateralization. It is an adequate method for orchidopexy of undescended testicle only if by this measure the scrotal position is indeed reached. If this procedure fails, the consequence of the operation will be orchidectomy, or another attempt to fix the testicle into the scrotum by the Fowler-Stephens maneuver or by autotransplantation. Both methods depend on undamaged vessel anastomoses. In this respect, the first procedure must avoid preparations near the upper testicular pole.

Fowler-Stephens' Long Loop Vas Orchidopexy. Fowler and Stephens (1959) presented a surgical method of orchidopexy of high undescended testes. If the vascular cord of the testicle is too short, even after maximal mobilization, they suggest dissecting the a. and v. spermatica. The vas generally is of sufficient length to reach the scrotal position. The vascular supply ought to be maintained by the a. ductus deferentis and the anastomoses to the lower spermatic artery. According to Fowler and Stephens and others, 25%–40% of testicular atrophy can be found after this maneuver, because of insufficient or undeveloped anastomoses between the spermatic artery and the vas. Consequently, the incidence of infertility is expected to be much higher. During surgery it may be helpful to perform a bleeding test as an attempt to determine the blood supply of the testis. After clamping the testicular vessels, an incision is made through the tunica albuginea, with arterial bleeding for several minutes after clamping indicating that there is a sufficient anastomotic supply.

Autotransplantation. Autotransplantation of the high undescended, especially the intra-abdominal testes, has become the method of choice to get the testicle into scrotal position (Silber 1981; Konrad et al. 1984, 1983; Konrad and Schwaiger 1984). The spermatic vessels are dissected high up at the main abdominal vessels and reanastomosed with the inferior epigastric ones. Until revascularization is performed, the basic arterial supply of the testicle and epididymis is provided by natural anastomoses. Transitional hypoxemy may occur where these anastomoses are weakly developed, nonexistant, or destroyed by previous surgery. Hypoxemy is minimized by quick microsurgical revascularization.

Further Surgical Interventions. Like the surgery for cryptorchism, other conventional operations contain the risk of damaging the arterial vessel supply. A most common operation, varicocelectomy is usually practised as a retroperitoneal dissection of the testicular vein. However, the small spermatic artery needs to be saved. In the lower region, the testicular artery may be injured by spermatocelectomy or epididymectomy. Biopsies of the testicles should be taken at the lateral side of the upper pole of the testis. At the medial part of the margo liber, injury to a testicularis propria beneath the tunica albuginea cuts off the main blood supply. It is valid for surgical interventions – repair of torsion or orchidopexy – to place sutures for fixation of the testicle. Injury of the spermatic propria artery means damage to the reproductive tissue or even partial atrophy of the testis.

Discussion

The findings of Hundeiker (1970, 1980), Krienen et al. (1981, 1982, Wurzer 1987), and others confirm clearly that there is a distinct testicular vascularization, and a large variety of vessel architecture and anastomosis.

The three arteries – spermatic, ductus deferentis, and cremasteric – are linked by anastomoses of fine calibers in three areas – spermatic cord, caput epididymis, and cauda epididymis. Hence, each artery of the testicle has its individual nutritional scope. After dissection of one artery, a basic blood supply can be maintained through the fine anastomoses. In approximately 25%–40%, after dissection of the testicular artery, atrophy of the testis occurs but a much higher incidence may be expected. Consequently, for a much higher percentage, the minimal blood supply through anastomoses is not at all sufficient for preserving the function of the reproductive tissue. In opposition to Hundeiker (1970) we found that the a. testicularis propria participates in the blood supply of the caput epididymis. Considering the tributaries of the spermatic artery, a loss of its blood supply does result in much more harm than a dissection of the a. ductus deferentis. The differences of the calibers of the arteries themselves as well as of their fine anastomoses illustrate that. Through clinical experience Palomo (1949), cited in Fowler and Stephens (1959) describes no testicular atrophy after high dissection of the testicular artery. Fowler and Stephens (1959) and Gibbons et al. (1979) found atrophy in 30% after high dissection of the testicular artery. Clatworthy (1972) had a rate of 10% atrophy by carefully sparing the regions of anastomoses. Maar et al. (1981) saw no atrophy but very often a noninfectious swelling of the epididymis in the spermatic cord region. Preparation of the spermatic cord vessels was followed by partial atrophy in 50%. A dissection of the spermatic artery does not allow any prediction as to whether an atrophy of the testicle or of the epididymis will result.

Silber (1981) emphasizes the importance of reanastomosing the testicular artery. He found no atrophy after autotransplantation of abdominal testicles. No reanastomosed testicles were atrophied in any case. Konrad and Schwaiger (1984) had a quota of success of 92% with autotransplantation, which demonstrates the main role of the testicular artery for testicular survival after surgical treatment.

References

Bevan AD (1899) Operation for undescended testicle and congenital inguinal hernia. JAMA 33:773
Clatworthy HW jr, Hollanbaugh RS, Grosfeld IL (1972) The long-loop-vas orchidopexy for the high undescended testis. Am Surg 38:69
Fowler R, Stephens FD (1959) The role of testicular vascular anatomy in the salvage of high undescended testes. Aust NZJ Surg (1959):92–106
Gibbons MD, Cromie WJ, Duckett JW Jr (1979) Management of the abdominal undescended testicle. J Urol 122:76–79
Hoechst B, Hadziselimovic F (1982) Zeitpunkt und Therapie der Kryptorchismusbehandlung. Z Kinderchirurg 37:15–19
Hundeiker M (1970) Untersuchungen über die Vaskularisation des Hodens. Habil, Gießen
Hundeiker M (1980) Anatomie der Gefäßversorgung des Hodens. Fortschritte der Fertil.forsch 8, Kongreßbericht Kiel 1979. Grosse Verlag, Berlin, pp 313–317
Konrad G, Schwaiger R (1984) Autotransplantation des Abdominalhodens und freie Hodentransplantation. Im Dienst der Chirurgie 49. Ethicon GmbH, Hamburg
Konrad G, Zabransky S, Schwaiger R, Alzin H, Neisius D (1984) Das freie Hodentransplantat bei eineiigen Zwillingen; ein Fallbericht. Extracta Paediatr 8(1):17–26
Konrad G, Schwaiger R, Neisius D, Kopper B, Ziegler M (1983) Abdominalhoden: Diagnostik und operative Therapie. In: Rodeck G (ed) Verhandlungsbericht der Deutschen Gesellschaft für Urologie, 35. Tagung. Springer, Berlin Heidelberg New York, pp 369–371
Krienen P, Notermans HP, Passia D, Hofmann N (1981) Über die Herstellung und Untersuchungen von Ausgußpräparaten mit Plastogen G. I. Mitteilung. Der Präparator Jg 27 [3]:109–113
Krienen P, Notermans HP, Passia D, Hofmann N (1982) Über die Herstellung und Untersuchungen von Ausgußpräparaten mit Plastogen G. II. Mitteilung. Der Präparator Jg 28. [1]:205–210
Maar K et al (1981) Untersuchungen zur Varicocelenoperation nach Palomo. Urologe [A] 20:365–369
Palomo A (1949) J Urol 61:604. In: Fowler R, Stephens FD (1959) The role of testicular vascular anatomy in the salvage of high undescended testes. Aust N Z J Surg (1959):92–106
Persky L, Albert DJ (1971) Staged orchidopexy. Surg Gynecol Obstet 132:43
Silber SJ (1981) The intraabdominal testes: microvascular autotransplantation. J Urol 125:329–333
Steinmann W, Frewein J (1982) Die Darstellung von Lymphgefäßen und Lymphkapillaren mittels Korrosion am Ganzpräparat des Stierhodens. Der Präparator Jg 28:355–359
Wurzer B (1987) Experimentelle Untersuchung über die Vaskularisation des Hodens und Nebenhodens. Inauguraldissertation

Alteration of Penile Ultrastructure in Impotence: Morphology and Clinical Correlation

C. PERSSON-JÜNEMANN[1,2], W. DIEDERICHS[2], and T. F. LUE[2]

Introduction

Within the past few years rapid advances have been achieved integrating the basic understanding of anatomy, physiology, and pharmacology in a concept of penile erection. Within this concept the smooth musculature of the corpus cavernosum has gained a central role.

This study was designed to reveal ultrastructural changes within the functional tissue of the corpus cavernosum in impotent men and to determine any correlation with the degree of clinical erectile dysfunction.

Patients and Methods

Thirty-two impotent patients (32–79 years) who underwent surgical implantation of a penile prosthesis were included in this study. Classification of their impotence was based on the erectile response to intracavernous injection of papaverine ($n = 25$), categorized from no response (E0) to full rigid erection (E5). In addition duplex ultrasonography and pulsed doppler analysis before and after papaverine ($n = 19$) was utilized for vascular evaluation.

At the time of prosthesis insertion, tissue samples were obtained from the mid-shaft of the corpus cavernosum. After proper preparation the ultrastructural examination was performed with a transmission electron microscope, and morphological findings were correlated with the preoperative clinical classification.

Results

Clinical Findings. Based upon the clinical evaluation, three pathogenetic categories were distinguished: nonvascular, mild to moderate arterial insufficiency, severe arterial insufficiency. The first group ($n = 3$, 36–57 years) showed a full, rigid erectile response (E5) to intracavernous papaverine injection and a normal functional evaluation of the penile arteries (Lue et al. 1985). Their impotence was classified as psychoneurogenic, and they served as the control group. Nineteen patients (42–71 years) were included in the second group with partial response to papaverine injection (E2–3) and evidence of a moderate degree of arterial disease in the duplex ultrasonography. Nine patients (47–69 years) classified as severe arterial insufficiency

[1] Urologische Klinik, Klinikum Mannheim der Universität Heidelberg, 6800 Mannheim 1, FRG
[2] University of California, S.F., Dept. Urology, School of Medicine, San Francisco, CA 94143, USA

Investigative Urology 3
Edited by H. Rübben et al.

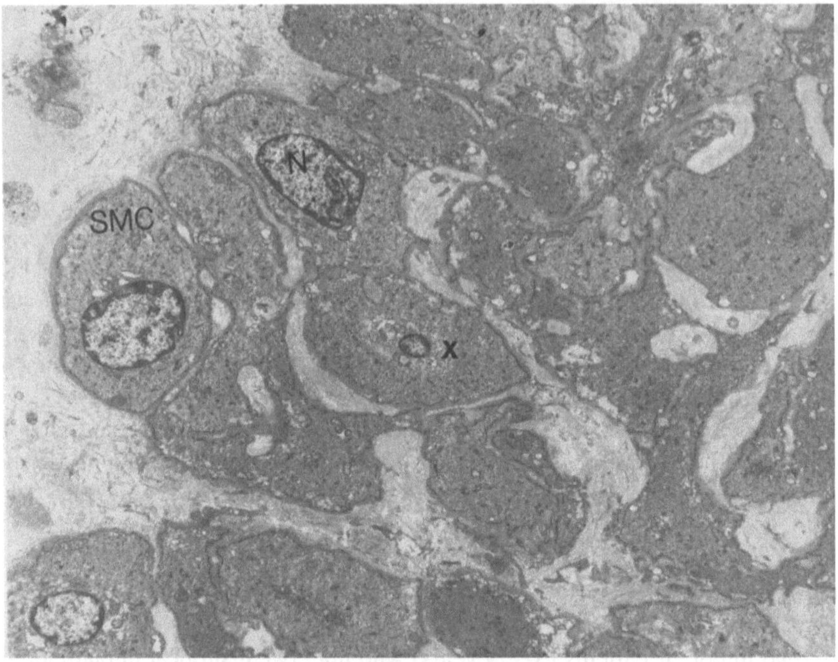

a

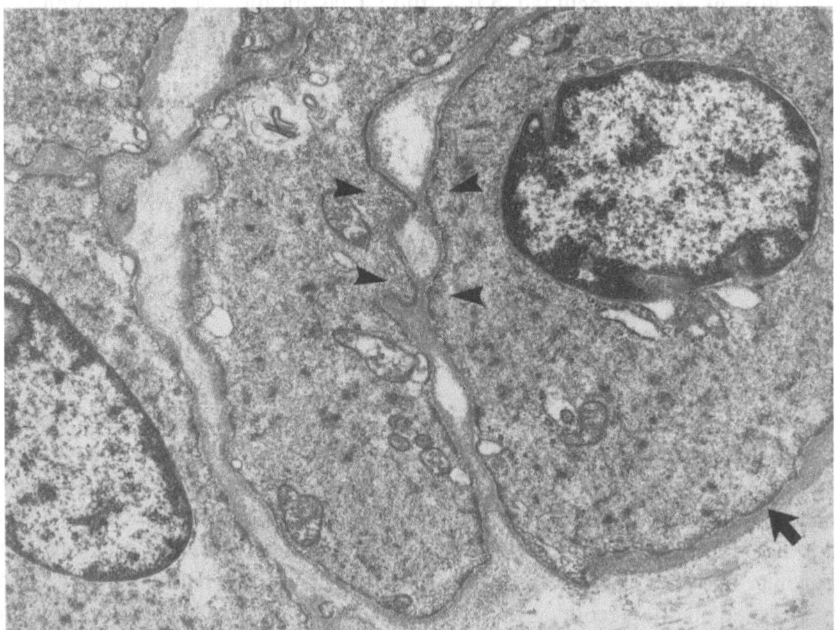

b

Fig. 1. a Normal trabecular ultrastructure with a bundle of intimately related smooth muscle cells *(SMC)* embedded in strands of fibroconnective tissue. Homogeneous cytoplasm containing densely packed myofilaments and perinuclear organelles *(x)*. Cell nucleus *(N)* with homogeneous chromatin network within a double membrane. × 3953. **b** Normal smooth muscle cell invested with distinct basement membrane *(arrow)* showing numerous sites of cell contact *(arrowheads)*. × 11992 (From Persson et al. (in press), with permission the *Journal of Urology*) showed a poor erectile response after papaverine, with mere penile elongation or moderate tumescence (E0–1). On ultrasonography the increase in arterial diameter was minimal, and peak-flow velocities reduced or not measurable.

Electron Microscopy

The specimens from patients forming the *control group* are morphologically similar and show the characteristic ultrastructure of penile tissue (Bossart et al. 1980; Goldstein et al. 1982; Benson et al. 1980; Leeson and Leeson 1965). Confluent sinusoids show an intact endothelial lining comprising large, attenuated cells with protruding nuclei. The endothelium rests upon a complete basement membrane and features vast pinocytotic activity.

Subjacent to the endothelium, smooth muscle cells are organized in small groups associated with surrounding connective tissue. The elongated nucleus consists of a fine homogeneous chromatin network within a double membrane. Cytoplasmic components include densely packed myofilaments and organelles; mitochondria, endoplasmic reticulum, ribosomes, and the golgi apparatus located in a limited perinuclear area (Fig. 1a). The cytoplasmic membrane shows regions of pinocytotic activity and dense thickenings opposed to corresponding regions of adjacent cells (nexus; Fig. 1b).

Nerve tissue consisting of bundles, preterminal, and terminal varicosities is embedded in connective tissue in close proximity to bundles of smooth muscle. Blood

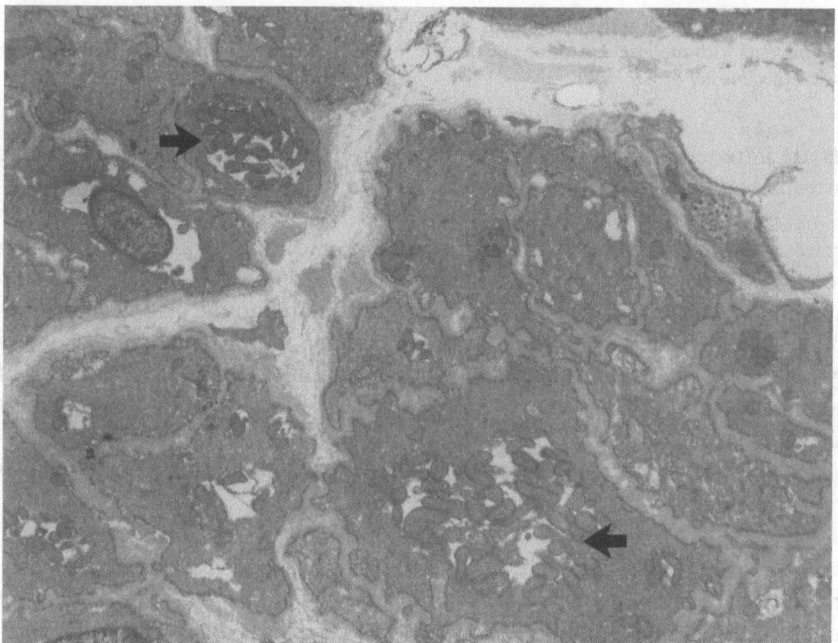

Fig. 2. Beginning alteration of intracellular smooth muscle cell structure in patient with moderate arteriogenic impotence. Pronounced increase and aggregation of mitochondria *(arrows)*. Morphological elements maintain normal distribution. × 4059 (From Persson et al. (in press), with permission the *Journal of Urology*)

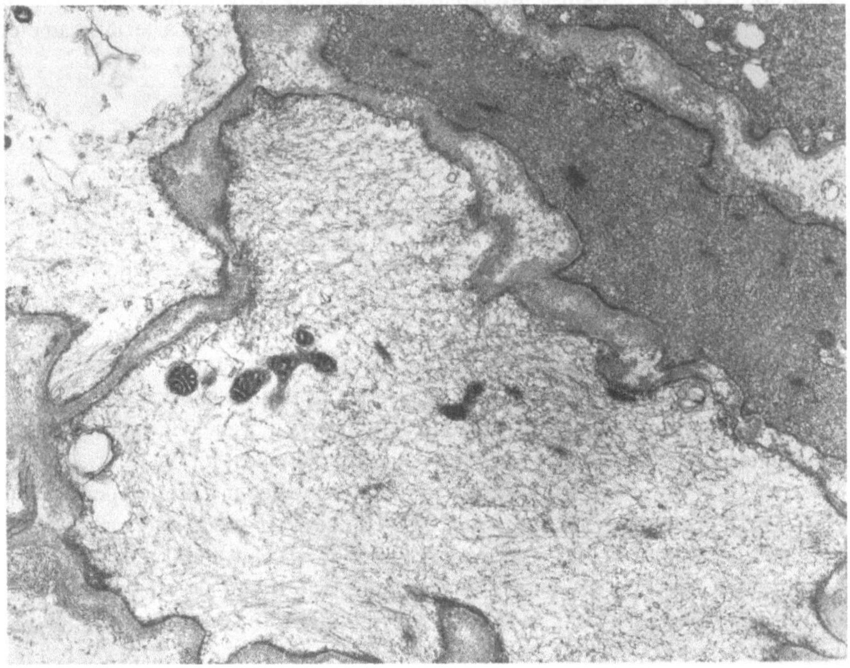

Fig. 3. Presence of light smooth muscle cells showing homogeneous intracellular loss of myofilaments in patients with moderate arteriogenic disease. ×12078 (From Persson et al. (in press), with permission the *Journal of Urology*)

vessels are infrequent, most being precapillary arterioles with an endothelial lining and surrounding pericyte or smooth muscle elements.

Moderate Arterial Disease. Regarding the number and distribution of the cellular components, the penile architecture of patients with moderate arterial disease is consistent with the control group. Primary changes are related to the cytoplasmic structure of the smooth muscle cell; pronounced increase and aggregation of mitochondria and cytoplasmic vacuolization containing glycogen granules (Fig. 2). The presence of light smooth muscle cells was seen in 10 patients (Fig. 3). In addition three patients revealed a quantitative loss of smooth muscle, replaced by connective tissue. Endothelial and vascular alteration was not encountered; axonal reduction in nerve bundles occurred in eight patients.

Severe Arterial Disease. The penile tissue in this group shows marked changes concerning cellular structure and distribution of the trabecular elements. Smooth muscle cells are reduced in number and replaced by dense connective tissue separating individual cells. Alteration of the smooth muscle cell includes an irregular contour with fragmentation and loss of the basal lamina and an increase of perinuclear organelles with displacement of the reduced contractile myofilaments to the periphery. The nuclei are pleiomorphic with unevenly distributed chromatin situated along the nuclear membrane (Fig. 4a). Cell-membrane contacts are reduced and in several

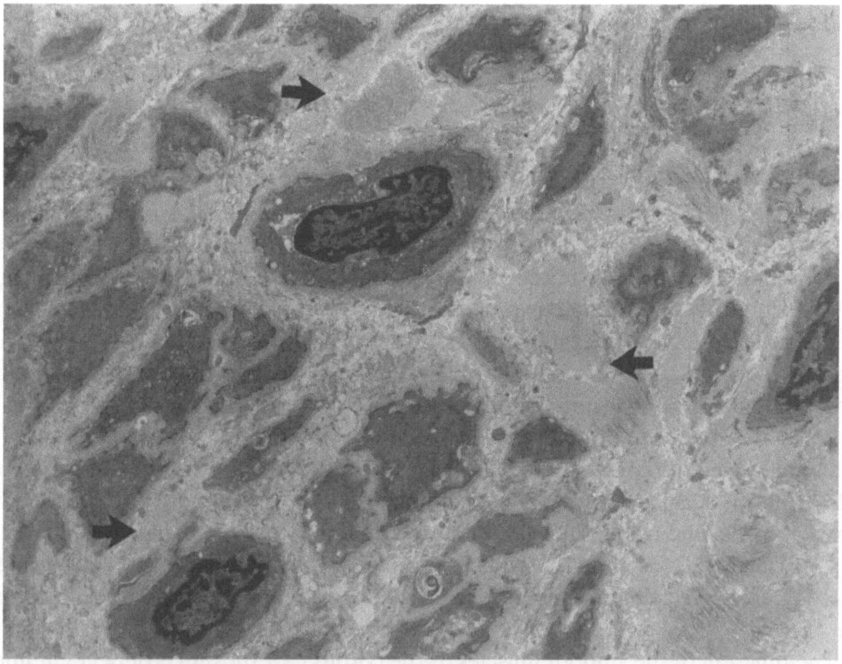

a

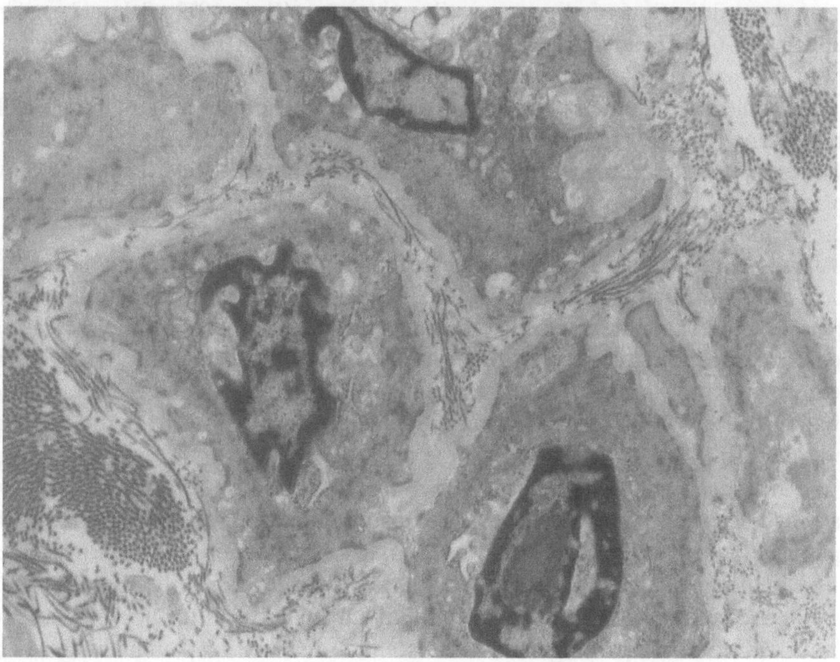

b

Fig. 4. a Ultrastructural alteration in patient with severe arteriogenic impotence. Increased mass of fibroconnective tissue *(arrows)* separating individual smooth muscle cells. Chromatin is unevenly distributed within irregular nucleoplasm. × 4133. **b** Irregular cell contour with fragmentation of basement membrane leading to loss of intercellular contacts in patients with severe arteriogenic impotence. × 11992 (From Persson et al. (in press), with permission the *Journal of Urology*) cases completely lost (Fig. 4b). Endothelial alterations are significant, resulting in major defects of the sinusoidal lining. Nerve bundles are less frequently encountered.

Discussion

The use of intracavernous injection of papaverine and duplex ultrasonography for evaluation of penile arterial function has proved to be feasible in clinical application (Lue et al. 1985; Virag et al. 1984; Wetzner et al. 1983). In this study we compared the morphological changes in the cavernous tissue in impotent men of various ages with the clinically determined degree of vascular insufficiency.

The morphological alteration of the cavernous ultrastructure in patients with arteriogenic impotence affects primarily the smooth muscle cells. The extent of morphological changes corresponds to the severity of arterial disease and the failure of the erectile response to intracavernous injection of papaverine.

In moderate arterial disease, early changes were found in the intracellular structure of the smooth muscle cell with a distinct increase and aggregation of mitochondria, consistent with findings in the smooth muscle cell of the iris in diabetes (Ishikawa et al. 1985). Together with cytoplasmic vacuolization, these changes could be interpreted as an active cellular attempt to respond to an altered environmental and nutritive situation.

The function of the smooth muscles of the corpus cavernosum is dependent upon the intact organization of the contractile apparatus (Bois 1973; Schoenberg and Needham 1976). The decrease of myofilaments found in severe arterial disease showed two patterns of manifestation. One is an homogeneous intracellular loss of the contractile myofilaments actin and myosin, resulting in light smooth muscle cells, a phenomenon previously described in diabetic patients and by Melman et al. (1981) in the penile tissue of patients with abnormal norepinephrine levels. The other shows displacement of the reduced mass of myofilaments to the periphery due to increase of the perinuclear organelles.

A fragmentation or loss of the basement membrane confinement of the smooth muscle cell is distinctive in patients with severe arterial disease. In addition to the increased amount of interspersed fibroconnective tissue, the resulting decrease of specific corresponding regions of pinocytotic activity and dense thickening of the basement membrane (nexus) could interfere with the intercellular transmission of excitation (Caesar et al. 1957; Bergmann 1956), possibly by impairing the diffusion of neurotransmitters.

The arteriosclerotic changes in impotent men reported by several authors (Ruzbarsky and Michal 1977; Cohen et al. 1980) were found in the major arteries of the corpus cavernosum and the dorsal artery. In our study, we examined morphological changes in the small arterioles and the capillaries. Therefore, arteriosclerotic changes were not encountered. Our study shows definite axonal loss in the nerve bundles of patients with known neurological disorders and a decrease in patients with severe arterial disease. The absence of nerve bundles in the specimens of several patients probably was due to degeneration of the nerves.

Previous studies have shown that the smooth muscle cell represents the structural basis for sinusoidal relaxation, a key factor in penile erection (Lue et al. 1983;

Juenemann et al. 1986; Fournier et al. 1987). Based upon our findings, we propose two explanations of erectile failure due to impairment of sinusoidal relaxation: a decreased number of intracellular myofilaments impairs the contractility of the individual smooth muscle cell, and in addition the loss of cell membrane contacts (nexus) results in failure of the tissue to interact as a unit.

Based upon the above findings, we believe that the success of surgical reconstructive procedures in patients with arterial insufficiency and venous incompetence depends upon the integrity of the penile tissue. In the future, the morphological examination of penile biopsies may prove helpful in determining patients who may profit from surgical intervention. Furthermore, the reliability of noninvasive tests such as duplex ultrasonography should be examined.

References

Benson GS, McConnell J, Lipschultz LI (1980) Neuromorphology and neuropharmacology of the human penis. J Clin Invest 65:506

Bergmann RA (1956) Proceedings of first European regional conference on electron microscopy, Stockholm

Bois RM (1973) The organisation of the contractile apparatus of vertebrate smooth muscle. Anat Rec 177:61

Bossart MI, Spjut HJ, Scott FB (1980) Ultrastructural analysis of human penile corpus cavernosum. Its significance in tumescence and detumescence. Urology 15:448

Caesar R, Edwards GA, Ruska H (1957) Architecture and nerve supply of mammalian smooth muscle tissue. J Biophys Biochem Cytol 3:867

Cohen MS, Sharpe W, Warner RS, Zorgniotti A (1980) Morphology of corporeal cavernosa arterial bed in impotence. Urology 16:382

Fournier Gr Jr, Juenemann K-P, Lue TF, Tanagho EA (1987) Mechanisms of venous occlusion during canine penile erection: an anatomic demonstration. J Urol 137:163

Goldstein AMB, Meehan JP, Zakhary R, Buckley PA, Rogers FA (1982) New observations on the microarchitecture of the corpora cavernosa in man and possible relationship to mechanism of erection. Urology 20:259

Ishikawa S, Bensaoula T, Uga S, Mukuno K (1985) Electron-microscopic study of iris nerves and muscles in diabetes. Ophthalmologica (Basel) 191:172

Juenemann K-P, Luo JA, Lue TF, Tanagho EA (1986) Further evidence of venous outflow restriction during erection. Br J Urol 58:320

Leeson TS, Leeson CR (1965) The fine structure of cavernous tissue in the adult rat penis. Invest Urol 3:144

Lue TF, Takamura T, Schmidt RA, Palubinskas AJ, Tanagho EA (1983) Hemodynamics of erection in the monkey. J Urol 130:1237

Lue TF, Hricak H, Marich KW, Tanagho EA (1985) Evaluation of arteriogenic impotence with intracorporeal injection of papaverine and the duplex ultrasound scanner. Sem Urol 3:43

Melman A, Bressler RS, Henry DP, Macadoo VK (1981) Ultrastructure of human penile tissue in patients with abnormal norepinephrine content. Invest Urol 19:46

Persson C, Diederichs W, Lue PS, Yen TSB, Fishman IJ, McLin PH, Tanagho E (in press) Correlations of altered penile ultrastructure with clinical arterial evaluation. J Urol

Ruzbarsky V, Michal V (1977) Morphological changes in the arterial bed of the penis with aging. Relationship to the pathogenesis of impotence. Invest Urol 15:194

Schoenberg CF, Needham PM (1976) A study of mechanism of contraction in vertebrate smooth muscle. Biol Rev 51:53

Virag R, Frydman D, Legman M, Virag H (1984) Intracavernous injection of papaverine as a diagnostic and therapeutic method in erectile failure. Angiology 35:79

Wetzner SM, Tutunjian J, Marich KW (1983) Duplex scanning: a vascular diagnostic technology. Am Rev Diagn 1:31

The Erection Ring – A New Treatment Approach in Venogenic Erectile Dysfunction

J. Steffens, H. Derouet, and M. Ziegler[1]

Introduction

Owing to a lack of successful results the treatment of venous erectile dysfunction of unclear etiology is presently passing through a dynamic phase (Lewis 1988). Previously the treatment of choice was venous ligature, the initial results of which have been encouraging. During a 1-year observation period success rates of between 28% and 75% have been reported (Buvat et al. 1986; Lewis 1988; Michal et al. 1986; Pfeiffer and Terhorst 1988; Wagenknecht et al. 1986; Wespes and Schulman 1985). However, other surgical procedures have proven disappointing, especially in complex venous leakage with drainage via the deep cavernous veins. Wespes et al. recently reported a 5-year success rate of 46% (Wespes et al. 1988). Nonsurgical alternative treatments have long been known. External erectile aids, in particular, have frequently been employed. The use of suction aids (Osbon-Erecaid system) to induce penile tumescence, which is then maintained by constriction bands at the root of the penis, is a recognized procedure for exceptional cases (Osbon 1983; Witherington 1988). Since 1917 different variations of these erectile aids have been patented in the United States of America (Fre-San Products Manufacturing Co. 1976; Jennings 1970; Jones 1974; Lederer 1917; Sell 1959; Sutherland and Isbister 1975; Wilson 1973). Similarly, numerous inflatable external erection systems have been patented in Europe since 1925 (Ekes 1929, 1932; Geyer 1987; Höflinger 1955; Kratzenstein 1926; Nadig 1985; Nitardy 1913; Skora 1933; Wu 1978).

Since 1987 an elastic inflatable erection ring which compresses the root of the penis has been available. The outflowing venous blood is thus congested, while the influx of arterial blood remains unaffected. This instrument is thus suitable for treating venogenic impotence. In this article we shall describe how the erection ring works and report on our initial clinical results.

Material and Methods

The erection ring (Rüsch, Waiblingen, FRG) consists of a soft, elastic, silicon tube with a built-in valve. The pressure within the tube can be increased by injecting air with a syringe (Fig. 1). Since the inside wall of the ring is not as thick as the outside wall, the main pressure after inflation is exerted on the center, and as the external wall is not so highly elastic the ring is only slightly broadened. This avoids substantial shortening of the penis.

[1] Urological Clinic of the University of the Saarland, 6650 Homburg/Saar, FRG

Investigative Urology 3
Edited by H. Rübben et al.

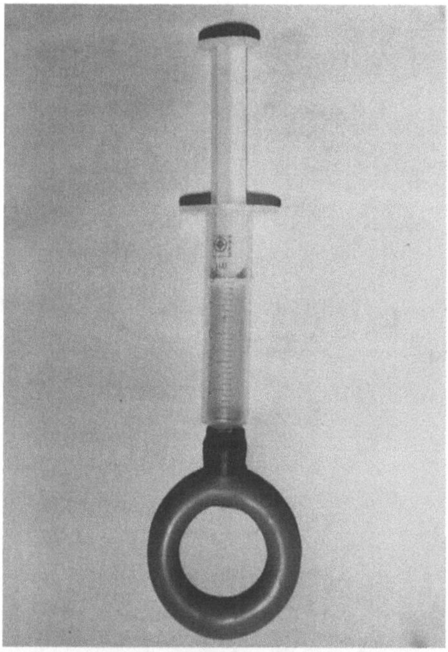

Fig. 1. The erection ring consisting of a soft, elastic, silicone tube, which is filled through a valve by means of a syringe

Between January and May 1988 20 patients with erectile dysfunction of venous origin were treated by passing an individually fitted erection ring (internal diameter 24, 27, 30, or 34 mm) over the flaccid penis and positioning it at the root. The rings were then filled with 5–10 cc air from a syringe inserted through the valve. The effects of the resulting constriction on venous drainage were investigated using dynamic and pharmaco-cavernosography and angiodynography. A color doppler device was used for the angiodynography, which represents an advance on duplex sonography and affords both a high resolution, real-time image of the soft tissue structures and simultaneous imaging of the blood flow over the entire surface of the B mode. The effects on arterial influx following inflation of the ring were evaluated by duplex sonography.

Results

During compression cavernosography showed a reduction in venous outflow in all cases (Fig. 2). Angiodynography revealed a dilated dorsal vein with reduced outflow (Fig. 3). Arterial influx was not affected at a therapeutic ring pressure (5–10 cc air), which was also evident in the duplex sonograms and angiodynograms. The lowest volume of air at which the deep penile arteries become compressed was 30 cc (Fig. 4).

Six out of 20 patients (30%) with venogenic erectile dysfunction were able to perform sexual intercourse at home after fitting the ring and sexual stimulation (Fig. 5). In 14 patients (70%) with complex venous leakage adequate rigidity was only ob-

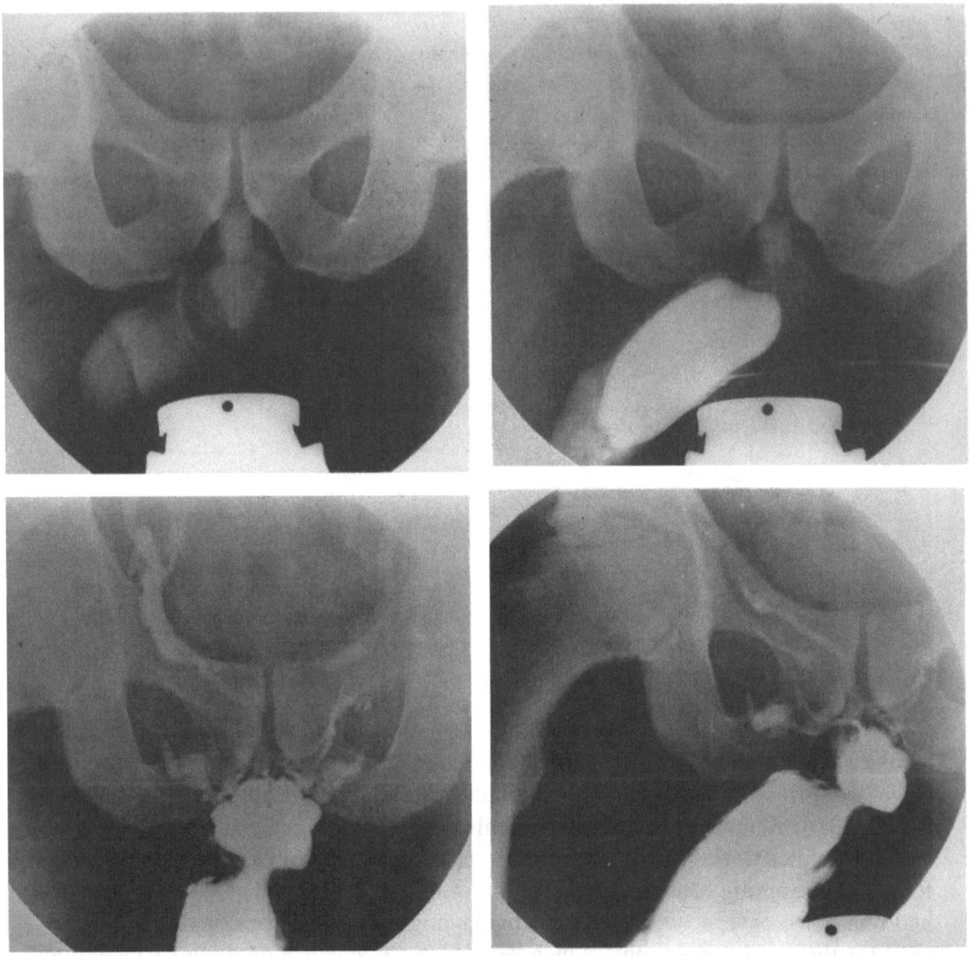

a b c d

Fig. 2. a Plain film before cavernosography: the erection ring positoned at the root of the penis and filled with 10 cc air. **b** Pharmaco-cavernosogram: complete interruption of venous outflow during the filling phase, the ring compressing the root of the penis. **c** and **d** Pharmaco-cavernosogram (antero-posterior and lateral): in the late phase incomplete interruption of venous outflow with the ring compressing the root of the penis

tained when the erection ring was combined with autoinjection therapy. The average dose of the papaverine-phentolamine mixture injected was 1 ml.

Acceptance of the erection ring was good, despite the fact that the valve proved difficult to handle. There were no complications. However, after frequent use of the ring air began to escape from it owing to material fatigue, and it therefore had to be frequently replaced.

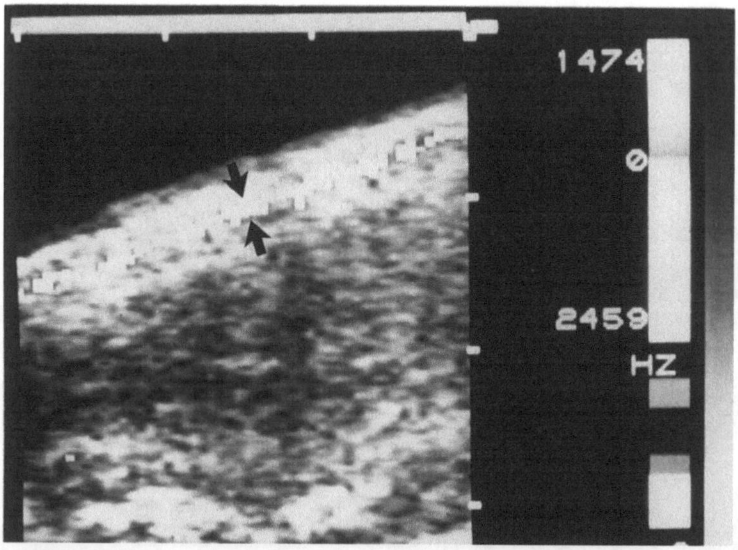

a

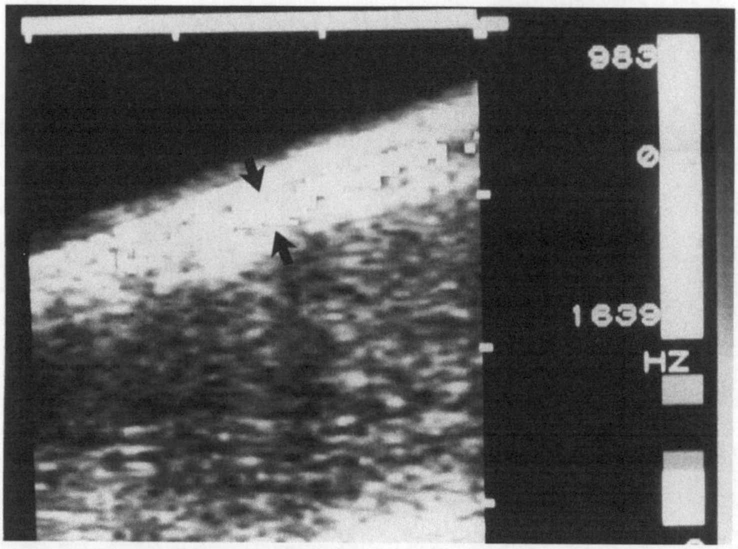

b

Fig. 3. a Angiodynography: normal lumen and normal flow rate in the dorsal vein before ring compression. **b** Angiodynography: dilated dorsal vein with reduced outflow of blood following ring compression (10 cc air)

Discussion

Externally applied erection aids have long been employed in the treatment of erectile dysfunction (Ekes 1929, 1932; Fre-San Products Manufacturing Co. 1976; Geyer 1987; Höflinger 1955; Jennings 1970; Jones 1974; Kratzenstein 1926; Lederer 1917; Nadig 1985; Nitardy 1913; Pfeiffer and Terhorst 1988; Sell 1959; Skora 1933; Sutherland and Isbister 1975; Wilson 1973; Wu 1978). The reduction of venous outflow by

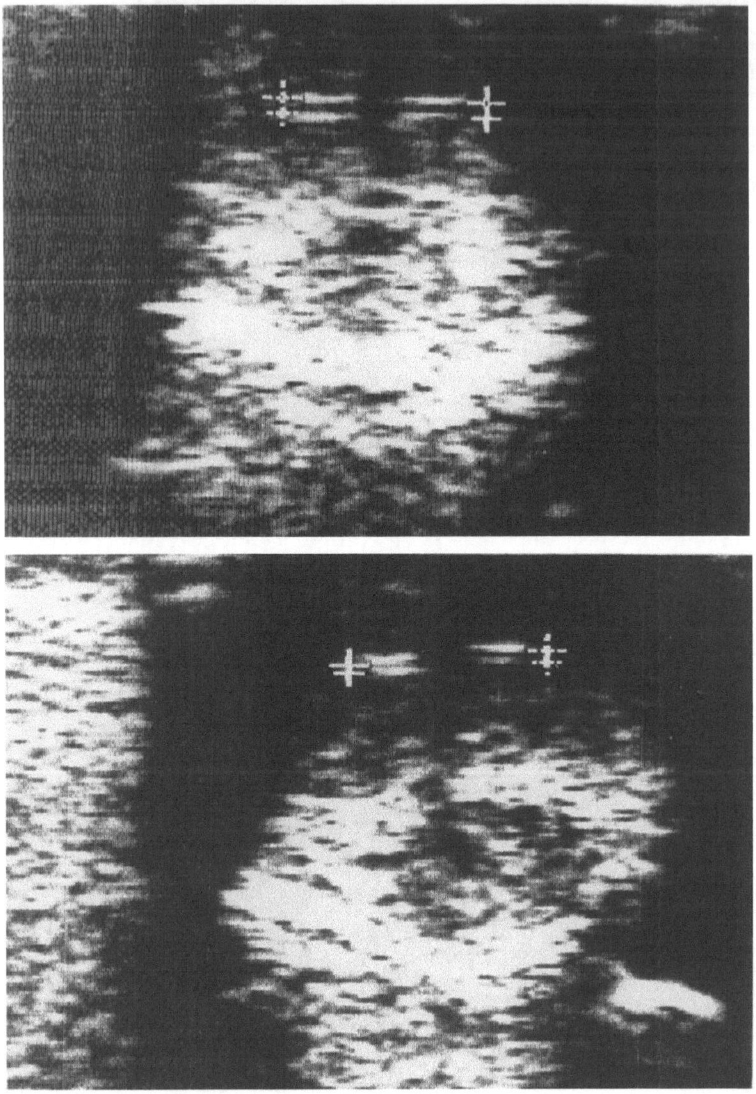

Fig. 4. **a** Duplex sonography: no compression of the deep penile arteries at a filling volume of 10 cc (diameter: 1.4 cm). **b** Duplex sonography: the lowest volume of air at which the deep penile arteries become compressed is 30 cc (diameter 1.1 cm)

means of an inflatable ring compressing the root of the penis was an idea first introduced by Kratzenstein in 1925 (Kratzenstein 1926). The main feature of the erection ring described here is the thinness of its inside wall, which means that when it is filled with 5–10 cc air the pressure is exerted mainly towards the center. The outer wall is not very elastic, and thus the penis is hardly shortened.

The way in which the ring works was demonstrated in our patients by modern imaging techniques. Cavernosography revealed that venous drainage is reduced but

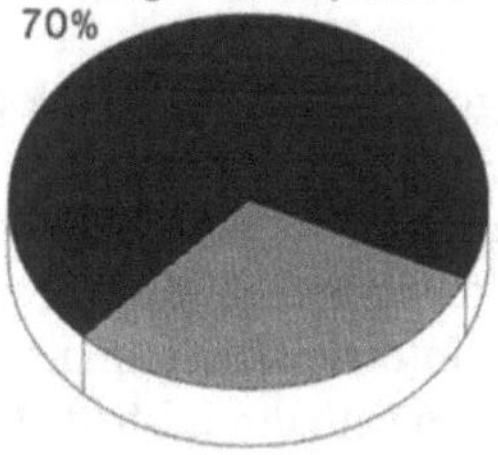

Fig. 5. Results of treatment in venogenic impotence ($n = 20$)

not completely interrupted when the ring is filled with 10 cc air. The ring is therefore also suitable for use in cavernosography conducted for diagnostic purposes. Angiodynography, a new imaging technique carried out after injection of papaverine, with which it is now possible for the first time to demonstrate arterial and venous blood flow in color, showed a dilated dorsal vein and reduced drainage of blood following application of the ring. When the ring was filled with the therapeutic volume of 5–10 cc air, duplex sonography showed no impairment of arterial influx.

Twenty patients with venogenic erectile dysfunction were treated with the ring. Of these men 30% were successfully treated with this externally applied erection aid as the sole method of treatment. In these patients the reduction in venous outflow was sufficient to obtain a degree of rigidity permitting coitus after sexual stimulation. In 70% of the patients with complex venous leakage it was necessary to combine the erection ring with autoinjection therapy, as the ring was not sufficient to support erection.

Although the ring was well accepted, the difficulty of handling the valve was a minus factor; moreover, after the ring had been used several times air began to escape from it due to material fatigue, and it therefore had to be replaced frequently. These unsatisfactory features leave room for improvement, which should, however, culminate in the development of a ring which is easy to handle and longer lasting.

To date we can consider our results with this successful, nonstressful, and complication-free method of treatment to be good, since in many cases of complex venous leakage we have been able to avoid using venous surgery, the results of which are at present disappointing (Buvat et al. 1986; Lewis 1988; Michal et al. 1986; Wespes et al. 1988). Michal et al. (1986) and Buvat et al. (1986) reported success rates of 25% and 28%, respectively, after the first postoperative year. With our own patients we had similarly poor results following venous ligature and have thus stopped conducting venous surgery for the present.

In view of the low success rate (46%) shown by the first 5-year results reported by Wespes et al. (1988), it is doubtful whether venous resection can at all be considered a causal therapy for venogenic impotence of unclear etiology. In contrast, the procedure described above – use of an erection ring in combination with autoinjection therapy – has proven efficient in all forms of venous insufficiency and would appear to be the treatment of choice for this form of erectile dysfunction, the management of which has caused so much difficulty in the past.

Summary

A new inflatable erection ring is described, the basic design of which was developed as early as 1925. It consists of a soft, elastic silicone tube which is slipped over the flaccid penis before intercourse and secured firmly at the root. It is then filled with 10 cc air through a valve. Cavernosography conducted after application of the ring showed venous outflow to be reduced but not completely interrupted at an air volume of 10 cc. Angiodynography revealed a dilated dorsal vein with diminished efflux of blood. In the pulsed duplex ultrasound image the arterial influx was seen to be unaffected at 10 cc air, but the deep penile arteries were compressed at 30 cc.

In a clinical trial of the erection ring in 20 patients with venogenic erectile dysfunction 30% of the men profited from this external aid as sole therapy, while 70% required a combination of the ring with autoinjection therapy. This simple and successful form of therapy is not associated with any complications, and in view of the disappointing results of venous surgery may be considered the treatment of choice in patients with venogenic impotence.

References

Buvat J, Lemaire A, Buvat-Herbaut M, Marcolin G, Desmons F, Rigot JM (1986) Erectile impotence with severe venous incompetence: results of treatments in 35 cases. Second world meeting on impotence, Prague
Ekes L (1929) German patent specification no. 476413, May 16
Ekes L (1932) German patent specification no. 565238, November 28
Fre-San Products Manufacturing Co. (1976) CTD special: a tremendous asset to the impotent male. Cleveland product brochure
Geyer A (1987) German patent specification G 8700174.8, May 21
Höflinger B (1955) German patent specification no. 923695, February 21
Jennings CC (1970) U.S. patent number 3, 495, 589, February 17
Jones A (1974) U.S. patent number 3, 820, 533, June 28
Kratzenstein G (1926) German patent specification no. 427488, March 31
Lederer O (1917) U.S. patent number 1, 225, 341, May 8
Lewis RW (1988) Venous surgery for impotence. Urol Clin North Am 15:115–121
Michal V, Krysl I, Klika JT, Fara P (1986) Revascularization of the cavernous bodies. Second world meeting on impotence, Prague
Nadig PW (1985) European patent specification no. 0148586, July 17
Nitardy E (1913) German patent specification no. 260938, October 15
Osbon GD (1983) U.S. patent number 4, 378, 008, March 29
Pfeiffer G, Terhorst B (1988) Chirurgische Therapie bei erektiler Impotenz vaskulär-venöser Genese. Urologe A 27:139–141
Sell FW (1959) U.S. patent number 2, 874, 698, February 24
Skora A (1933) German patent specification no. 574684, April 19
Sutherland J, Isbister T (1975) U.S. patent number 1, 497, 441, September 27
Wagenknecht LV (1986) Ergebnisse eines neuen Operationsverfahrens bei erhöhter Venendrainage mit erektiler Impotenz. Verl Dt Ges Urol 39. Tag. Springer, Berlin Heidelberg New York, pp 451–452
Wespes E, Schulman CC (1985) Venous leakage: surgical treatment of a curable cause for impotence. J Urol 133:796–798
Wespes E, Delcroix C, Struyren J, Schulman CC (1988) Five years' experience in the diagnosis and treatment of patients with caverno-venous leakage. Abstract EAU, London, p 120
Wilson EM (1973) U.S. patent number 3, 744, 486, July 10
Witherington R (1988) Suction device therapy in the management of erectile impotence. Urol Clin North Am 15:123–128
Wu AC (1978) German patent specification no. GM 78 22 298, July 5

Inhibitory Presynaptic Alpha-Adrenoceptors in the Human Corpus Cavernosum

H. VAN AHLEN[1], G. J. MOLDERINGS[2], H. PORST[1], and M. GÖTHERT[2]

Introduction

From many clinical investigations and from earlier histological studies, we know that noradrenaline plays an important role in penile tumescence, probably causing the normal, unerect, flaccid state of the penis. In radioligand studies adrenergic alpha-receptors were shown to outnumber beta-receptors in the human corpus cavernosum (Levin and Wein 1980), and high concentrations of noradrenaline were found (Melman and Henry 1980). Global stimulation of these intracavernosal receptors by injecting noradrenaline or other alpha adrenergic drugs will lead to detumescence by contraction of the smooth muscle cells (de Meyer and De Sy 1986; Block et al. 1987). This treatment has been well established for the therapy of prolonged erections and priapism.

From other human tissues it is, however, well-recognized that there are presynaptic inhibitory alpha-adrenoceptors at the sympathetic nerve ending itself, modulating the release of noradrenaline from these vesicles (Starke 1981; Göthert et al. 1984). We wanted to evaluate whether such receptors could also be found in human corpora cavernosa and to which subtype they belonged.

Material and Methods

Pieces of human corpus cavernosum were obtained from patients undergoing surgery for a congenital penile deviation or for Peyronie's disease. No patient suffered from concomitant erectile dysfunction. The pieces were cut into strips of approximately 3 by 15 mm and were incubated for 60 min at a temperature of 37°C in a physiological salt solution, containing [^{3}H]noradrenaline (0.1 µmol/l). Subsequently, the preparations were mounted vertically in an organ bath between two platinum electrodes (tension 0.5 g) and were then superfused with noradrenaline-free physiological salt solution, containing desipramine (0.6 µmol/l) and corticosterone (40 µmol/l) to block neuronal and extraneuronal noradrenaline uptake.

The superfusate was collected in 3-min fractions: Five 6-min periods of transmural electrical stimulation (0.66 Hz) were applied to each of the preparations after 93 (S_1), 117 (S_2), 141 (S_3), 165 (S_4), and 189 (S_5) min after the superfusion. The tritium overflow in the superfusate and in the solubilized preparations was determined by liquid scintillation counting.

Tritium efflux was calculated as the fraction of tritium present in the strip at the time of the onset of each collecting period. Basal tritium efflux was expressed as the

[1]Department of Urology and [2]Institute of Pharmacology and Toxicology, University of Bonn, FRG

Investigative Urology 3
Edited by H. Rübben et al.

ratio of the fractional rate during the collecting period immediately before S_3, S_4, and S_5 (t_3, t_4, t_5) over that immediately before S_2 (t_2). Stimulation-evoked overflow was calculated by subtraction of the basal efflux from the total efflux during 12 min subsequent to the onset of stimulation. Evoked tritium overflow was given as a fraction of tissue tritium at the onset of stimulation, and the ratios of the overflow evoked by S_3, S_4, and S_5 over that evoked by S_2 wer determined.

Results are given as means ± SEM; Student's *t*-test was used for statistical evaluation and comparison of the mean values.

Results

Basal and Stimulation-Evoked Tritium Outflow. In control experiments basal tritium efflux decreased gradually with time (Table 1, Fig. 1). Electrical stimulation of the preparations at a frequency of 0.66 Hz increased this outflow, and the ratio of this showed constant quantities (Table 2, Fig. 1). Tetrodotoxin, a Na^+ channel blocker, added to the superfusion fluid in a concentration of 1 µmol/l, strongly inhibited this electrically evoked tritium overflow by about 90% ($P < 0.05$) (Fig. 2). The evoked tritium outflow was completely abolished when the tissues were superfused with Ca^{2+}-free solution 9 min before S_3 to 13 min after S_4. However, after Ca^{2+} was reintroduced following S_4 the electrically evoked overflow was again detectable (Fig. 3).

Neither the addition of tetrodotoxin nor superfusion with Ca^{2+}-free solution changed the basal efflux to any extent. To evaluate the subtype of the assumed pre-

Table 1. Control values for basal tritium efflux

t_2 (nCi/min)	Fractional rate (min^{-1})	t_3/t_2	t_4/t_2	t_5/t_2
1.54 ± 0.22	0.0004 ± 0.0001	0.93 ± 0.03	0.90 ± 0.05	0.85 ± 0.04

t_1–t_5 represent the 4-min periods of superfusate sampling immediately before the respective stimulation periods. Basal efflux during t_3–t_5 is given as ratio over the respective t_2 value. The efflux of tritium per minute is expressed as fraction of tissue tritium. Means ± SEM of seven experiments

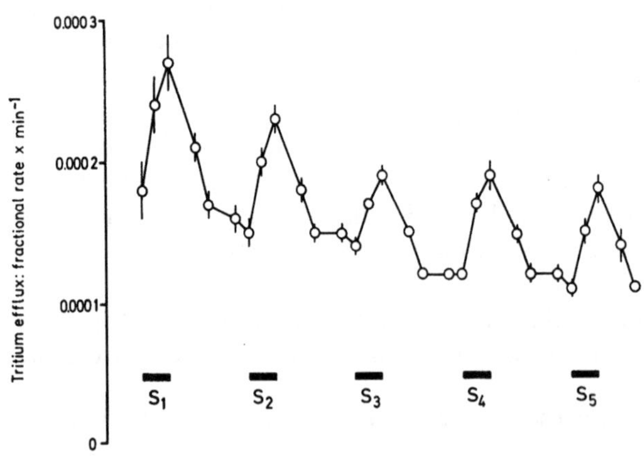

Fig. 1. Tritium efflux from human corpus cavernosum under five periods of electrical stimulation (*S_1–S_5*; 0.66 Hz). Efflux of tritium per minute, expressed as fraction of tissue tritium at the onset of the respective collection period

Table 2. Evoked tritium overflow above basal efflux after transmural electrical stimulation (S_1–S_5)

S_2 (nCi/min)	Percentage of tissue ^3H	S_3/S_2	S_4/S_2	S_5/S_2
1.63 ± 0.44	0.38 ± 0.06	0.92 ± 0.06	0.94 ± 0.03	0.92 ± 0.07

Overflow evoked by S_3–S_5 is given as ratio over the respective S_2. The overflow is expressed as percentage of tissue tritium. Means ± SEM of seven experiments

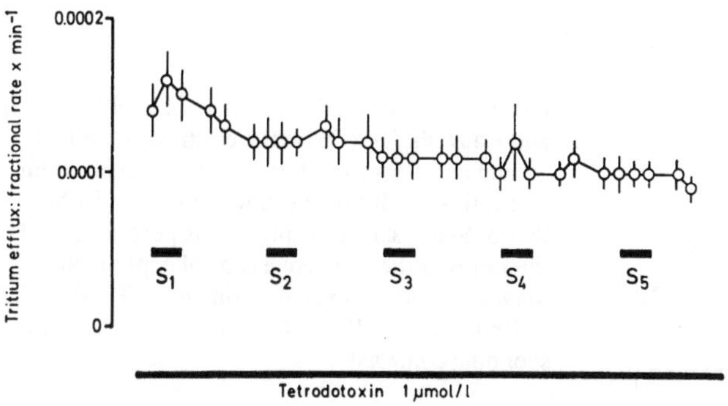

Fig. 2. Same experiments as in Fig. 1 but after the addition of tetrodotoxin (1 μmol/l) during the time indicated by the *horizontal bar*

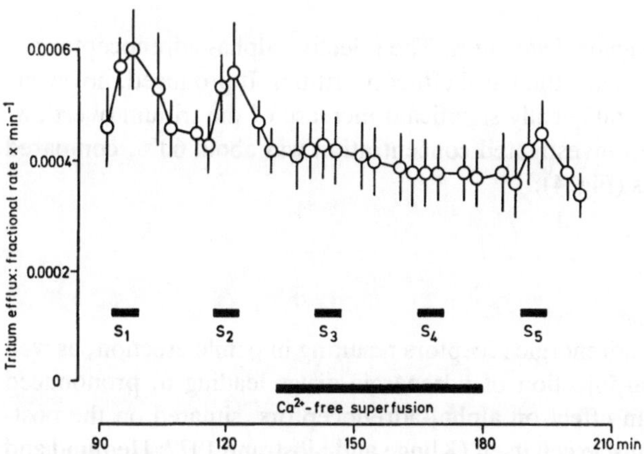

Fig. 3. Same experiments as in Fig. 1 but with omission of Ca^{2+} during the time indicated by the *horizontal bar*

synaptic receptor at the site of the noradrenergic vesicle we performed the same experiments, adding specific $alpha_2$ agonists and antagonists.

Effects of Alpha-Adrenoceptor Agonists. Basal efflux was not affected by the specific $alpha_1$ agonist methoxamine nor by the specific $alpha_2$ agonist B-HT 920 (6-allyl-2-amino-5,6,7,8-tetrahydro-4H-thiazolo-5,4-D-azepine dihydrochloride). Methoxamine did not significantly alter the measured overflow after electrical stimulation (Fig. 4). The selective $alpha_2$-adrenoceptor agonist B-HT 920 produced a dose-dependent, statistically highly significant decrease of the electrically stimulated tritium overflow (Fig. 4). The inhibition obtained with the highest concentration of B-HT 920 reached almost 80%, compared with the control experiments.

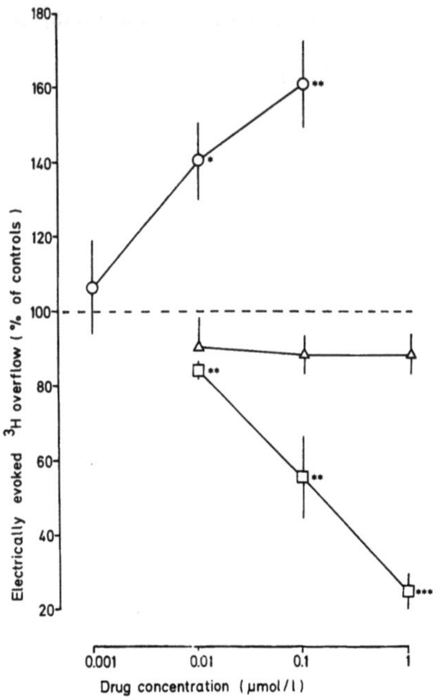

Fig. 4. Effects of methoxamine (△), B-HT 920 (□) and Rauwolszine (○) on the electrically evoked tritium overflow from human corpus cavernosum. The ratios of tritium overflow evoked by S_3–S_5 to that of S_2 are shown, expressed as percentages of the ratios in the respective control experiments. Means ± SEM of seven experiments. * $P<0.05$; ** $P<0.025$; *** $P<0.001$ (compared with corresponding controls)

Effect of an Alpha₂-Adrenoceptor Antagonist. The selective alpha$_2$-adrenoceptor antagonist Rauwolszine did not alter the basal efflux of tritium. It produced, however, a concentration-dependent, statistically significant increase of the tritium overflow. The facilitation at the highest investigated concentration was about 60%, compared with the control experiments (Fig. 4).

Discussion

The local blockade of alpha adrenergic receptors resulting in penile erection, as well as their stimulation by local injection of adrenergic drugs leading to pronounced detumescence, are due to an effect on alpha$_1$-adrenoceptors, situated on the post-synaptic membrane of the muscle cell itself (Klinge and Sjöstrand 1977; Hedlund and Andersson 1985; Dail et al. 1987). Alpha$_1$-adrenoceptor stimulation will not influence noradrenaline release, as could be demonstrated with the specific alpha$_1$-adrenoceptor agonist methoxamine in our own experiments.

Our results provide evidence that additional inhibitory presynaptic alpha$_2$-adrenoceptors are, however, present on the sympathetic nerve terminals in human corpus cavernosum. Their stimulation leads to a modulation of the electrically evoked noradrenaline release. Under the described experimental conditions and according to the control experiments we can assume that the measured, electrically evoked tritium overflow reflects the physiological, potential-induced, noradrenaline release in this tissue.

Stimulation of these alpha$_2$-adrenoceptors causes an inhibition of the noradrenergic transmission, decreasing the excitatory noradrenaline release. Blockade increases noradrenaline release, probably due to a disinhibition, e.g., by the antagonism versus endogenous noradrenaline at the presynaptic alpha$_2$-adrenoceptor (Göthert et al. 1984). Therefore, alpha$_2$-adrenoceptors may play an important role in the regulation of the erectile process, and our results give additional support to the theory that sympathetic activity greatly influences this process.

References

Block T, Sturm W, Ernst G, Schmiedt E (1987) The intracavernous application of alpha adrenergic drugs in the treatment of priapism. World J Urol 5:178–181

Dail WG, McGuffee I, Minorsky N, Little S (1987) Responses of smooth muscle strips from penile erectile tissue to drugs and transmural nerve stimulation. J Auton Pharmacol 7:287–293

Göthert M, Schlicker E, Hentrich F, Rohm N, Zerkowski HR (1984) Modulation of noradrenaline release in human saphenous vein via presynaptic alpha 2 adrenoceptors. Eur J Pharmacol 102: 261–267

Hedlund H, Andersson KE (1985) Comparison of the responses to drugs acting on adrenoceptors and muscarinic receptors in human isolated corpus cavernosum and cavernous artery. J Auton Pharmacol 5:81–88

Klinge E, Sjöstrand NO (1977) Comparative study of some isolated mammalian smooth muscle effectors of penile erection. Acta Physiol Scand 100:354–367

Levin RM, Wein AJ (1980) Adrenergic alpha receptors outnumber beta receptors in human penile corpus cavernosum. Invest Urol 18:225–226

Melman A, Henry D (1980) The possible role of the catecholamines of the corpora in penile erection. J Urol 121:419–421

Meyer JM de, De Sy WA (1986) Intracavernososus injection of noradrenaline to interrupt erections during surgical intervention. Eur Urol 12:169–170

Starke K (1981) Alpha adrenoceptor subclassification. Rev Physiol Biochem Pharmacol 88:199–206

Intratesticular Concentration of Etoposide: An Experimental Study

T. Stein[1], S. Krege[2], G. Heimann[3], and H. Rübben[2]

Introduction

The efficiency of systemic chemotherapy on intratesticular germ cell tumors is a subject of controversy. Different studies support the existence of a blood-testis barrier, preventing chemotherapeutic agents from reaching all areas of the testis: 26 patients with advanced germ cell cancer underwent chemotherapy followed by delayed orchiectomy. Of these 17 had a complete remission of intratesticular tumor at the time of orchiectomy, but 9 still had viable tumor in the testis despite extensive remission of metastatic disease. In all cases either metastases were not destroyed entirely, or complete remission was not confirmed by histologic exploration (Chong et al. 1986; Fowler and Whitmore 1981; Snow et al. 1983).

Other studies agree on the effectiveness of chemotherapy of intratesticular germ cell tumors: Autopsy findings in 103 leukemic patients treated by chemotherapy imply that the chemotherapeutic agents penetrated into the testis, because no advancement of the testicular disease was noted (Kuhjda et al. 1982). Taking biopsies from normal contralateral testis during treatment of patients with primary nonseminomatous germ cell tumors, no areas of carcinoma in situ were found after chemotherapy in contrast to those patients not receiving chemotherapy (Skakkebaek 1985). Experimental data demonstrated the transport of cyclophosphamide and vincristine across the blood-testis barrier (Forrest et al. 1981).

As etoposide is an effective agent in the treatment of advanced germ cell tumors, and detection of etoposide in plasma and various organs is standardized in comparison with detection of cisplatinum and bleomycin, the aim of this study is to measure the concentration of etoposide in testicular tissue and to compare it with concentrations reached in other tissues after intravenous application.

Materials and Methods

Etoposide (10 mg/kg body weight) was injected intravenously into 45 healthy Wistar rats (250 g of body weight). Groups of three rats were narcotized with high-dose ether after 7, 15, 30, 45, 60, 75, 90 min or 2, 3, 4, 5, 6, 7, 8, 12 h. After thoracotomy a blood sample was taken by intracardial puncture of the left ventricle. Heparin diluted in sodium chloride (12500 IE) was given to prevent blood clotting, followed by systemic perfusion with 250 ml of Ringer's solution. Testicles, liver, right kidney, and muscle of the right hind leg thigh were removed. A control group of three ani-

[1]Dept. Clinical Chemistry, [2]Dept. Urology, and [3]Dept. Pediatrics, Med. Faculty Rheinisch-Westfälische Technische Hochschule Aachen (RWTH), Pauwelsstr., 5100 Aachen, FRG

Investigative Urology 3
Edited by H. Rübben et al.

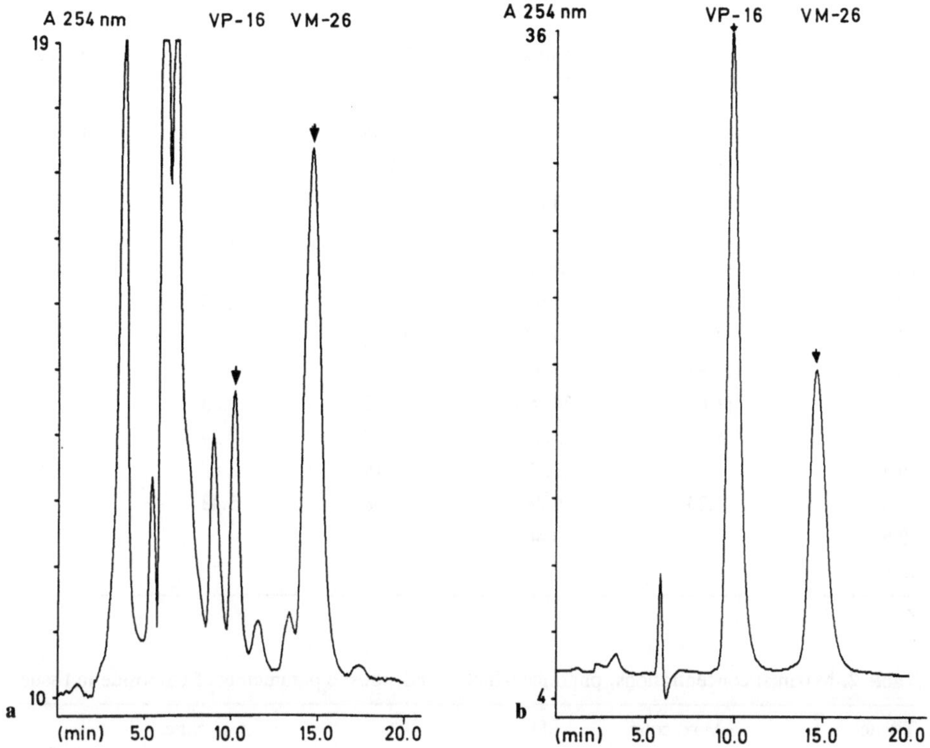

Fig. 1a, b. Data of the standard and testicular analysis

mals was not treated with etoposide. From three animals treated with etoposide urine samples were collected after 6, 12, 24, 48, and 72 h.

Proteolysis of tissue and plasma samples by papain digestion was followed by chloroform extraction. The method was used to release the strongly protein-bound drug completely. The organic phase was dried under nitrogen, and the samples were resolved in the mobile phase. Measurement of etoposide was performed by high performance liquid chromatography (HPLC), using teniposide as internal standard (Farina et al. 1981). A Lichrosorb RP-8 (5 μm) column from Merck-Darmstadt was used; separation was achieved with an isocratic solvent system of methanol (55%) and water (45%) at a flow rate of 1 ml/min according to D'Incalci et al. (1982), and analysis performed with a Bruker LC equipped with a 254-nm absorbance detector. Data of the standard and testicular analysis are given in Fig. 1.

Results

Tissue and plasma concentrations of etoposide at different times are shown in Table 1. The concentration of etoposide is related to 1 g wet weight or 1 ml of plasma. Extraction recovery for tissue is 73%, for plasma 57%. Table 2 and Fig. 2 give a summary

Table 1. Etoposide concentration in various organs and plasma (μg/g wet weight or μg/ml plasma)

Time	Liver	Kidney	Testis	Muscle	Plasma
7 min	11.11	35.34	11.73	4.86	0.96
15 min	11.41	41.33	12.45	0.10	0.29
30 min	11.66	36.00	18.56	11.95	0.28
45 min	17.66	34.03	16.28	12.15	0.21
60 min	19.50	32.36	16.36	12.00	0.06
75 min	12.41	33.36	16.36	13.07	–
90 min	19.91	31.91	16.39	12.40	0.02
2 h	12.88	24.02	16.20	10.73	–
3 h	12.91	35.43	16.26	10.79	–
4 h	11.62	34.09	15.62	9.33	–
5 h	8.56	25.39	11.67	10.54	–
6 h	7.60	22.07	7.19	8.68	–
7 h	3.33	9.34	0.98	5.43	–
8 h	–	0.46	–	–	–
12 h	–	–	–	–	–

Table 2. Maximal concentrations, pharmacokinetic, and statistic parameters of etoposide in tissue

Tissue	Max. conc. (μg)	SD	CC	$t_{max.}$ conc. (min)	t_{50} (min)
Testicle	18.56	2.37	0.93	10–28	356.67
Liver	14.80	2.45	0.895	44	281.81
Kidney	37.60	4.24	0.94	18	460.38
Muscle	12.30	0.88	0.97	53	626.38

SD, standard deviation; CC, coefficient of correlation

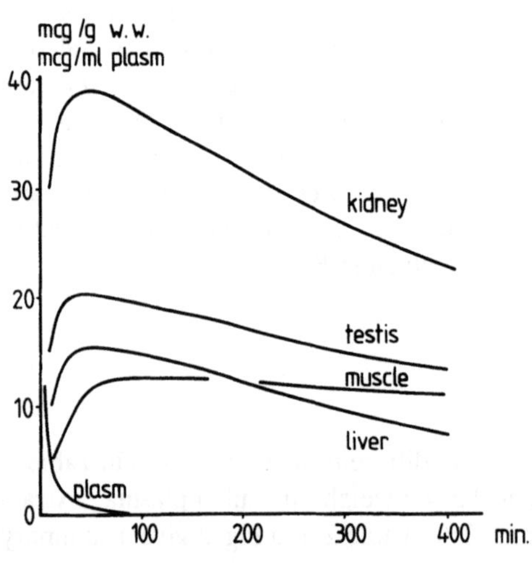

Fig. 2. Etoposide concentration in tissue and plasma

of the maximal concentrations and pharmacokinetic as well as statistic parameters of etoposide in tissue. A maximum concentration of 0.96 µg etoposide/ml plasma was found after 7 min; this low concentration indicates that after bolus injection the drug is distributed very quickly. The t_{50} was found to be 10.54 min. Extraction recovery in plasma was 57%, SD 0.16; CC 0.90.

Monitoring the concentration of etoposide in urine with an extraction recovery of 82% leads to the finding of 54.5 µg/ml in the first 6 h after etoposide injection. The high amount of etoposide in the 6-h urine correlates well with the decrease of the drug in tissue during the first 6 h.

Discussion

The concept of a blood-testis barrier was described initially by Ribbert (1904) and Bouffard (1906). Electron microscopic studies led to the conclusion that peritubular myoid and Sertoli's cell layers may be responsible for the barrier (Fawcett et al. 1970).

From the pharmacological point of view there have been different experiences about the capability of drugs to cross the barrier: actinomycin D, ascorbic acid, and various contrast materials show less penetration into the testis compared with other tissue (de Bruyn et al. 1950; Ro and Busch 1965; Hammarström 1966). After i.v. cisplatinum injection comparison of liver-, kidney-, and testis-tissue concentrations showed less accumulation in the testis (Litterst et al. 1976). In contrast cyclophosphamide and vincristine can penetrate the barrier rapidly (Forrest et al. 1981).

Also, clinical experiences concerning the efficiency of chemotherapy on primary testicular germ cell tumors are controversial. Eight patients with disseminated, nonseminomatous, testicular germ cell tumor received various courses of chemotherapy. At the time of delayed orchiectomy seven of them were considered free of the tumor by computed tomography. Three orchiectomy specimens still revealed carcinoma. Only six patients had retroperitoneal lymph node dissection, and one had thoracotomy. In one case lymph nodes showed teratoma as did the thoracotomy. Two patients showed progression of their metastatic disease within 10 months (Snow et al. 1983). Some 16 patients with advanced germ cell cancer underwent chemotherapy followed by orchiectomy. Criteria for a complete remission consisted of radiographic findings of disease and normalization of serum biomarkers. In four patients the orchiectomy specimen revealed viable tumor; three of them were said to have a complete remission of distant metastases. In nine the orchiectomy specimens did not show viable tumor; only seven of them were in complete remission (Chong et al. 1986).

In the case of an 18-year-old man with a testicular tumor and retroperitoneal, mass, neck, pulmonary, as well as liver metastases, most of the tumor foci were excised after chemotherapy. The patient underwent orchiectomy, retroperitoneal lymph node dissection with left pelvic lymphadenectomy, partial hepatectomy and 2 months later excision of a remaining pulmonary nodule and five additional pulmonary lesions resembling metastastic carcinoma. Residual carcinoma was found in a pelvic lymph node, the remaining pulmonary nodule, and the testis (Fowler and Whitmore 1981). In contrast to the conclusion of the authors mentioned above we do not see any clear-cut evidence for the failure of chemotherapy on intratesticular tumor alone.

The study by Skakkebaek (1985) underlines the intratesticular efficiency of chemotherapeutic agents. Biopsies from the clinically normal contralateral testis of patients with nonseminomatous germ cell tumors did not show carcinoma in situ in contrast to those taken from patients not receiving chemotherapy.

Experimental studies show different data for various agents after systemic application. Cisplatinum was administered intravenously into rats (5 mg/kg bw). Plasma levels and the concentration in liver, kidney, and testis were measured. After 60 min 0.50 ± 0.02 µg Pt/g wet weight was found in the testis; at 24 h there was 0.32 ± 0.06 µg in the testis, 2.89 ± 1.41 µg in the liver, and 11.61 ± 0.27 µg in the kidney (Litterst et al. 1976). In our study etoposide is administered intravenously to rats. Results indicate that the tissue concentration of etoposide in the testis is comparable to concentrations in the liver and muscle: testis, 18.56 µg/g wet weight; liver, 14.80 µg; muscle, 12.30 µg. These are the maximal concentrations reached in each tissue. The kidney as the excretion organ shows the highest level of etoposide with 37.60 µg/g. Thus, our study does not support the existence of a blood-testis barrier for etoposide.

The fact that some chemotherapeutic agents, effective in the treatment of testicular germ cell tumors, reach a similar concentration in the testis to that in other tissues might be of relevance in the discussion about treatment of extragonadal testicular germ cell tumors (ETGCT). ETGCT are histopathologically identical with testicular tumors and occur in mediastinal (71%), retroperitoneal (25%), pulmonary (1%), esophageal (1%), pineal (< 1%), and presacral (< 1%) locations (Kühn and Weißbach 1985). If the testicles, unsuspicious at clinical examination, are removed and investigated histologically, one-third shows normal tissue, one-third scars as a result of burnt-out tumors, and one-third microcarcinomas. Thus it is still a point of discussion whether testes which are normal at clinical examination should be removed. As therapy of ETGCT consists in the majority of patients of systemic chemotherapy, polychemotherapy including etoposide may be able to destroy possible microfoci of cancer. If these experimental results are confirmed by clinical observation, bilateral orchiectomy of clinically unsuspicious testicles will be unnecessary.

References

Boufford G (1906) Injection des couleurs de benzidine aux animaux normaux: etude expérimentale et histologique. Ann Inst Pasteur 20:539

Bruyn PPH de, Robertson RC, Farr RS (1950) In vivo affinity of diaminocridines for nuclei. Anat Rec 108:279

Chong C, Logothetis CJ, von Eschenbach A, Ayala A, Samuels M (1986) Orchiectomy in advanced germ cell cancer following intensive chemotherapy: a comparison of systemic to testicular response. J Urol 1221

D'Incalci M, Farina P, Sessa C, Molina P, Mangioni C, Jancovick M, Masera G, Beer M, Cavalli F (1982) Pharmacokinetic of VP-16 in humans. Chemioterapia 1:126–129

Farina P, Marzillo G, D'Incalci M (1981) High-performance liquid chromatography determination of 4′-dimethyl-epipodophyllotoxin-9-4,6-0-ethylidene-beta-D-glucopyranoside (VP-16-213) in human plasma. J Chromatogr 222:141

Fawcett DW, Leak LV, Heidger PM (1970) Electron microscopic observations on the structural components of the blood-testis-barrier. J Reprod Fertil [Suppl 10] 21:105

Forrest JB, Turner TT, Howards SS (1981) Cyclophosphamide, vincristine and the blood-testis-barrier. Invest Urol 18:443
Fowler JE, Whitmore WF (1981) Intratesticular germ cell tumors: observations on the effect of chemotherapy. J Urol 126:422
Hammarström L (1966) Autoradiographic studies on the distribution of ^{14}C-labelled ascorbic acid and dehydroascorbic acid. Act Physiol Scand [Suppl 289] 70:3
Howards SS, Jessee SJ, Johnson AL (1976) Micropuncture studies of the blood-seminiferous tubule barrier. Biol Rep 14:264
Kuhjda FP, Haupt HM, Moore GW, Hutchins GM (1982) Gonadal morphology for patients receiving chemotherapy for leukemia. Am J Med 72:759
Kühn MW, Weißbach L (1985) Localization, incidence, diagnosis and treatment of extratesticular germ cell tumors. Urol Int 40:166
Litterst CL, Torres IJ, Guarino AM (1976) Plasma levels and organ distribution of platinum in the rat, dog and dogfish shark following single intravenous administration of *cis*-dichlorodiamino-platinum (II)
Ribbert H (1904) Die Abscheidung intravenös injezierten gelösten Karmins in den Geweben. Z Allgemein Physiol 4:201
Ro TS, Busch H (1965) Concentration of ^{14}C-actinomycin D in various tissues following intravenous injection. Biochem Biophys Acta 108:317
Skakkebaek NE (1985) Carcinoma in situ of the testis: diagnosis and management. (Am Urol Assoc) J Urol 133A
Snow BW, Rowland RG, Donohie JP, Einhorn LH, Williams SD (1983) Review of delayed orchiectomy in patients with disseminated testis tumor. J Urol 129:522

III. BPH-Prostate Cancer

Diagnostic Studies Using Human BPH Tissues Transplanted on Thymus-Dysplastic Mice

P. G. Fabricius[1], F. Rommel[1], F. Sinowatz[2], V. Permanetter[3], and C. Hammer[4]

Introduction

The nude mouse model may be considered as established for studies of malignant human tumors (Scheidhauer et al. 1987). With xenotransplantation of human BPH preparations, autonomous growth cannot be expected (Fabricius et al. 1987). However, a spontaneous human prostatic hyperplasia would be available for the purpose of several studies.

Material and Methods

A total of 150 male BALB/c mice (Bomholtgard, Dk) received transplanted human BPH tissue (adenomectomy preparations) into their sides (right and left, three tumors per animal maximum). After the end of the test (maximum observation time 24 weeks after surgery) the tumor size (measurement calipers, all three perpendicular diameters, formula: $V = 0.52 \times D_1 \times D_2 \times D_3$), the histology, and the PSA levels in the serum of the *nu/nu* mice were evaluated. In addition, tumor-bearing nude mice were subjected to immunoscintigraphy using ^{131}I-labeled monoclonal antibodies (MoAb) against PSA (Tandem-PSA, Hyrbritech).

Results

The 150 *nu/nu* mice received a BPH xenograft. The behaviour of the tumor volume after transplantation is shown in Fig. 1. After a brief tumor enlargement phase, the graft shows a detectable shrinkage of 30% by day 28 p.o. Histologic examinations show that vascularization of the graft from the host animal is detectable from day 3 p.o. Nevertheless, necrosis develops which recedes only after 4 weeks (Fig. 2). The most sensitive reaction to the changes induced by the xenograft is that of the glandular epithelium. A squamous metaplasia was detected from day 3 p.o. which receded slowly from day 14 p.o. The whole stromal tissue developed fibrosis which was observed in all grafts from the 2nd week. Independent of the tissue selected for graft removal, the reactions to PAP (prostatic specific acid phosphatase) and PSA (prostatic specific antigen) were positive as per the immunoperoxidase technique (Fig. 3). The PSA measurements in the serum of the host animals yielded the following findings:

[1]Department of Urology, [3]Institute of Pathology, [4]Institute of Surgical Research, Klinikum Großhadern, and [2]Institute of Animal Anatomy, Ludwig Maximilians University, Munich, FRG

Investigative Urology 3
Edited by H. Rübben et al.

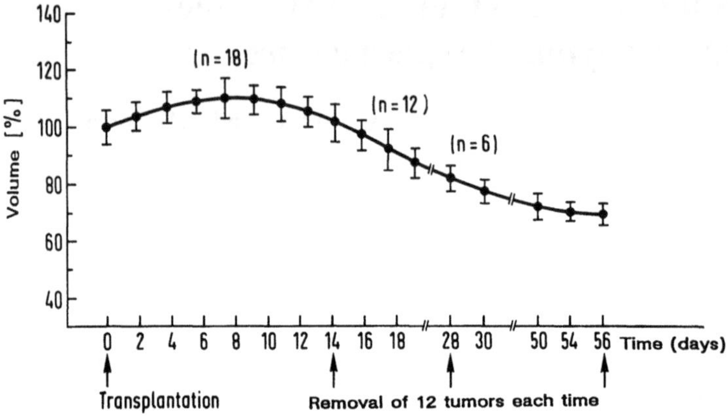

Fig. 1. Volume changes in untreated BPH human grafts in the thymus-dysplastic mouse: 30 tumors were observed over 28 days and 6 tumors up to 112 days after transplantation. The size determination was based on caliper measurements, the volume was calculated according to the formula of an ellipsoid ($0.52 \times D_1 \times D_2 \times D_3$). The initial volume of about 70 mm^3 was selected

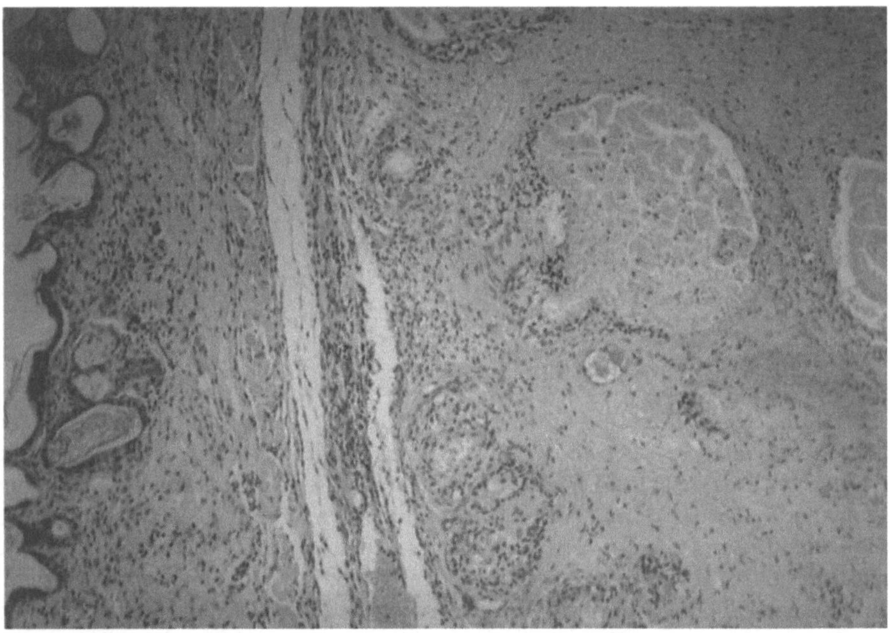

Fig. 2. Central necrosis in BPH tissue 7 days postimplantation. H & E staining, × 157

Control animals had no measurable PSA concentrations; BPH tumor-bearing animals showed quite different PSA values, depending on the tissue used for blood collection and the volume of the BPH tissue. Immediately after transplantation, very high PSA levels were measured. During the following days there was an exponential decrease of PSA concentration in serum (Fig. 4). The PSA values were found to be

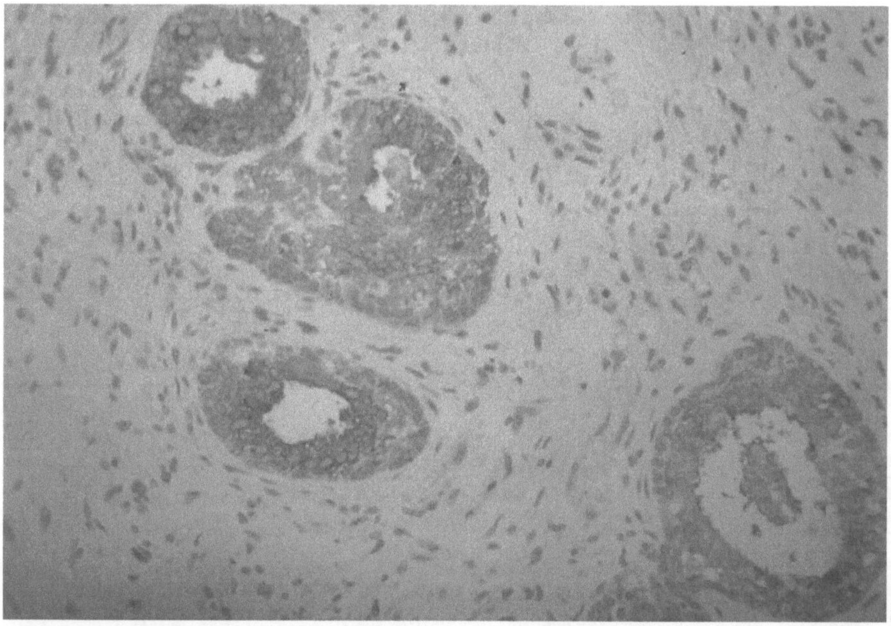

Fig. 3. Squamous metaplasia of the central glandular tubes which have partly already recovered 28 days postimplantation. H & E staining, × 175

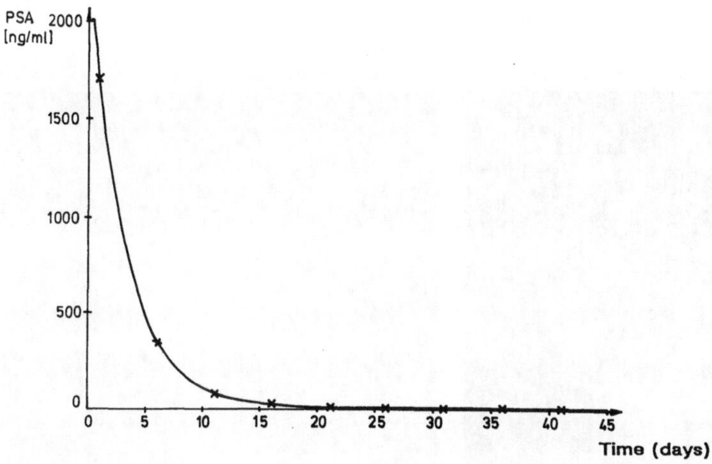

Fig. 4. Decrease in PSA concentration in the serum of nude mice postimplantation of human BPH tissue as a function of time. Mean values of about six experimental animals have been recorded in each case

dependent upon the volume (Fig. 5). The volumes vary by a factor of 3.1 and the PSA concentrations, by a factor of 3.4.

Some 30 min after mechanical irritation of the subcutaneous BPH graft, the nude mouse showed an increase of the PSA concentration by more than 320% of the initial value (Fig. 6). This PSA increase was significant ($P < 0.01$).

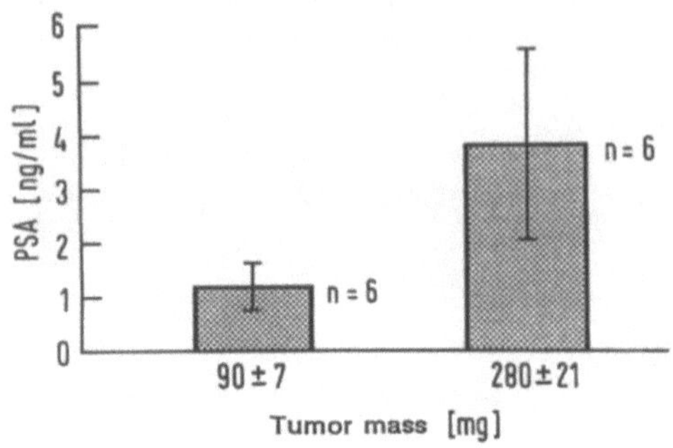

Fig. 5. PSA concentration of nude mice with one or three transplanted human BPH tumors. The difference between both is significant with $P < 0.01$

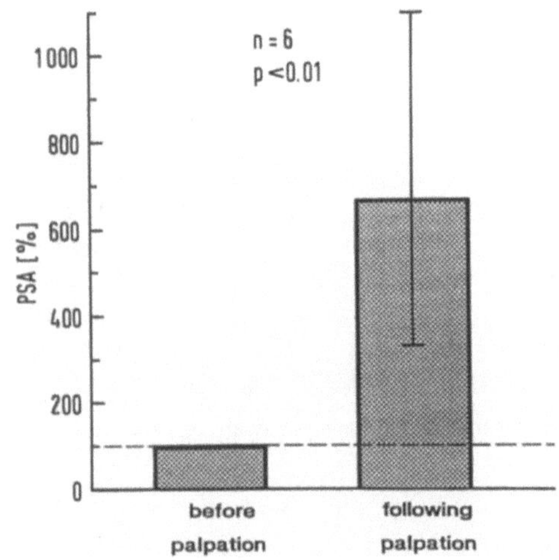

Fig. 6. PSA level 30 min after palpation of the subcutaneously transplanted BPH tumors on day 14 following xenotransplantation as compared with the initial concentration

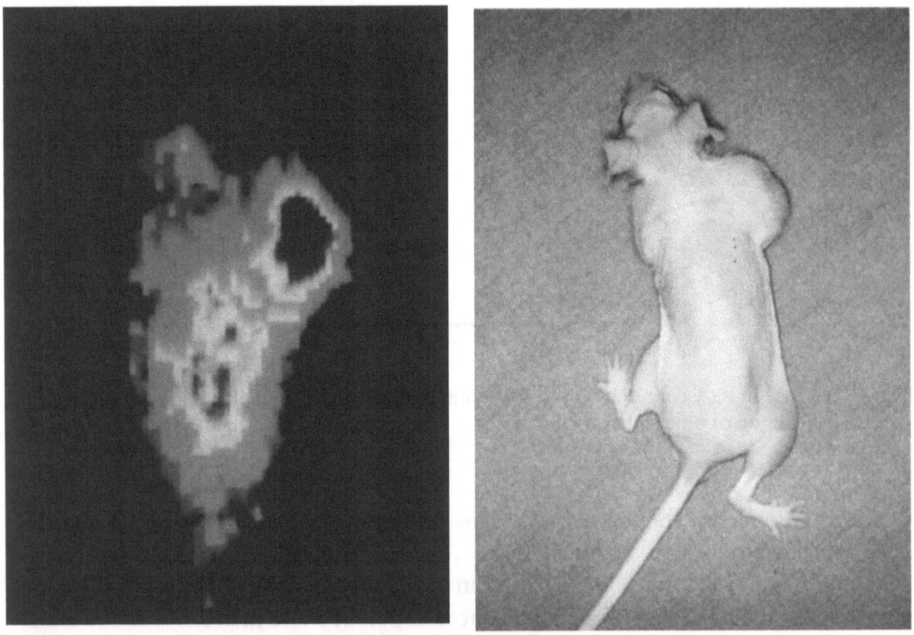

Fig. 7. Prostatic tumor bearing *nu/nu* mouse *(above right shoulder)* and immunoscintigraphy of the tumor (7 days postinjection of ^{131}I-labeld MoAb against PSA)

Table 1. Biokinetic distribution studies of ^{131}I-MoAb against PSA. Any tumor-bearing nude mouse was injected the labeled antibody via a tail vein. After 4, 7, and 12 days, six animals were killed each time, and the activity in the blood, the tumor, and different organs was measured. The percentage of ^{131}I-MoAb against PSA per g tissue is indicated

Day p.i.	Blood	Tumor	Tu/ blood	Heart	Liver	Prostate
4	8.04 ± 0.9	8.12 ± 2.5	1.01	2.13 ± 0.2	2.51 ± 0.5	1.37 ± 0.8
7	3.31 ± 0.8	3.24 ± 0.4	0.98	0.86 ± 0.2	1.01 ± 0.06	0.67 ± 0.1
12	1.75 ± 0.2	3.47 ± 1.8	1.98	0.49 ± 0.2	0.56 ± 0.05	0.35 ± 0.1

The immunoscintigraphic image of a subcutaneous BPH xenograft is given in Fig. 7. Although this figure permits a clear localization of the tumor, the tumor/blood ratio was only 1.98 on day 12 after injection of the nuclide (Table 1).

Discussion

The question was whether human BPH tissue transplanted to the *nu/nu* mouse maintains a part of the human morphological and biochemical properties and thus may be used for diagnostic, possibly also therapeutic studies. Since we transplanted tissue sections, the solid tumor structure of the original preparation was not changed.

Histology reveals reactions to insufficient nutrition and ischemia of the BPH tissue immediately after transplantation. However, these reactions as measured after 4 weeks in the epithelium were only of minor extent.

Wagner et al. reported no degenerated glandular structures in similar experiments. This might be due to the fact that they conducted no examinations in this early phase. However, a stroma fibrosation was found by them as well (Wagner et al. 1987). Since the morphologic findings were difficult to standardize, an evaluation of the therapeutic effects could only be done to a limited extent by histology.

The histological examinations of PAP and PSA activity clearly identified the xenograft as prostatic tissue even after 16 weeks. The solid human prostatic tumor was found to be appropriate, for cultivation in the nude mouse proved that it is sufficiently vascularized. If the morphological changes in the epithelium cells and the stroma after incubation in the culture medium are compared, the establishment of primarily solid tumors in the nude mouse appears to offer more advantages (McMahon and Thomas 1973; Schröder and Mackensen 1974).

The behavior of the PSA concentration in the serum of nude mice, depending on the time elapsed after surgery, revealed that great PSA quantities are released due to tissue trauma, initially as a result of diffusion. The processes of cell transformation also result in epithelium tissue death, thus causing an above-average PSA expression by the BPH tissue. Different tumor markers are known to show a correlation of the serum level and the tumor mass (Staab et al. 1985). It is not surprising that such a relation could be detected for the organ marker PSA as well.

Manipulations of the prostate cause a brief PAP rise in the serum which is no longer detectable after 48 h. The same phenomenon could be shown experimentally for the PSA concentrations. The influence of tumor mass and mechanical manipulations on the PSA behavior in the periperal blood showed that increased PSA values in patients have to be evaluated critically from the clinical point of view. MoAb enables the use of tumor tissue for scintigraphic imaging (Scheidhauer et al. 1987). Although there are already established procedures for some colorectal and gynecological tumors as well as for melanoma, the practical use is difficult. In the case of the prostate only PAP labeling has been used for scintigraphy up to now (Babain et al. 1987).

In the case of results presented here, it is possible to show the correlation between prostatic soft tissue, as detected immunologically using ^{131}I-labeled MoAb, and PSA. However, it remains unclear how the MoAb after i.v. application reached the intracellular PSA or whether only a high PSA concentration within the vessels of the graft was responsible for imaging.

Acknowledgement. These studies were kindly supported by the Stiftung Bohnewand/Gravenhorst.

References

Babain RJ, Murray JL, Lamki LM, Haynie TP, Hersh EM, Rosenblum MG, Glenn HJ, Unger MW, Carlo DJ, Eschenbach AC v (1987) Radioimmunological imaging of metastatic prostatic cancer with 111-Indium labeled monoclonal antibody PAY 276. J Urol 137:439–443

Czapo Z, Schrott KM, Brand K, Walter R (1987) Vergleichende experimentelle Untersuchungen der Tumormarker PAP/RIA and PSA/RIA anhand menschlicher Nacktmaustumormodelle. In: Ackermann R (ed) Verhandlungsbericht der Deutschen Gesellschaft für Urologie. Springer, Berlin Heidelberg New York Tokyo, pp 205–207

Fabricius PG, Sturm W, Amselgruber W, Rommel F, Fornara P (1987) Transplantation of hypertrophied prostatic tissue (BPH) into the nude mouse – its value and possibilities for therapeutic studies. J Endocrinol Invest 10:68

McMahon MJ, Thomas GH (1973) Morphological changes of benign prostatic hyperplasia in culture. Br J Cancer 27:323–335

Scheidhauer K, Landthaler M, Denecke H, Stefani FH, Schumacher U, Leinsinger G, Eiermann W, Moser E, Lissner J (1987) Radioimmunszintigraphie mit monoklonalen Antikörpern. Digit Bilddiagn 7:134–140

Schröder FH, Mackensen SJ (1974) Human prostatic adenoma and carcinoma in cell culture. Invest Urol 12:176–181

Staab HJ, Anderer FA, Schindler AE, Ahlemann LM, Zwirner M (1985) Optimizing tumor markers in breast cancer: monitoring, prognosis and therapy control. Cancer Detect Prev 8:35

Wagner B, Otto U, Becker H, Klöppel G, Klosterhalfen H (1987) Kann die benigne Prostatahyperplasie hormonell induziert werden? Transplantation von menschlichem Prostatagewebe auf die NMRI *nu/nu* Maus. In: Ackermann R (ed) Verhandlungsbericht der Deutschen Gesellschaft für Urologie. Springer, Berlin Heidelberg New York, pp 456–458

Age-Dependency and Regional Distribution of Enkephalinergic Nerves in the Human Prostate

T. JUNGBLUT[1], G. AUMÜLLER[2], B. MALEK[3], and H. MELCHIOR[1]

Introduction

Numerous studies have been made of the autonomic innervation of the prostate in different mammals, including humans (e.g., Sjöstrand 1965; Norberg et al. 1967; Vaalasti and Hervonen 1979, 1980). These studies have revealed a dual adrenergic and cholinergic autonomic innervation of this organ. Since the first reports of the existence of enkephalin-immunoreactive nerves in the male urogenital tract (Vaalasti et al. 1980; Alm et al. 1981), the presence of these nerves has been confirmed (Del Fiacco 1982; Vaalasti et al. 1986). The enkephalins may act as neurotransmitters in concert with the classical transmitters (Burnstock 1986; Fried et al. 1986; De Potter et al. 1987). In spite of this, close to nothing is known about the histotopography, the chemical diversity, and the hormone sensitivity or age dependency of these peptidergic nerves.

We have used a plethora of antisera against different proenkephalin-, prodynorphin-, or proopiomelanocortin-derived opioid sequences which were applied to paraffin sections of juvenile and adult (normal or pathologic) human prostates to gain some insights into the regional distribution and age-dependent chemoarchitecture of prostatic peptidergic nerves.

Material and Methods

Human Tissue. A part of the tissue specimens was kindly provided from the Department of Pathology of Philipps University (Prof. Dr. C. Thomas) and were taken from autopsies of traffic accident victims or unexpected child death cases. Fixation was performed in 4% formaldehyde or in a few cases in Bouin's fluid. The age distribution was as follows: 1 1-year-old boy, 1 5-year-old boy, 1 15-year-old boy, 1 17-year-old young man, 1 27-year-old man, 1 47-year-old man, and 5 elderly men (62–75 years) suffering from BPH or prostatic cancer (Bouin-fixed prostatectomy specimens).

Antisera and Immunohistochemistry. Several polyclonal antisera against different compounds of opioid-derived polypeptides, as specified in Table 1, were used. Immunoreactions were performed on 5-µm thick paraffin sections mounted on chromalaun-gelatin-coated glass slides after deparaffinization with xylene and hydration by in-

[1] Klinik für Urologie der Städtischen Kliniken Kassel, FRG
[2] Institut für Anatomie, Philipps-Universität Marburg, FRG
[3] Klinik für Dermatologie, Justus-Liebig-Universität Gießen, FRG

Investigative Urology 3
Edited by H. Rübben et al.

Table 1. Details of antisera used

Antigen	Abbreviation	Host	Dilution	Reference
Alpha-neoendorphin	None	Rabbit	1:4000	Weber et al. 1982
Heptapeptide	MRF (= ME + arg + phe)	Rabbit	1:4000	Weber et al. 1983
Dynorphin A	None	Rabbit	1:3000	Weihe et al. 1985
Beta-endorphin	None	Rabbit	1:2000	Weber et al. 1982
Octapeptide	MRGL (= ME + arg + gly + leu)	Rabbit	1:8000	Weber et al. 1983
Beta-neoendorphin	None	Rabbit	1:4000	Weber et al. 1983
Leu-enkephalin	Leu-Enk	Rabbit	1:4000	Weihe et al. 1985
Met-enkephalin	Met-Enk or ME	Rabbit	1:4000	Weber et al. 1983

cubating the sections for 48 h at 4°C with the respective diluted antisera. The immunoreaction was visualized using the immunoperoxidase method (Sternberger 1974). Control incubations were made by diluting the primary antibody to final replacement by nonimmune serum. All controls were negative. Antisere were kindly provided by Prof. Dr. E. Weihe (Johannes-Gutenberg-Universität Mainz, FRG).

Results

Table 2 gives a survey of the regional distribution of immunoreactive nerves with the different antisera tested. There were considerable differences in the intensity of immunoreactions of the different specimens studied. While in infant and juvenile glands immunoreactivity was homogenously and relatively densely distributed (Figs. 1–3), it was extremely sparse and heterogenous in specimens from adults or elderly

Table 2. Regional distribution of enkephalinergic nerves in the human prostate

Prostatic compartment	Antibody			
	MRF	MRGL	Leu-Enk	Met-Enk
Capsule				
Vessels	(+)	(+)	(+)	(+)
Smooth muscle	–	(+)	–	–
Stroma				
Vessels	–	+	+	+
Smooth muscle	+	++	+	++
Periurethral				
Vessels	(+)	+	+	+
Smooth muscle	(+)	(+)	(+)	(+)

Subjective rating scale of immunoreactivity: – absent, (+) rare, + frequent, ++ very frequent

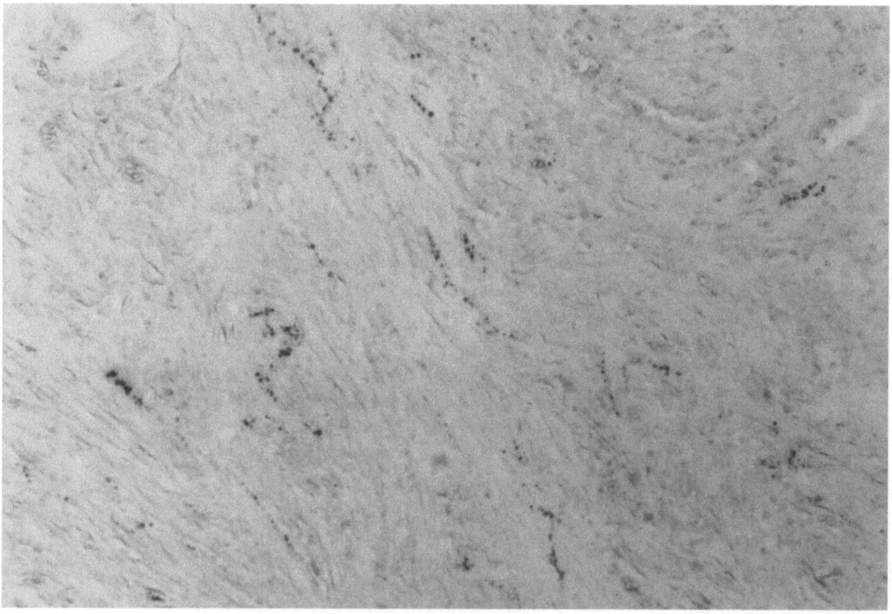

Fig. 1. One-year-old boy, stroma, MRGL immunoreactivity. ×125

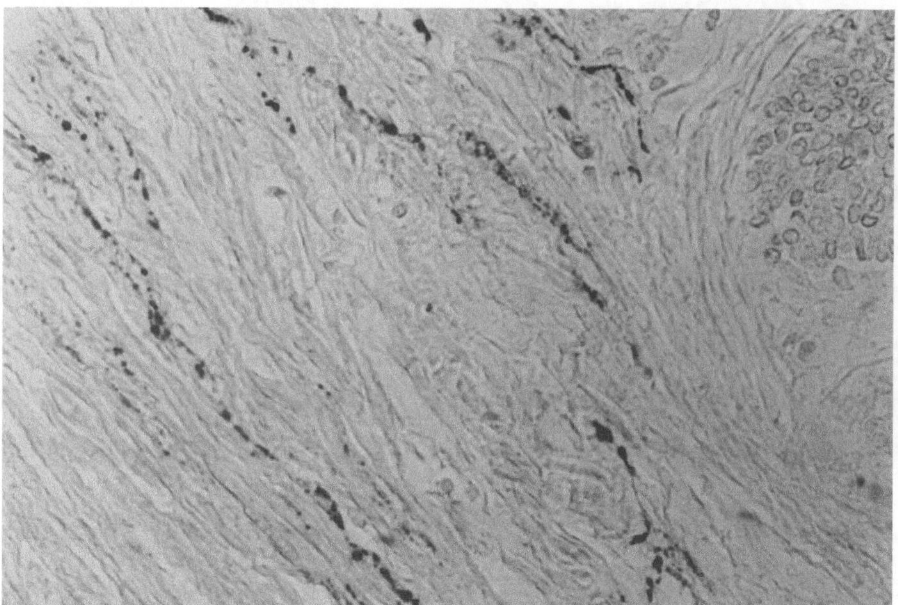

Fig. 2. Five-year-old boy, stroma, MRGL immunoreactivity. ×313

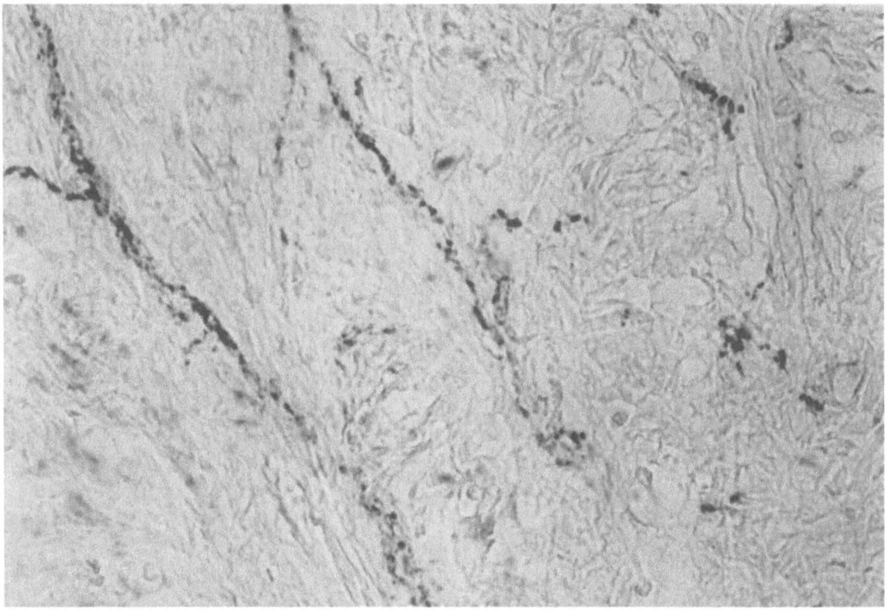

Fig. 3. Five-year-old boy, stroma, ME immunoreactivity. × 313

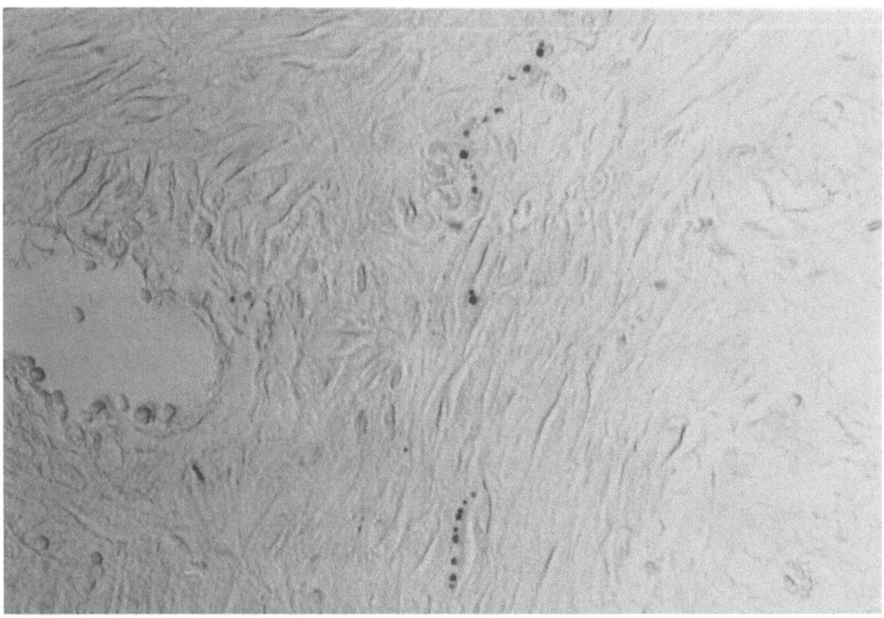

Fig. 4. Elderly man (62 years), stroma, Leu-enkephalin immunoreactivity. × 313

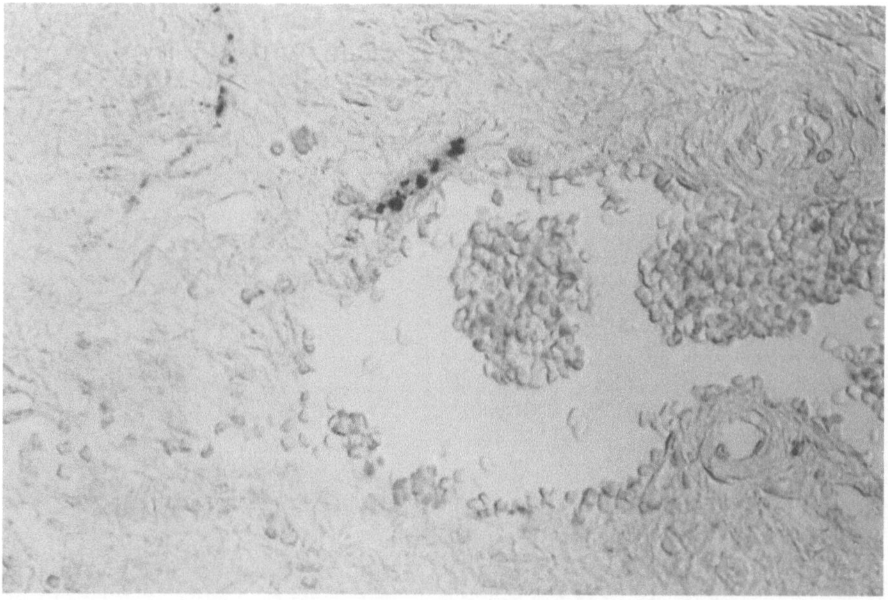

Fig. 5. Elderly man (68 years), stroma (vessels), MRGL immunoreactivity. × 313

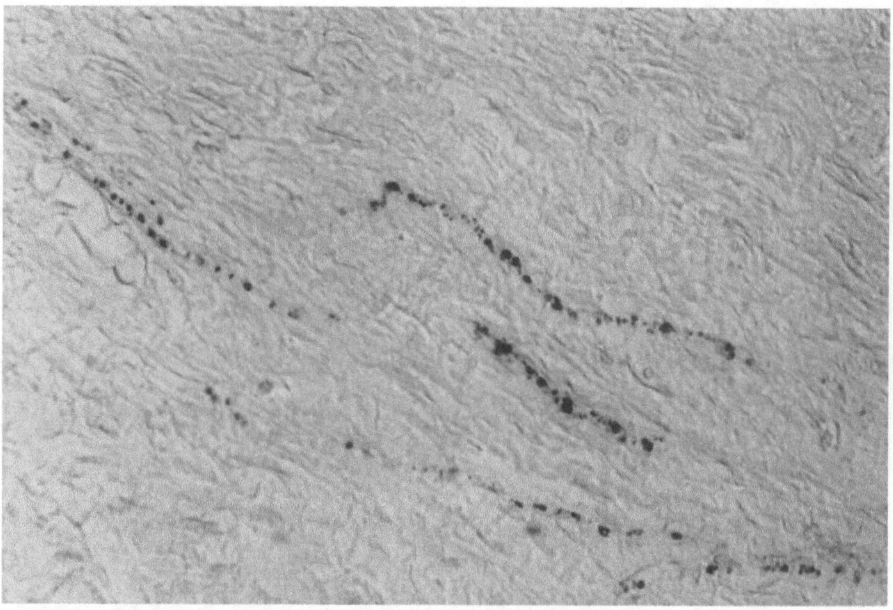

Fig. 6. Fifteen-year-old boy, stroma, MRF immunoreactivity. × 313

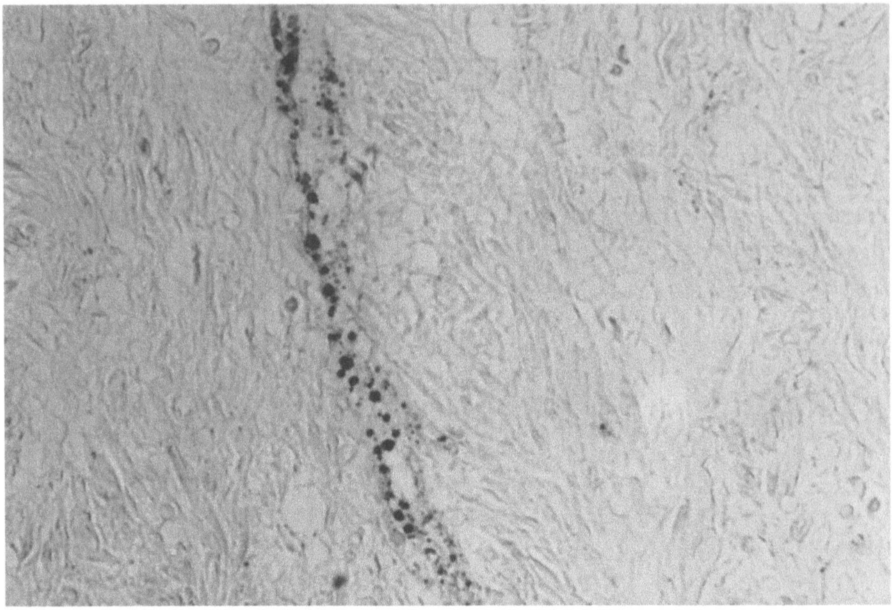

Fig. 7. Twenty-seven-year-old man, stroma MRGL immunoreactivity. × 313

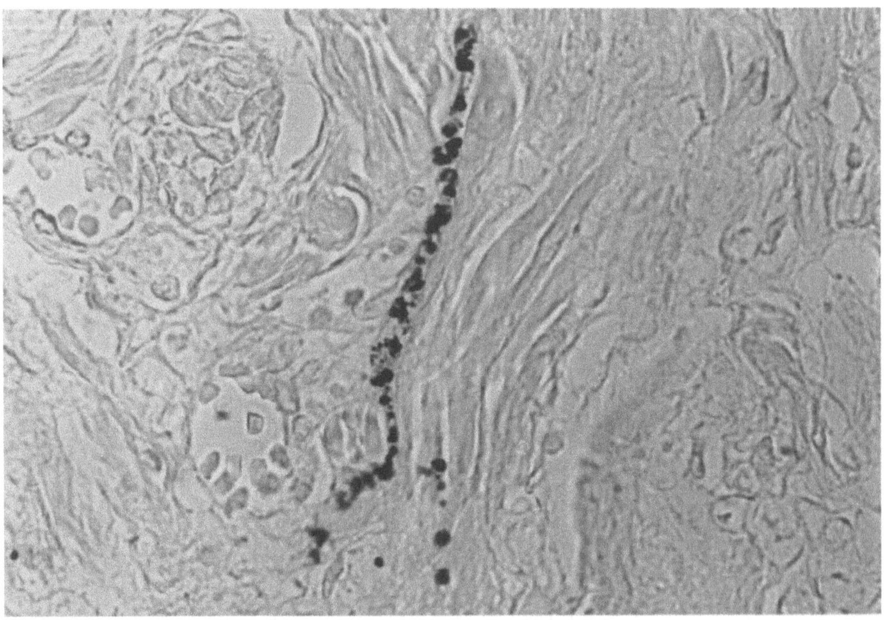

Fig. 8. Forty-seven-year-old man, vessels, MRGL immunoreactivity. × 313

men (Figs. 4, 5). Immunoreactive nerves, occasionally arranged in bundles in the periphery of the gland and branching within the stroma, could be traced in parallel with smooth muscle (Figs. 6, 7) and with blood vessels (Fig. 8).

Occasionally some ganglionic cells reacting with antiserum against octapeptide were found only in the infantile specimens in the space between the dorsolateral capsule of the prostate and the seminal vesicles. Antisera against beta-endorphin, alpha-neoendorphin, beta-neoendorphin, and dynorphin A gave no positive immunoreaction with prostatic nerves.

Discussion

In the present study a characteristic age-dependence and histotopography in the chemoarchitecture of enkephalinergic nerves of the human prostate has been found. Previous studies (Vaalasti et al. 1980, 1986; Del Fiacco 1982) have reported a rather irregular and heterogenous distribution of enkephalin-immunoreactive nerves in the human prostate, contrasting with the dense and homogenous network of VIP-immunoreactive nerves. MRF- and MRGL-immunoreactive nerves of the human prostate are first described in the present study. Others (e.g., Gu et al. 1983) were unable to find enkephalin-immunoreactive nerves in the human prostate. These differences may be due either to technical reasons or to the fact that in older specimens the immunoreaction for enkephalin is greatly reduced as compared with younger specimens. Such an age dependency of prostatic innervation has been previously suggested by neurohistologists (Casas 1958; Jabonero et al. 1963; Bacsich 1969).

Contrary to the findings of Vaalasti et al. (1986) we have found some ganglionic cells in the human prostatic capsule reacting with enkephalin antisera. They were found in the infantile specimens in the space between the dorsolateral capsule portion of the prostate close to the seminal vesicles. The MRGL immunoreactivity was mainly found in the small cells of the ganglion. According to Gosling (1983) the large neurons are rich in acetylcholinesterase but lack catecholamines, while the small cells, which are mostly lacking in older specimens, are rich in catecholamines and are devoid of acetylcholinesterase. They give rise to short adrenergic nerves innervating prostatic stromal smooth muscle cells.

According to Gosling (1983) there is an age-dependent reduction of afferent corpuscles in adult prostate. Gu et al. (1983) suggest the presence of substance P in afferent prostatic nerve fibers; at least in our studies no dynorphin- or beta-endorphin-like immunoreactivity has been found in prostatic nerves or pelvic viscera as had been presumed (Basbaum et al. 1986). Recently, it has been suggested (Kawatani et al. 1986) that the high percentage of visceral neurons containing VIP may function as afferent pathways from the pelvic organs. On the other hand, it has been proposed that VIP is present in cholinergic nerves and may function in the control of secretion and blood flow (Gu et al. 1983; Vaalasti et al. 1986). The coexistence of classic transmitters with peptidergic ones seems to be accepted (Millhorn et al. 1987; Stjernquist et al. 1987). Since the definitive mode of prostatic smooth muscle contraction is not yet established the possible function of enkephalinergic nerves, which are found closely related to smooth muscle cells, should be considered.

Enkephalin-like immunoreactivity is also present, though less strongly, in the periurethral zone, where it is mostly related to the vessels. Hence, the nervous substrate for myovascular reflexes is present.

In consideration of the fact that immunoreactivity decreases in older specimens and that the periurethral zone shows a less strong immunoreactivity, a possible role of the enkephalins on the pathogenesis of BPH seems improbable.

Summary

Nerves displaying immunoreactivity of met-enkephalin, leu-enkephalin, heptapeptid and octapeptid were detected in the dorsolateral stroma closely related to smooth muscle predominantly of juvenile glands. A less strong immunoreactivity were present around stromal vessels and periurethal. Subepithelial periacinar nerves showing leu-enkephalin, met-enkephalin, octa- and heptapeptid immunoreactivity were found in a few instances. The most prominent immunoreaction was achieved with octapeptid antiserum, followed in decreasing order by met-enkephalin, leu-enkephalin and heptapeptid. Their density decreased with age. Antisera against beta-endorphin, alpha-neo-endorphin, beta-neoendorphin and dynorphin A gave no positive immunoreaction with prostatic nerves. The regional distribution pattern described is in favour of a postsynaptic peptidergic sympathetic and parasympathetic innervation of prostatic stroma acting with classical neurotransmitters. A detailed examination of the regional distribution demonstrated octapeptid immunoreactivity inside some ganglionic cells of the prostatic capsule of juvenile organs.

References

Alm P, Alumets J, Hakanson R, Owman C, Sjöberg NO, Stjernquist M, Sundler F (1981) Enkephalin-immunoreactive nerve fibres in the feline genitourinary tract. Histochemistry 72:351–355

Bacsich P (1969) On the presence of Timofeew's sensory corpuscles in the autonomic plexuses of the human prostate and seminal vesicles. J Anat (London) 104:182–183

Basbaum AI, Cruz L, Weber E (1986) Immunoreactive dynorphin B in sacral primary afferent fibres of the cat. J Neurosci 6:127–133

Burnstock G (1986) The changing face of autonomic neurotransmission. Acta Physiol Scand 126: 67–91

Casas AP (1958) Die Innervation der menschlichen Vorsteherdrüse. Z Mikrosk Anat Forsch 64: 608–633

De Potter WP, Coen EP, De Potter RW (1987) Evidence for the coexistence and corelease of Met-enkephalin and noradrenaline from sympathetic nerves of the bovine vas deferens. Neurosci 20:855–866

Del Fiacco (1982) Enkephalin-like immunoreactivity in the human male genital tract. J Anat (London) 135:649–656

Fried G, Terenius L, Brodin E, Efendic S, Dockray G, Fahrenkrug J, Goldstein M, Hökfelt T (1986) Neuropeptide Y, enkephalin and noradrenaline coexist in sympathetic neurons innervating the bovine spleen. Cell Tissue Res 243:495–508

Gosling JA (1983) Autonomic innervation of the prostate. In: Hinman FJ (ed) Benign prostatic hypertrophy. Springer, Berlin Heidelberg New York, pp 348–360

Gu J, Polak JM, Probert L, Islam KN, Marangos PJ, Mina S, Adrian TE, McGregor GP, O'Shaughnessy DJ, Bloom SR (1983) Peptidergic innervation of the human male genital tract. J Urol 130: 386–391

Jabonero V, Genis MJ, Santos L (1963) Beobachtungen über die osmiumzinkjodidaffinen Elemente der Vorsteherdrüse. Z Mikrosk Anat Forsch 69:167–194

Kawatani M, Nagel J, de Groat WC (1986) Identification of neuropeptides in pelvic and pudendal nerve afferent pathways to the sacral spinal cord of the cat. J Comp Neurol 249:117–132

Millhorn DE, Hökfelt T, Terenius T, Buchan A, Brown JC (1987) Somatostatin- and enkephalin-like immunoreactivities are frequently colocalized in neurons in the caudal brain stem of rat. Exp Brain Res 67:426–428

Norberg KA, Risley PL, Ungerstedt U (1967) Adrenergic innervation of the male reproductive ducts in some mammals. I. The distribution of adrenergic nerves. Z Zellforsch 76:278–286

Sjöstrand NO (1965) The adrenergic innervation of the vas deferens and the accessory male genital glands. Acta Physiol Scand [Suppl 257] 65

Sternberger LA (1974) Immunocytochemistry. Prentice-Hall, Engelwood Cliffs

Stjernquist M, Owman C, Sjöberg NO, Sundler F (1987) Coexistence and cooperation between neuropeptide Y and norepinephrine in nerve fibres of guinea pig vas deferens and seminal vesicle. Biol Reprod 36:149–155

Vaalasti A, Hervonen A (1979) Innervation of the ventral prostate of the rat. Am J Anat 154:231–245

Vaalasti A, Hervonen A (1980) Nerve endings in the human prostate. Am J Anat 157:41–47

Vaalasti A, Linnoila I, Hervonen A (1980) Immunohistochemical demonstration of VIP, met- and leu-enkephalin immunoreactive nerves in the human prostate and seminal vesicles. Histochemistry 66:89–98

Vaalasti A, Tainio H, Pelto-Huikko M, Hervonen A (1986) Light and electron microscope demonstration of VIP- and enkephalin-immunoreactive nerves in the human male genitourinary tract. Anat Rec 215:21–27

Weber E, Roth KA, Barchas JD (1982) Immunohistochemical distribution of alpha-neoendorphin/dynorphin neuronal systems in rat brain. Proc Natl Acad Sci USA 79:3062–3066

Weber E, Evans CJ, Barchas JD (1983) Multiple endogenous ligands for opioid receptors. TINS August:333–336

Weihe E, Hartschuh W, Weber E (1985) Prodynorphin opioid peptides in small somatosensory primary afferents of guinea pig. Neurosci Lett 58:347–352

Tumor Marker Characterization in the Serially Transplantable PC-EW Human Prostatic Carcinoma Line in Nude Mice*

Z. Csapo, K. M. Schrott, and R. Walther[1]

Introduction

Prostatic acid phosphatase (PAP) and prostate specific antigen (PSA) are organ-specific substances. Although neither PAP nor PSA are tumor specific, their serum values in patients with prostate cancer frequently appear markedly elevated as compared with the values of healthy subjects or patients affected by malignancies of non-prostatic origin (Foti et al. 1977; Wang et al. 1979; Kuriyama et al. 1982). Since successful therapy causes a decrease in the serum levels of both substances, they can be regarded as useful tumor markers. Clinical findings during the past few years show that serum PSA can frequently be raised when the serum PAP is normal (Chu and Murphy 1986; Siddal et al. 1986; Ahmann and Schifman 1987). Preliminary studies in patients with prostate cancer have shown a correlation between the frequency of pathological PSA levels and disease stage, grade, and activity (Csapo et al. 1987). However, little data are available for comparing the indicator value of PSA with PAP.

The present study describes experimental results comparing the indicator value of serum PSA levels with PAP levels of the PC-EW tumor model. This serially transplantable human prostatic carcinoma line in the nude mouse has been developed through heterotransplantation of tumor tissue from a lymph node metastasis (Höhn et al. 1984). It is androgen dependent and is similar to the original tumor in terms of histological pattern (Fig. 1). On account of the histological similarity, hormonal dependence, as well as PAP and PSA production, the PC-EW nude mouse tumor line can be considered as an ideal experimental model for the tumor marker characterization of prostatic cancer.

Our study revealed that serum values of both PAP and PSA in untreated mice bearing the PC-EW tumor are dependent on the tumor volume. A close correlation between the two tumor markers was found, but the indicator value of PSA was 2^4–2^6 times higher than that of PAP. This means that PSA signalled tumor growth between four and six tumor doubling cycles earlier than PAP. In animals treated with different treatment modalities in cases of histologically and growth-kinetically verified tumor regression, the tumor markers investigated point to a decreasing or arrested tumor activity. The biochemical tumor activity was associated with an unchanged histological picture of the original tumor. During an androgenoprive therapy the parameters studied were found to have changed as expected. Arrest of growth and/or decrease in volume were associated with falling PSA and PAP values (often within

* Supported by the Wilhelm Sander Foundation Grant 85.029.1.

[1] Department of Urology, Medical Faculty, University of Erlangen-Nürnberg, Krankenhausstr. 12, 8520 Erlangen, FRG

Investigative Urology 3
Edited by H. Rübben et al.

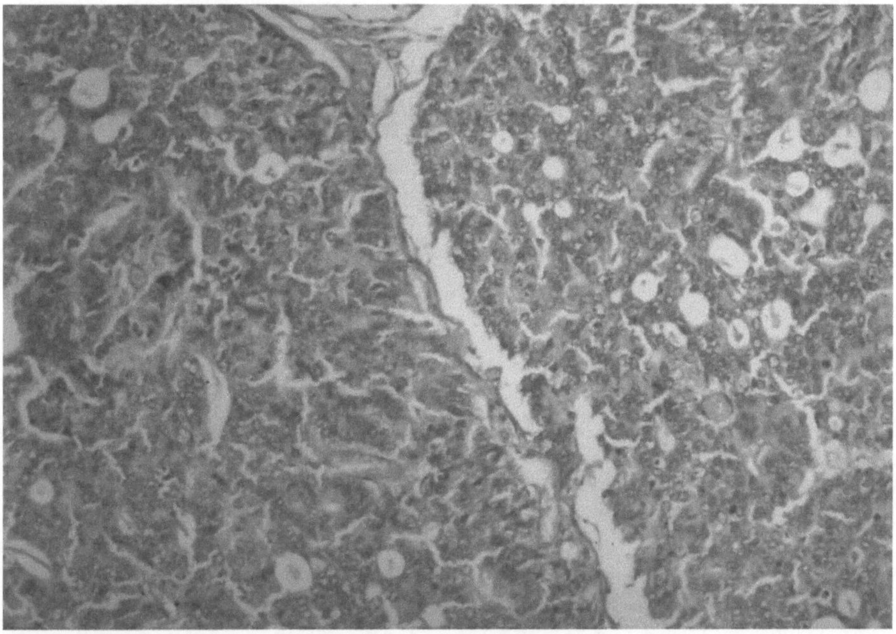

Fig. 1. Histology of the PC-EW tumor line at the 24th animal passage. × 188

the normal range), and with regressive histology. However, the PSA values appear to follow the decline of the PAP values to the basal level with a certain delay.

Material and Methods

Tumor Material. Male *nu/nu* nude mice from our own BALB/c line breed received a transplant of a 2–4 mm^3 particle from the PC-EW tumor at an age of 6–8 weeks. The fragments were grafted surgically into the dorsal subcutaneous space of the animals under ether anesthesia as described by Höhn et al. (1980). The macroscopic tumor size was determined by means of a slide caliper with dial gauge. Two diameters of the developing tumors, i.e., the largest diameter and the one perpendicular to it, were monitored daily. Tumor volume was calculated according to a formula established by van Steenbrugge et al. (1983). For the investigations tumors from the 24th–31st mouse transplant generation were used.

Treatment of the Animals. Therpay studies were started during the exponential growth phase of the tumors. The absolute measured diameter values were converted into percentages, and later, when therapy was applied, the tumor diameter was taken to be equivalent to 100%. This allowed direct comparison between the various tumors and the efficiency of the different therapy modalities (Fig. 6). Each tumor measured was analyzed histologically. Estrogen therapy using different doses (20 and 40 μg/day) in the form of 17-β-estradiol and a 5-alpha-reductase-inhibitor (6-methylen-

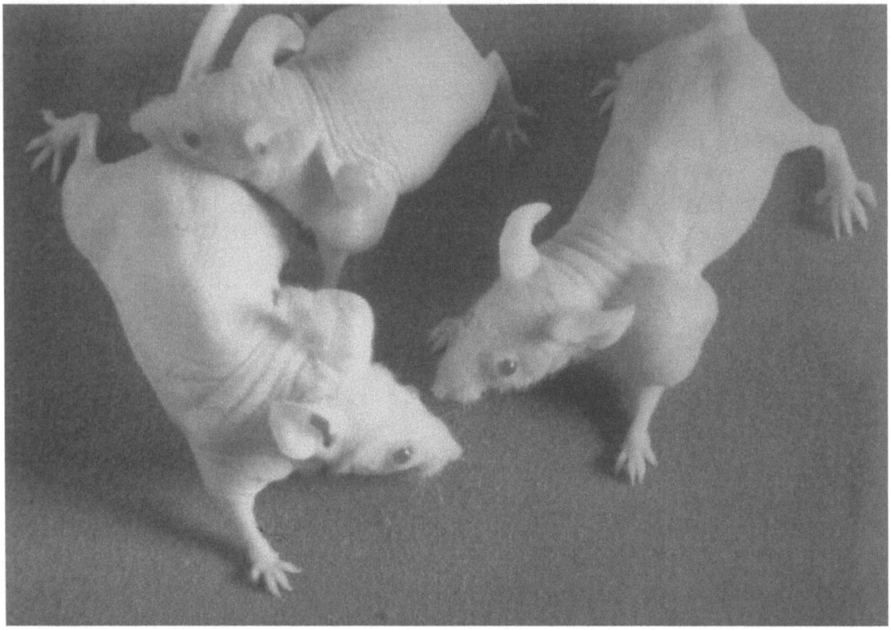

Fig. 2. PC-EW tumor-bearing male nude mice with different tumor volumes in the dorsal subcutaneous space

progesterone) with doses of 200 and 400 μg/day (10 and 20 mg/kg/day) were administered intraperitoneally for 20 days on average. Orchiectomy was carried out via the scrotal route under ether anaesthesia.

Serum Specimens. Tumor-bearing animals without therapy ($n = 47$) were killed at various points in time after transplantation. Serum values were determined in these animals with different end volumes of the tumor nodules (Fig. 2). The serum parameters from 23 treated mice were examined after a treatment period of 20 days on average. Blood was withdrawn after cervical section by opening the carotid arteries under ether anesthesia. In order to prevent hemolysis, the blood was briefly cooled down and the serum obtained by centrifugation for 2 min at 6000 rpm. Subsequently, the serum was deep-frozen or analyzed on the same day.

Radioimmunoassay Procedures. The tumor markers were determined by radioimmunoassay techniques. For the quantitative determination of PAP levels in serum the GammaDab (^{125}I) PAP Radioimmunoassay Kit (Travenol Genentech Diagnostics) was used. This procedure is a competitive binding assay which utilizes a precipitating antiserum reagent to separate antibody-bound tracer from unbound tracer. The PAP concentrations of the samples were interpolated from a standard curve. In case of high values, the sera were diluted up to ten times.

PSA was determined using a double antibody radioimmunoassay (PROS-CHECK PSA, Yang Laboratories) based on radioactive PSA (^{125}I) competitive binding principles, too. The antigen bound to the antibody following the incubation period was separated from the free components by the use of a precipitation solution containing the second antibody. With the calibration curve applied, this test is able to determine concentrations up to 50 ng/ml with a sensitivity of at least 0.2 ng/ml. Since the PSA values compared to the PAP values were often extremely elevated, the serum specimens had to be diluted 100- to 1000-fold.

Results

PAP and PSA in Serum of Control and Tumor-Bearing Male Nude Mice Without Therapy

For controls serum samples from 10 male nude mice without tumor were determined. They had a measurable PAP basal value of 0.5 ± 0.3 ng/ml and a PSA basal value of 0.6 ± 0.3 ng/ml. For the tumor-bearing animals a normal upper limit of 1.4 ng/ml for PAP and of 1.5 ng/ml for PSA ($\times \pm 3 \times$ SD) was defined.

In the 47 animals investigated it was possible to determine the serum level of the tumor markers within a broad tumor volume spectrum from 143 to 5630 mm^3. In 19 cases the tumor size was smaller than 1000 mm^3, in 7 animals it varied between 1000 and 2000 mm^3, in 8 cases between 2000 and 3000 mm^3, in 6 animals from 3000 to 4000 mm^3 and in 7 cases it was over 4000 mm^3. With this volume spectrum the PSA value was true-positive, i.e., within the pathological range in all instances. The values exceeded the upper normal limit by at least a factor of 32 in all cases. In 44/47 cases (94%) the value was more than 100 times, in 42/47 cases (89%) more than 200 times and in 24/47 (51%) it was even 1000 times higher than the normal upper limit. In the PAP determination 5 false-negative findings (= 11% of the total figure) were established among the first 13 animals (38%), with a tumor volume up to 637 mm^3.

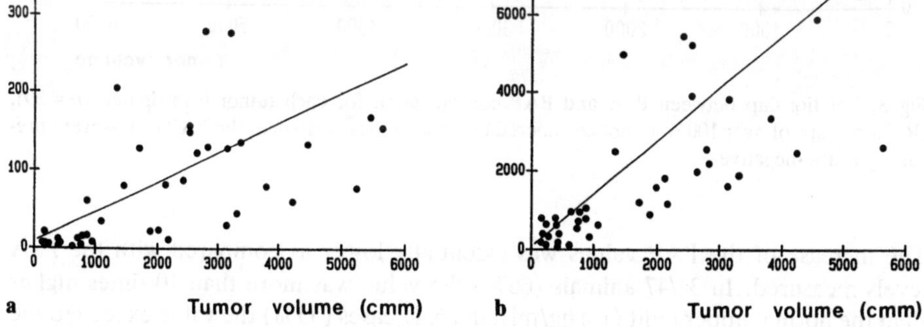

Fig. 3a, b. Serum values of PAP and PSA in relation to the actual PC-EW tumor volumes in untreated male nude mice with regard to all data ($n = 47$)

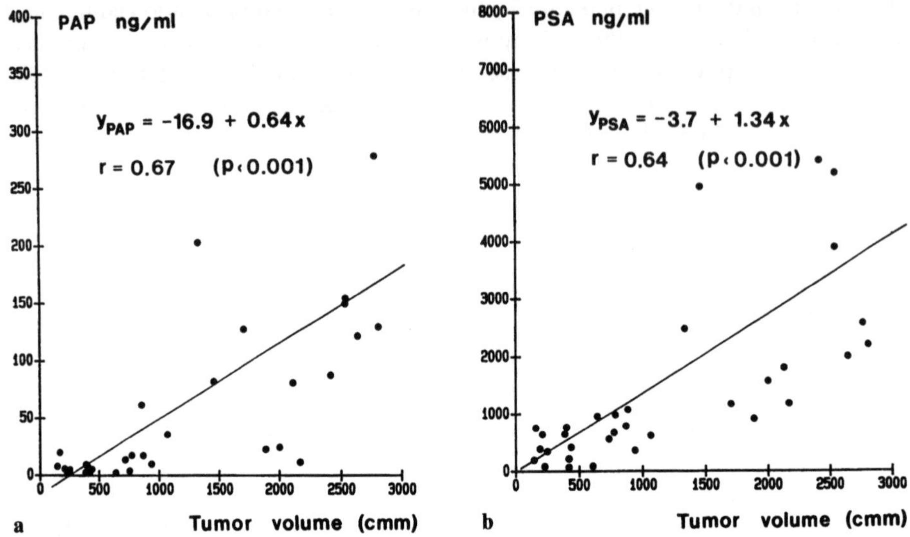

Fig. 4a, b. Correlation of serum PAP and PSA with the tumor volume in untreated nude mice bearing the PC-EW tumor smaller than 3000 mm^3 in volume ($n = 34$)

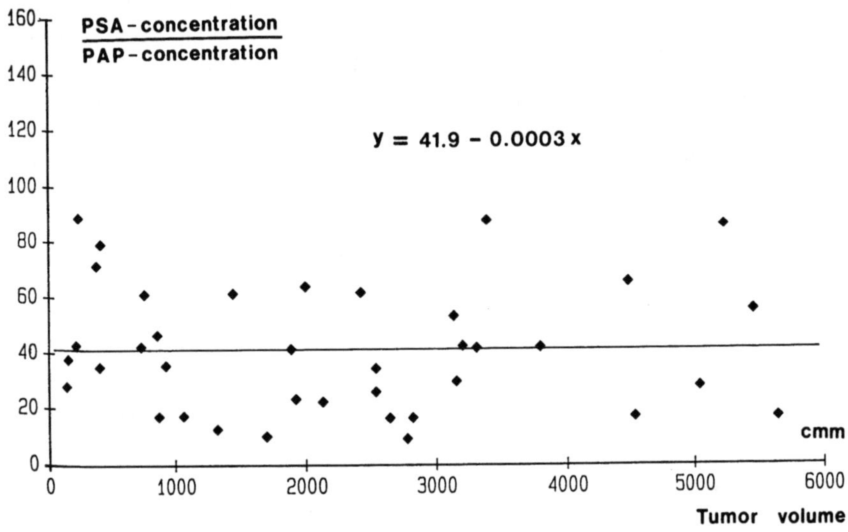

Fig. 5. Relationship between PSA and PAP concentration for each tumor investigated ($n = 39$). (Relationships of over 100 were not considered because in these instances the PAP results were prevailingly false-negative)

The increase of the PAP values was essentially lower as compared with the PSA levels measured. In 31/47 animals (66%) the value was more than 10 times higher than the normal upper limit (1.4 ng/ml), in 26/47 cases (55%) the value exceeded the limit by more than 20 times, and only in 10/47 cases (21%) was the PAP level over the 100 times limit. The highest PAP value was 360 ng/ml which means a 257-fold increase, whereas the maximum PSA value of 11.869 ng/ml meant an increase by the factor of almost 8000.

Figure 3 shows the serum values of PAP and PSA in relation to the actual PC-EW tumor volumes in the untreated male nude mice with regard to all data ($n = 47$). The serum values of both PAP and PSA proved to be strictly dependent on the tumor volume measured. However, the gradient of the regression straight line remained 36.3. This means that a certain tumor volume is related to a PSA serum level (roughly 36.3 times higher than that of PAP). However, with respect to tumor volumes up to 3000 mm^3 ($n = 37$) this ratio is 20.9 and thus somewhat lower (Fig. 4). This points to a levelling off of the PSA regression straight line for smaller tumor volumes.

Figure 5 demonstrates the relationship between PSA and PAP concentration for an investigated lesion. Since the upper limit of the normal ranges hardly differ (factor 0.93), the relationship between the actual measured PSA and PAP concentrations was analyzed. Relationships of over 100 ($n = 8$) were not considered because in the instances the PAP results were prevailingly false-negative. It can be clearly seen that the regression straight line thus computed followed an almost horizontal course ($y = 41.9 - 0.0003x$). The mean value of the PSA/PAP relationship was 41.2 ± 22.4 (median equal to 39.8!).

Influence of Different Treatment Modalities on the Concentration of PAP and PSA in the Serum of Tumor-Bearing Animals

Twenty days after the beginning of therapy, the PAP and PSA values were determined in 23 tumor-bearing mice with different tumor growths as shown by the growth curves of Fig. 6. (The blood samples could not be examined in all animals under treatment, which were measured for the presentation of the growth curves in

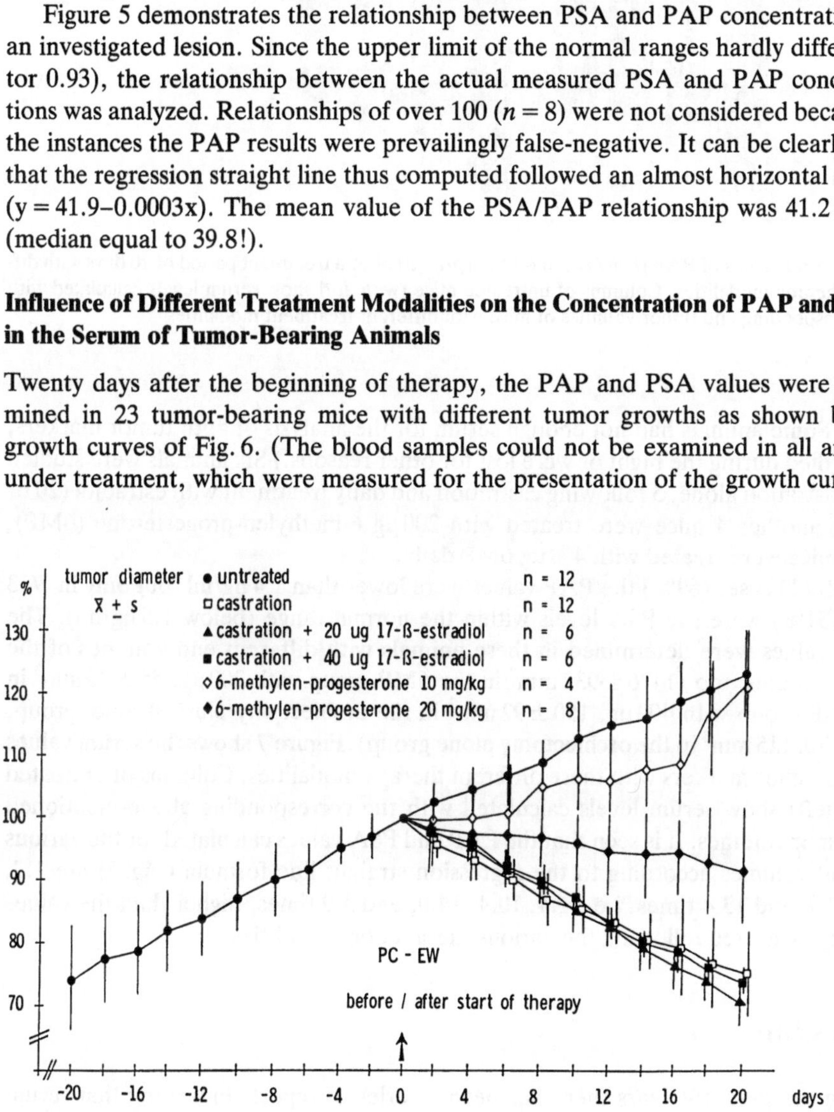

Fig. 6. Diameters of untreated and treated PC-EW tumors during the exponential growth phase. Tumor diameter on first day of therapy calculated to be 100%. Standard deviations are indicated

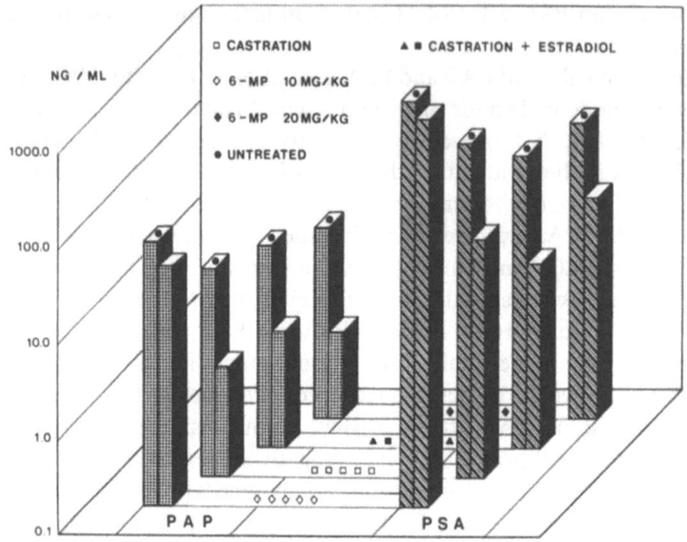

Fig. 7. Serum values of PAP *(hatched)* and PSA *(striped)* after a treatment period of 20 days with different therapy modalities. Columns of untreated mice *(with dot)* show serum levels calculated with the corresponding end tumor volumes of mice with different treatment modalities

Fig. 6. Some animals had not enough serum for the analysis of both tumor markers, others died during the night or were lost for other reasons.) Six animals were studied after castration alone, 5 following castration and daily treatment with estradiol (20 or 40 μg), another 4 mice were treated with 200 μg 6-methylen-progesterone (6MP), and 8 mice were treated with 400 μg 6MP daily.

In 16/23 cases (69%) the PAP values were lower than 1.4 ng/ml, but only in 7/23 cases (31%) were the PSA levels within the normal range (below 1.5 ng/ml). The serum values were determined in these animals with different end volumes of the tumor nodules, too (1476 ± 932 mm^3 in the 6MP group with 200 μg, 55 ± 33 mm^3 in the 6MP group with 400 μg, 150 ± 92 mm^3 in the orchiectomy plus estradiol group, and 220 ± 115 mm^3 in the orchiectomy alone group). Figure 7 shows the serum values of both tumor markers with these different therapy modalities. Columns of untreated mice (left) show serum levels calculated with the corresponding above-mentioned end tumor volumes. It is seen that the PAP and PSA values calculated for the various residual volumes according to the regression straight line formula (Fig. 3) are 1.7, 17.0, 7.9, and 13.4 times, i.e., 1.4, 10.4, 14.0, and 5.9 times, higher than the values actually measured following the various therapeutic modalities.

Discussion

During the past few years there has been a series of reports indicating that serum PSA levels can provide a specific test for monitoring carcinoma of the prostate. Since PSA is biochemically and immunologically distinct from PAP, the expression of

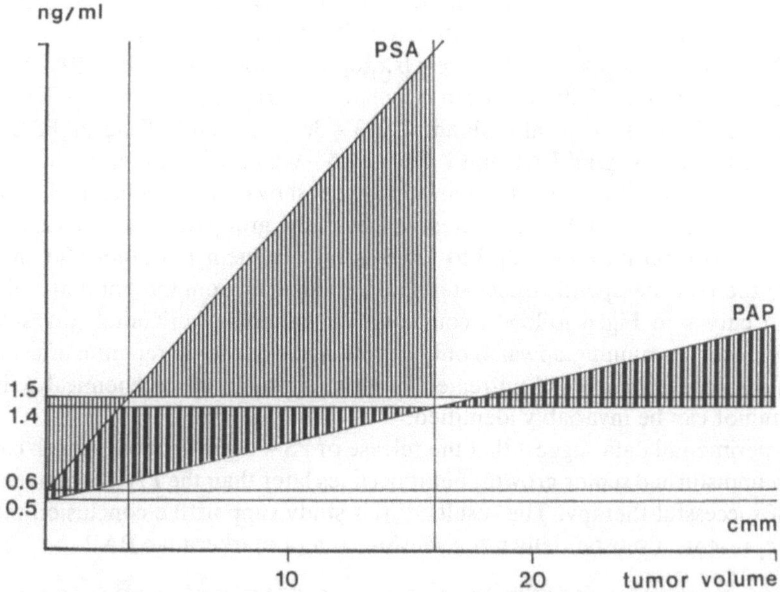

Fig. 8. Theoretical relationship between PAP and PSA secretion in smaller tumor volumes with visualization of the false-negative areas

these two organ-specific proteins may be unique parameters in combination tests for an increased rate in the serologic detection of prostate cancer.

In order to clarify in detail the efficiency of PAP and PSA in the diagnosis and follow-up of prostate cancer, comparative animal experiments were performed for the study of the PAP and PSA serum values in the hormone-sensitive human nude mouse prostatic carcinoma line PC-EW. Our data confirm that serum values of both PAP and PSA in untreated mice bearing the PC-EW tumor are dependent on the tumor volume (Figs. 3 and 4). A close correlation between the tumor markers and the tumor size was found, but the indicator value of PSA was 41.2 ± 22.4 times higher than that of PAP under these experimental conditions. This means that the PSA values indicate a tumor when its volume is 2^4–2^6 times smaller and thus are capable of signalling a lesion 4–6 tumor-doubling cycles earlier than the PAP serum values. PAP values were false-negative in 11% of the animals in the investigated volume spectrum, although the significant increase of the serum PSA almost indicates the tumor correctly. In our study all animals had already a subcutaneous tumor, readily measurable by means of calipers. Animals with yet smaller tumors (1–143 mm^3) could have also yielded false-negative PSA values. Figure 8 shows the theoretical relationship between PAP and PSA production in smaller tumor volumes with visualization of the false-negative areas.

Our findings are in agreement with the observations of Ahmann and Schifman (1987). Their results show that in contrast to acid phosphatase activity and PAP antigen the PSA values in clinically responsive patients generally remained substantially elevated. This suggests that PSA levels may be able to detect a smaller tumor burden than the other prostatic tumor markers.

In our treated animals both markers were found to decrease. Arrested growth and tumor regression were associated with falling PAP and PSA serum levels or with levels within normal ranges. The PAP levels dropped parallel with the PSA levels after a treatment period of 20 days from calculated pretreatment average values of 64.7 – 17.0 – 14.3 and 10.7 ng/ml PAP and 2.093 – 360 – 134 and 132 ng/ml PSA to 37.0 – 1.0 – 1.8 and 0.8 ng/ml PAP and 1.476 – 34.6 – 9.6 and 22.4 ng/ml PSA. During this 3-week period, however, the tumor markers showed no significant changes with respect to the calculated pretreatment values in the group of 6MP – 200 μg/day (PAP: 64.7 to 37.0 ng/ml, PSA: 2.093 to 1.476 ng/ml). In the light of these findings, we can see the real therapeutic effect starts no earlier than from the point at which the growth curves in Fig. 6 follow a course which is largely horizontal (arrest of growth). The curves running upwards only denote a low-grade therapeutic effect as compared with control curves of untreated animals, although the biochemical activity of the tumor can be invariably identified.

Our experimental data suggest that the release of PSA occurs not only much earlier during undisturbed tumor growth, but it declines later than the PAP serum level in cases of successful therapy. The results of this study support the conclusion that the PSA represents a substantially more sensitive tumor marker than PAP.

Acknowledgements. We thank Mr. M. Meyer, Institute of Medical Statistics and Documentation, University Erlangen-Nürnberg for the statistical analysis, Dr. I. Csuzda for his valuable technical assistance, and Dr. H. Pucher, Messrs Siemens, for his assistance in the English translation of the present paper.

References

Ahmann FR, Schifman RB (1987) Prospective comparison between serum monoclonal prostate specific antigen and acid phosphatase measurement in metastatic prostatic cancer. J Urol 137: 431–434

Chu TM, Murphy GP (1986) What's new in tumor markers for prostate cancer? Urology 27: 487–491

Csapo Z, Sigel A, Brand K (1987) Significance of prostatic acid phosphatase (PAP) and prostate specific antigen (PSA) in the diagnosis and follow-up of prostate cancer. Urologe B 27: 238–245

Foti AG, Cooper JF, Herschmann H, Malvarez RR (1977) Detection of prostate cancer by solid phase radioimmunoassay of serum prostatic acid phosphatase. N Engl J Med 297: 1357–1361

Höhn W, Schröder FH, Riemann JF, Jöbsis AC, Hermanek P (1980) Human prostatic adenocarcinoma: some characteristics of a serially transplantable line in nude mice (PC-82). Prostate 1: 95–104

Höhn W, Wagner M, Riemann JF, Hermanek P, Williams E, Walther R, Schrüffer R (1984) Prostatic adenocarcinoma PC-EW. A new human tumor line transplantable in nude mice. Prostate 5: 445–452

Kuriyama M, Wang MC, Lee CL, Killian CS, Papsidero L, Inaji H, Loor RM, Lin MF, Nishiura T, Slack NH, Murphy GP, Chu TM (1982) Multiple marker evaluation in human prostate cancer with the use of tissue-specific antigens. J Natl Cancer Inst 68: 99–105

Siddal JK, Cooper EH, Newling DWW, Robinson MRG, Whelan P (1986) An evaluation of the immunochemical measurement of prostatic acid phosphatase and prostatic specific antigen in carcinoma of the prostate. Eur Urol 12: 123–130

van Steenbrugge GJ, Blankenstein MA, Bolt-de Vries J, Romijn JC, Schröder FH, Vihko P (1983) Effect of hormone treatment on prostatic acid phosphatase in a serially transplantable human prostatic adenocarcinoma (PC-82). J Urol 129: 630–633

Wang MP, Valenzuela LA, Murphy GP, Chu TM (1979) Purification of a human prostate specific antigen. Invest Urol 17: 159–163

IV. Bladder Cancer

DNA Histogram of Invasive Bladder Carcinoma: Comparison of Flow Cytometry and Automated Image Analysis*

M. Stöckle[1], H. J. Tanke[2], G. Voges[1], H. Riedmiller[1], and R. Hohenfellner[1]

Introduction

Invasive bladder carcinoma is characterized by a considerable interindividual heterogeneity. The natural course of the disease as well as sensitivity of the tumors to various treatment modalities are thus unpredictable. Searching for more accurate characteristics of tumor biology than those presently available, the DNA histograms of 65 paraffin-preserved bladder carcinomas from cystectomy specimens were analyzed. Flow cytometry and automated image analysis, two competing methods, were compared.

Material and Methods

Preparation and Staining for Image Analysis. Paraffin-preserved tumor material of 75 bladder carcinoma patients who had undergone radical cystectomy was chosen for analysis. H & E-stained reference slides were used for the identification of tumor areas within the paraffin material. Of the 75 tumors, 65 showed enough tumor tissue for image analysis. Tumor areas of at least 3–4 mm in diameter normally were sufficiently large. A 50-μm section (two sections in relatively small tumors) was dewaxed (Histo-Clear, National Diagnostics, Summerville, New Jersey, USA), rehydrated in alcohol of decreasing concentration, and treated enzymatically by 0.05% pronase in 0.15 *M* phosphate buffered saline, pH 7.4, at 37°C for 30 min. The cell suspension was then sucked repeatedly through a Pasteur pipette and filtered through a 70-μm nylon mesh. The cells were centrifuged, resuspended in 50% ethanol containing 2% polyethylene glycol and diluted to a concentration of 10000/ml (Driel-Kulker et al. 1985). Standard smears were prepared by centrifugation of 1 ml of this suspension on glass slides using a cytospin technique. The slides were air-dried and consecutively stained using the Feulgen-SITS technique for quantitative staining of DNA (Tanke et al. 1979).

DNA Image Analysis. Automated image analysis for DNA cytometry was performed using the computer-controlled TV analysis system LEYTAS (Leiden Television Analysis System) (Ingen et al. 1980). This essentially consists of a computer-controlled

* Supported by Grant Sto. 177/2-2 of the Deutsche Forschungsgemeinschaft

[1] Department of Urology, Johannes Gutenberg University Mainz, Medical School, Langenbeckstr. 1, 6500 Mainz, FRG

[2] Institute for Cytochemistry and Cytometry, Rijks Universiteit, Wassenaarseweg, 2330 Leiden, The Netherlands

Investigative Urology 3
Edited by H. Rübben et al.

microscope with automated focusing and movement of the slides. The microscope image is screened and analyzed using the TV camera.

Image analysis was performed with the use of the TAS-image analysis software program (Leitz, Wetzlar, FRG), which allowed the predominant selection of Feulgen-stained nuclei of epithelial morphology. These were then measured for DNA content. An extensive artefact rejection, based on mathematical morphological criteria (Meyer 1979) is part of the program. Thus, only single nuclei were analyzed. Overlapping nuclei, dirt, and artefacts as well as most of the stroma and inflammatory cells could be excluded from analysis. Digitized images of the selected cells were stored in a memory buffer allowing visual control of the selected object. Selection and measurement are fully automated.

DNA Flow Cytometry. Of those tumors containing enough material, 43 were also analyzed by DNA flow cytometry, which requires a minimal amount of tumor, 3–4 times higher than that needed for image analysis. Hedley's (Hedley et al. 1983) technique was used to isolate the cells from the paraffin blocks which were stained with ethidium bromide. Flow cytometry was performed using a FACS-IV cell sorter (Becton-Dickinson, Mountain View, CA, USA). Interpretation of the flow cytometry DNA histograms was performed by an independent operator without knowledge of the image analysis results.

Results

Of the 75 paraffin blocks analyzed, 65 contained tumor material. Three main types of invasive bladder tumors could be distinguished according to the image-analysis DNA histogram.

Diploid tumors have a tumor cell peak showing the same DNA content (2c) as the nontumorous epithelial cells surrounding the tumor. Some cells show an increased DNA content, reaching a value of 4c, probably corresponding to S- and G2M-phase cells of the mitotic cell cycle. Tumor cells with a higher DNA content than 4c could not be found (Fig. 1). The DNA histograms of these tumors can hardly be distinguished from those of a nontumorous epithelial population. Thus, all smears of diploid tumors were checked by experienced cytologists to make certain that the histograms were really based on tumor cells.

Aneuploid tumors have a stem-cell line with a DNA content higher than the diploid value. Diploid tumor cells could not be found. Again, those tumor cells with an increased DNA content, i.e., up to double the value of the stem-cell line, probably represent S- and G2M-phase cells of the aneuploid line. Within the group of aneuploid tumors the DNA content of the stem-cell line allowed further subtyping:

1. Hypotriploid tumors have a stem-cell line with a DNA content of less than 3c (Fig. 2a).
2. Hypertriploid tumors (Fig. 2b) have a stem-cell line with a DNA content of more than 3c. In contrast to the hypotriploid tumors, more than 20% of all tumor cells found in these tumors have a DNA content higher than the stem-cell line, thus suggesting a high proliferation rate.

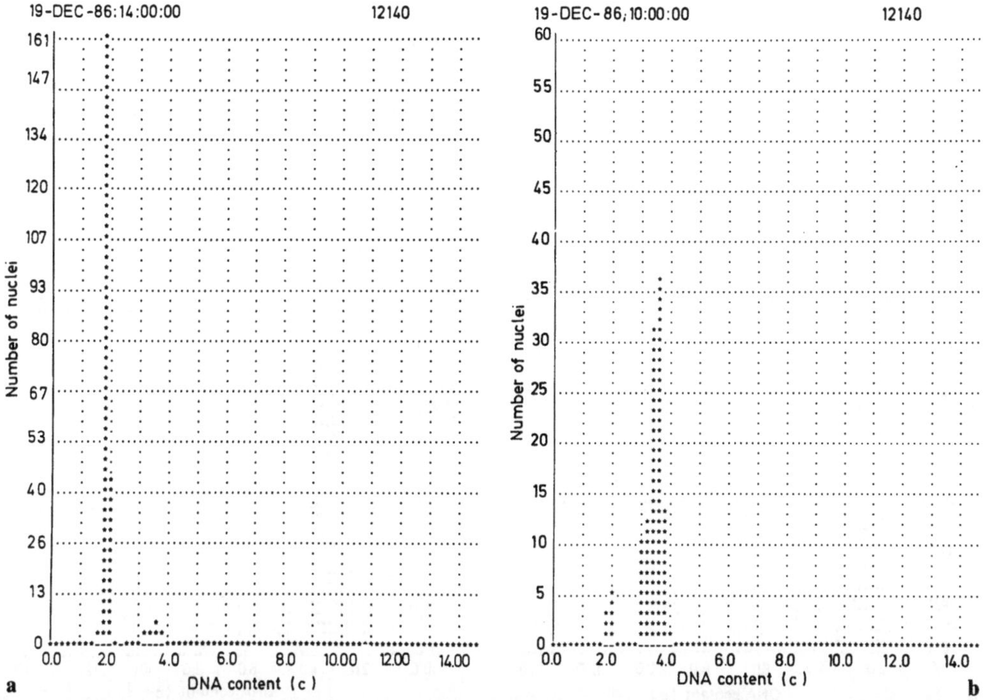

Fig. 1. a Diploid DNA histogram of an invasive bladder cancer. The tumor is characterized by a stem-cell line with diploid DNA content. Some cells have increased their DNA content, reaching values up to 4c, and it is assumed that these represent S- and G2M-phase cells of the mitotic cell cycle. The percentage of cells with a higher DNA content than the stem-cell line was normally low in diploid tumors, suggesting a low proliferation rate. **b** Measurement with altered selection criteria, selectively searching for cells with an increased DNA content. No cells with a DNA content higher than 4c can be found (the difference to Fig. 3c should be noted)

3. Hypertetraploid tumors, found in only 2 of 65 cases, had a stem-cell line with a DNA content of more than 4c (Fig. 2c).

A third main type of invasive bladder tumor is characterized by three peaks in the diploid, tetraploid, and octoploid region (Fig. 3a). Disregarding the diploid cells, we initially interpreted this tumor type as being a special subtype of aneuploidy, calling it tetraploid or hypotetraploid (Stöckle et al. 1987). With further experience, we ascertained that this special type always contains a high content of diploid cells. Comparing ploidy patterns of different areas of these tumors we even found that a nearly diploid pattern could frequently be found (Fig. 3b). In these cases only a modified selection program searching especially for cells with an increased DNA content was able to demonstrate the nondiploid character of the tumor (Fig. 3c). Having thus learned that the percentage of tetraploid and octoploid tumor cells could vary considerably within the same tumor, whereas the amount of diploid tumor cells remained constantly high, we decided to classify this tumor type as polyploid.

The different types of invasive bladder carcinomas as characterized by the DNA histogram derived from image analysis show significant prognostic differences concerning the long-term survival of the patients after radical cystectomy (Fig. 4).

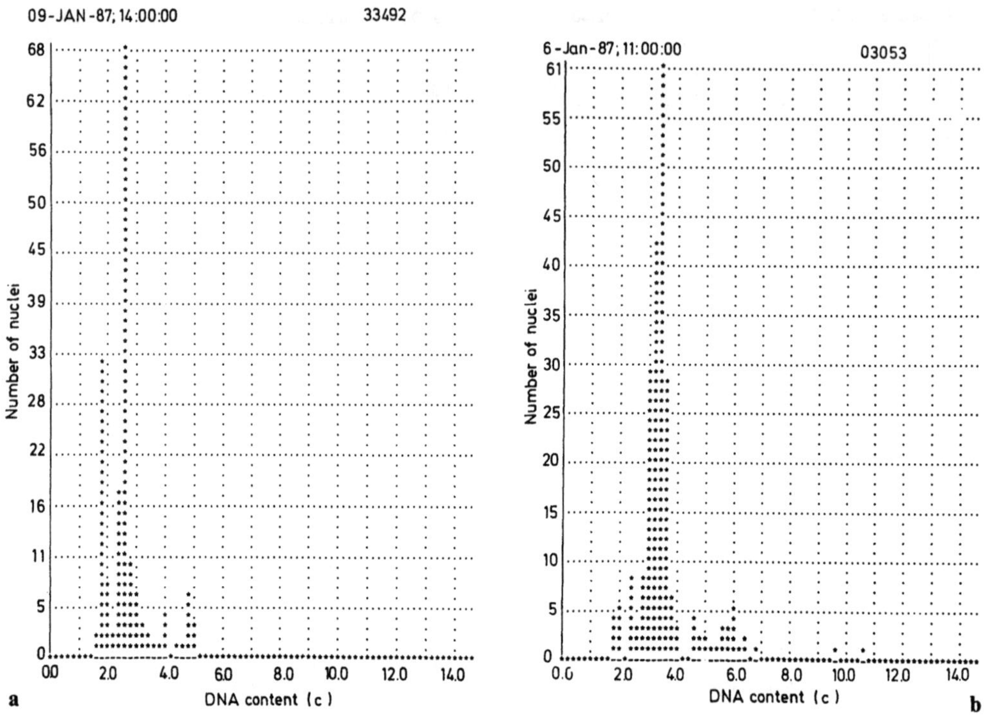

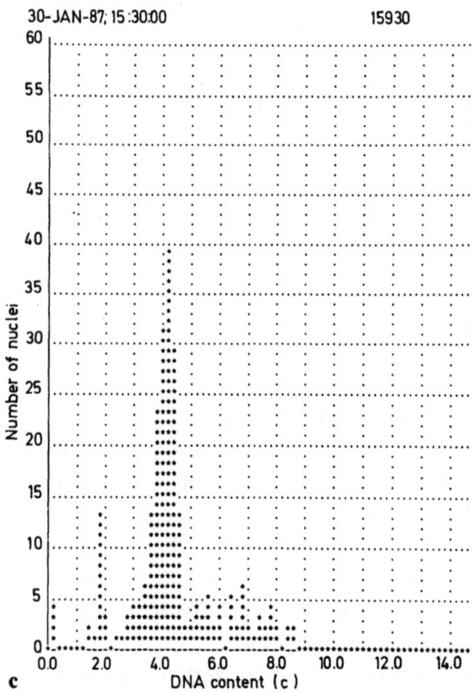

Fig. 2a–c. Aneuploid tumors characterized by a stem-cell line with a DNA content higher than 2c. Diploid cells are found infrequently and represent nontumorous epithelial nuclei surrounding the tumor. DNA content of the stem-cell line allows further subtyping of the tumor: **a** hypotriploid tumor, **b** hypertriploid tumor, **c** hypertetraploid tumor

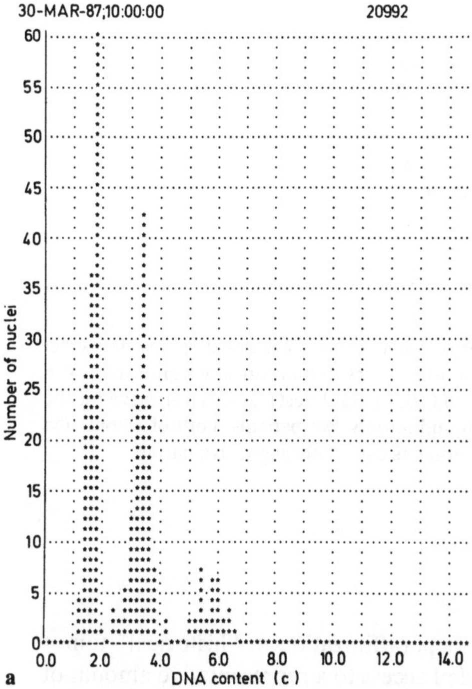

a

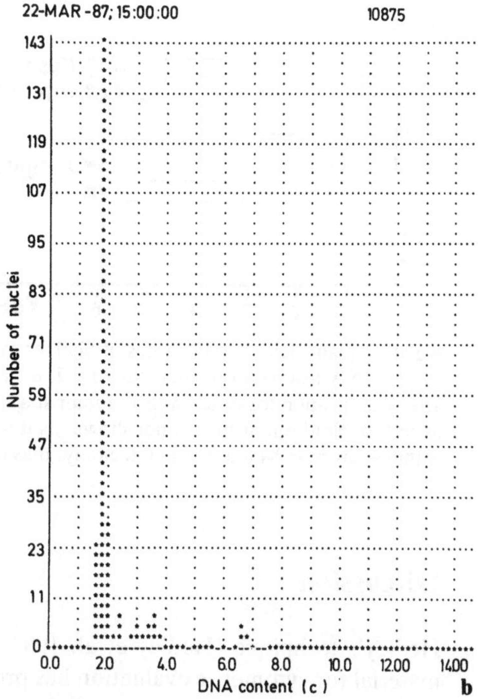

b

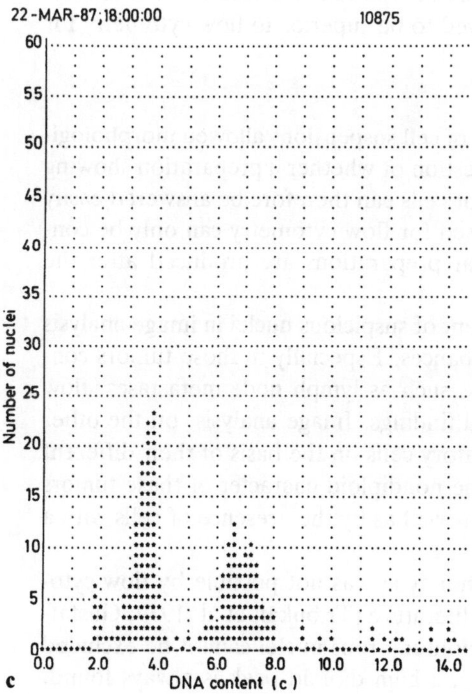

c

Fig. 3. a Polyploid tumor characterized by three peaks in the diploid, tetraploid, and octoploid range. **b** Polyploid tumor with a "nearly diploid" pattern. Only three cells in the octoploid range indicate the nondiploid character of the tumor. **c** Same tumor as in Fig. 3b, analyzed according to the same selection criteria as in Fig. 1b (selection search for nuclei with increased DNA content): the nondiploid character of the tumor is now indicated undoubtedly by the presence of an octoploid tumor cell peak

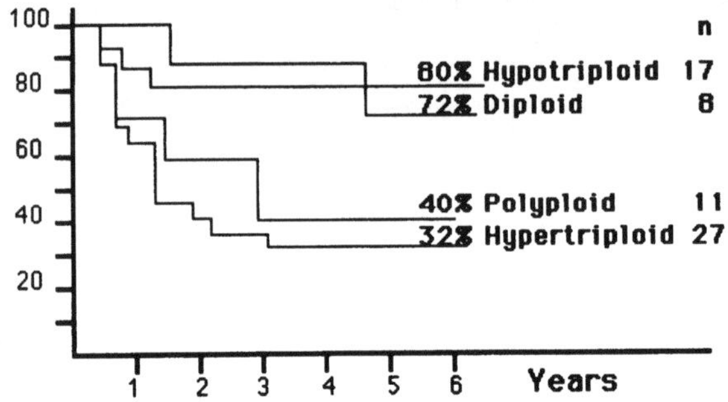

Fig. 4. Kaplan-Meier survival rates of bladder cancer patients after radical cystectomy with respect to the DNA histogram of their tumors. The survival differences are statistically significant, even after stratification for differences in tumor stage ($P = 0.009$, log-rank test). A survival curve for the hypertetraploid tumor type is not shown, as it was found in only two patients, both of whom died within a few months following cystectomy, thus indicating its extremely aggressive nature

Discussion

Hedley's technique (Hedley et al. 1983) of deparaffinization of "historical" tumor material for cytometric evaluation has provided access to a representative amount of identically treated tumors for preliminary studies, as shown in this investigation. Furthermore, the prognostic relevance of each tumor type can be calculated without further delay. In our study image analysis proved to be superior to flow cytometry for three reasons:

1. The use of smear preparations instead of cell suspensions allowed morphological rechecking of the analyzed cells. The question of whether a preparation showing a diploid DNA ploidy pattern contains tumor cells can therefore be answered easily in image cytometry. The cell suspensions used for flow cytometry can only be controlled morphologically, if cytological smear preparations are produced after the measurement.

2. The possibility of selective measurement of suspicious nuclei in image analysis makes this system less susceptible to disturbances. Especially in those tumors containing high amounts of inflammatory cells, such as lymph node metastases, flow cytometry commonly results in false diploid findings. Image analysis, on the other hand, by disregarding most of the inflammatory cells on the basis of their different morphology, unequivocally demonstrates the nondiploid character of these tumors by the proof of a nondiploid stem-cell line as well as by the presence of cells with a DNA content higher than 4c.

3. Characterization of the polyploid tumor type was not possible by flow cytometry and has not yet been described in the literature (Tribukait et al. 1979; Gustafson et al. 1982; Coon et al. 1986). As the nontumorous nuclei cannot be excluded from DNA measurement in flow cytometry, a high diploid peak is always found. Therefore, those polyploid tumors with a large amount of tetraploid and octoploid cells (Fig. 3a) were generally interpreted as aneuploid-tetraploid tumors. Other parts

of polyploid tumors showing fewer tetraploid and octoploid elements (Fig. 3b) were judged as being diploid in most instances.

Comparing DNA patterns of various sites of identical tumors, the DNA histogram was found to be a stable tumor characteristic, a finding that corresponds well with the cytogenetic analysis of Summers et al. (1981). This suggests that invasive bladder cancer is a disease of clonogenic nature.

Ljungberg et al. (1986), analyzing DNA patterns of metastasizing renal cell carcinoma, found diploid metastases of an aneuploid primary tumor in some cases, and vice versa. They interpreted this finding as an expression of a polyclonal disease, each clone having the possibility of invasive growth and metastases. The existence of a polyploid type of renal cell carcinoma, on the other hand, could also be a possible explanation for these controversial findings.

Future investigations are currently being planned that will aim at more individualized treatment strategies for invasive bladder cancer. It remains to be determined whether tumor characterization by DNA histogram allows prediction of tumor sensitivity to various treatment modalities.

Summary

In a retrospective analysis, the DNA-histograms of 65 paraffin-preserved bladder carcinomas from cystectomy specimens (stage pT1 to pT4a, pNo, pN1, pN2) were analyzed, comparing flow cytometry and automated image analysis.

Automated image analysis was able to characterize invasive bladder carcinoma as being either diploid, polyploid or aneuploid. Within the group of aneuploid tumors, the DNA content of the stem-cell-line allowed further subtying of the tumors: hypotriploid, hypertriploid and hypertetraploid tumors could be distinguished.

Comparing different sites of identical tumors, the DNA histogram was found to be a stable and reproducible tumor characteristic. Tumor types characterized in such a way differed significantly in prognosis.

Flow cytometry, on the other hand, often showed false diploid findings, especially in tumors containing large amounts of inflammatory cells. Characterization of the polyploid tumor type was not possible by flow cytometry.

References

Coon JS, Schwartz D, Summers JL, Miller AW, Weinstein RS (1986) Flow cytometric analysis of deparaffinized nuclei in urinary bladder carcinoma. Comparison with cytogenetic analysis. Cancer 57:1594–1601

Driel-Kulker AMJV, Mesker WE, Velzen IV, Tanke HJ, Feichtinger J, Ploem JS (1985) Preparation of monolayer smears from paraffin-embedded tissue for image cytometry. Cytometry 6: 268–272

Gustafson H, Tribukait B, Esposti PL (1982) The prognostic value of DNA analysis in primary carcinoma in situ of the urinary bladder. Scand J Urol Nephrol 16:141–146

Hedley DW, Riedlander ML, Taylor IW, Rugg CA, Musgrove EA (1983) Method for analysis of cellular DNA content of paraffin-embedded pathological material using flow cytometry. J Histochem Cytochem 31:1333–1335

Ingen EMv, Verwoerd N, Ploem JS (1980) LEYTAS-2: a hybrid system for the analysis of cytological preparations, using both hardware and software methods. Microscopica Acta [Suppl] 4: 73–81

Ljungberg B, Stenling R, Roos G (1986) Prognostic value of deoxyribonucleic acid content in metastatic renal cell carcinoma. J Urol 136:801–804

Meyer F (1979) Iterative image transformations for automative screening of cervical smears. J Histochem Cytochem 27:128–135

Stöckle M, Tanke HJ, Mesker WE, Ploem JS, Jonas U, Hohenfellner R (1987) Automated DNA-image cytometry: a prognostic tool in infiltrating bladder carcinoma. World J Urol 5:127–132

Summers JL, Falor WH, Ward R (1981) A 10-year analysis of chromosomes in noninvasive papillary carcinoma of the bladder. J Urol 125:177–178

Tanke HJ, Ingen EMV v, Ploem JS (1979) Acriflavine-Feulgen Stilbene staining: a procedure for automated cervical cytology with a television based system (LEYTAS). J Histochem Cytochem 27:84–86

Tribukait B, Gustafson H, Espasti P (1979) Ploidy and proliferation in human bladder tumors as measured by flow-cytofluorometric DNA-analysis and its relations to histopathology and cytology. Cancer 43:1742–1751

Automatic Identification of Bladder Tumor Cells by Multiple Parameters in Flow Cytometry

H. LEYH[1], G. VALET[2], and A. LEHMER[1]

Introduction

Despite clear improvements in evaluating flow-cytometric DNA examinations, present identification rates in bladder cancer are not sufficient as a basis for clinical decisions.

Therefore, the aim of our study is to improve the sensitivity and specificity of conventional DNA analysis by means of simultaneous measurement of several tumor cell-associated parameters and by additional cell distinction through measuring antigenic determinants of the cellular surface with monoclonal antibodies.

Material and Methods

Material. The following evaluation consists of 181 samples from patients with histologically proven transitional cell carcinoma of the bladder and of 131 control samples from people without clinical evidence of bladder tumor. The material of the 312 samples was obtained by bladder biopsies from tumor site or normal mucosa ($n = 60$), by bladder washings ($n = 138$), and by spontaneously voided urine ($n = 114$).

Preparation of Samples. Bladder biopsies were chopped with a McIlwain tissue chopper several times, and the suspension was filtered through a 80 × 80 µm nylon mesh sieve. All samples were then divided into two groups for further analysis.

(a) Measurement of DNA and biochemical cell parameters: In the first group additional to DNA determination the functional state of unfixed cells was judged from intracellular pH and esterase activity: 206 cell samples were stained with ADB (1,4-diacetoxy-2,3-dicyano-benzene) and PI (propidium iodide) for 5 min at room temperature for simultaneous determination of intracellular esterase activity and cytoplasmic pH in living cells as well as of DNA in dead cells. ADB traverses the cell membrane easily and is cleaved into DCH (2,3-dicano-hydrochinon) and acetate by intracellular esterases. The intensity of the blue fluorescent DCH is proportional to the intracellular esterase activity, and the color is a measure of intracellular pH in vital cells. Dead cells do not concentrate DCH, but their cell nucleus is stained by the DNA stain PI with a bright fluorescence. Finally NH_2-group-bearing, porous, and monosized particles prestained with a DCH solution were added as an internal concentration, fluorescence, and size standard.

[1] Urologische Klinik und Poliklinik der TU München, Klinikum rechts der Isar, Ismaningerstr. 22, 8000 München 80, FRG
[2] Max-Planck-Institut für Biochemie, 8033 Martinsried, FRG

Investigative Urology 3
Edited by H. Rübben et al.

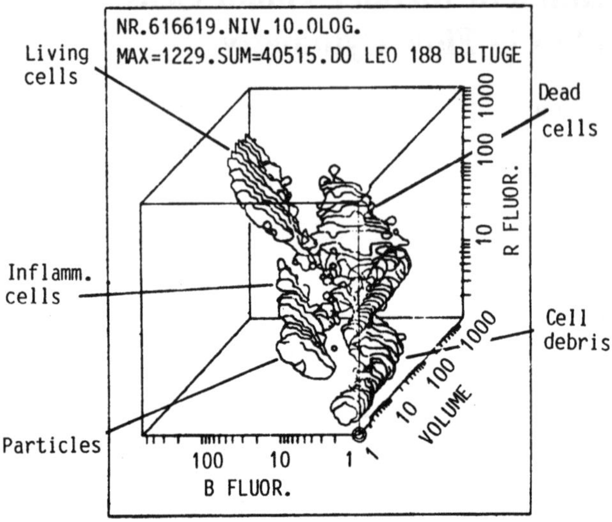

Fig. 1. Display of a simultaneous three-parameter measurement: cell volume, esterase activity (*b*lue *fluor*escence), and DNA distribution (*r*ed *fluor*escence)

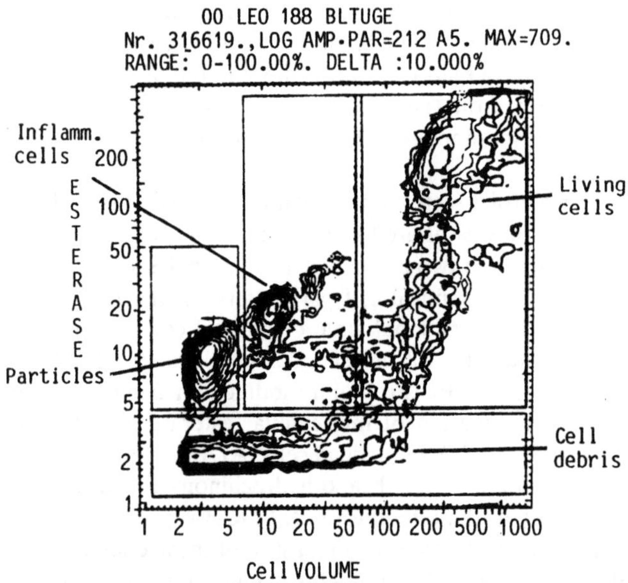

Fig. 2. Two-parameter histogram of esterase activity and cell volume. The three-dimensional cube representation shows that standardization particles, cell debris, inflammatory, dead, and living epithelial cells can be distinguished. The projection of the cube data onto the cell volume versus esterase plane gives a good tool for the quantitative evaluation of the data

(b) Evaluation of DNA and cell surface antigens: For further cell separation 106 ethanol-fixed samples were incubated first with monoclonal Lewis blood-group antibodies for 24 h and afterwards with a fluorescein-isothiocyanate (FITC)-labelled IgG fraction of a rabbit mouse-specific antiserum for a further 24 h as well as with PI for DNA determination. The dye cocktail additionally contained monosized NH_2-group-bearing, fluorescein-isothiocyanate-stained, porous, latex particles as an internal standard.

Flow-Cytometry. Simultaneous measurement of cell volume and two different fluorescence signals of the stained cells were performed with a three-parameter flow-cytometer (Fluvo-Metricell/HEKA). The digitized amplitudes of the obtained signals of each cell were collected on magnetic tape.

Data Evaluation. Data preparation and display were accomplished by Fortran computer programs, which allow one to plot three-dimensional views of the histograms and calculate the percentage of particles in limited areas (Figs. 1, 2). Recognition of abnormal cell samples was done automatically.

Results

Some 220 of the samples submitted for analysis (including 146 tumor samples) showed a sufficient number (at least 200) of epithelial cells for further evaluation. Table 1 contains the histological tumor categories of the examined bladder tumors.

DNA Determination. Of the tumor samples 40% showed one or more aneuploid or tetraploid peak.

Measurement of DNA and Functional Cell Values. Adding the analysis of biochemical cell parameters to DNA determination the identification rate of bladder tumor samples was 83%, the rate of false positive results 19%.

Evaluation of DNA and Cell Surface Antigens. Flow-cytometric identification rate for abnormal cells was improved also by the use of Lewis blood-group antibodies.

Table 1. Histological tumor stage (T_A, T_{1-3}) and differentiation grade (G_{1-3}) of the examined bladder tumors ($n = 146$)

	G_1	G_2	G_3	
T_A	15	60	–	75
T_1	2	32	4	38
T_2	–	3	22	25
T_3	–	–	8	8
	17	95	34	146

Table 2. Flow-cytometric identification of bladder tumor cells

	Flow-cytometric tumor identification	
	Right positive	False positive
DNA analysis (aneuploidy)	36%	2%
DNA analysis + biochemical cell parameters	83%	19%
DNA analysis + cell surface antigens	88%	21%

Table 3. Influence of cell preparation on tumor identification rate

Sample	Flow-cytometric tumor identification	
	Right positive	False positive
Bladder biopsy	91%	14%
Bladder washing	84%	15%
Voided urine	77%	26%

Table 4. Tumor identification rate depending on histological tumor category

Tumor category	Flow-cytometric tumor identification
$T_{A,1}$	80%
$T_{2,3}$	92%
$G_{1,2}$	81%
G_3	93%

Of the tumor samples 88% could be recognized, with a false positive rate of 21% (Table 2).

Influence of Cell Preparation on Tumor Identification Rate. The correlation between flow-cytometric and histological/clinical results was somewhat increased in bladder biopsies and bladder washings as compared with voided urine (Table 3).

Tumor Identification Rates Depending on Histological Tumor Category. The tumor identification rate by flow cytometry was nearly as high in superficial and low-grade tumors as in muscle-infiltrating or high-grade tumors (Table 4).

Discussion

Flow-cytometric measurements of bladder tumor samples have shown aneuploidy as a good and prognostically reliable indicator of malignancy. On the other hand a lot of tumor samples could not be recognized due to missing aneuploidy, especially in highly differentiated tumors (Tribukait 1987; Valet et al. 1986). Sensitivity in flow-cytometric tumor identification was improved by considering an elevated proliferation activity of the cells, represented by an increased proportion of S-phase in the cell cycle. Yet this improvement was achieved at the expense of a greater quantity of false positive results due to a wrong interpretation of inflammatory cell samples (de Vere White 1986).

In the present approach we tried to improve identification rates of bladder tumor cells by assessment of multiple, further, cell-related, biochemical parameters and by additional use of monoclonal antibodies in flow cytometry. Maintenance of the intracellular pH within narrow limits is an important requirement for correct functioning of the cellular metabolism. In tumor cells the intracellular pH frequently moves to acidic values. With ADB it is possible to determine intracellular pH and at the same time esterase activity of single cells by flow cytometry (Valet et al. 1981).

In comparison to that measurement, which requires only a short period of incubation, immunological investigations need longer incubation times (about 1–2 days). One can identify a certain portion of bladder tumors by determination of blood groups on the cell surface. Instead of the often misleading ABO blood group antibodies we have used antibodies against Lewis blood groups A and B, which are detectable in more than 95% of the population (Juhl et al. 1986). Compared with sole DNA examination, identification rates of bladder tumor cells can be improved by evaluation of multiple parameters in flow cytometry (Valet et al. 1984). By additional measurement of biochemical cell parameters and by determination of cell surface antigens a correlation between cytological and positive histological results was found in 83% and 88%, respectively. The rate of false positive results in the controls was about 20% on average.

The combination of all three methods (DNA analysis, measurement of tumor cell related biochemical parameters, and additional use of monoclonal antibodies) is likely to increase tumor identification rates. Flow cytometry then could be very valuable as a screening examination for urine samples in the future.

Summary

Compared to sole DNA examination flow-cytometric assessment of 312 samples from patients with bladder tumors respectively from healthy controls shows a distinct improvement of tumor identification rate by evaluating further biochemical cell parameters and by additional use of monoclonal antibodies. Transitional cell carcinoma was correctly identified in 84% of all bladder biopsies, bladder washings or voided urines with a false positive rate of 20%.

References

Juhl BR, Hartzen SH, Hainau B (1986) Lewis a antigen in transitional cell tumors of the urinary bladder. Cancer 58:222–228

Tribukait B (1987) Flow cytometry in assessing the clinical aggressiveness of genito-urinary neoplasms. World J Urol 5:108–122

Valet G, Raffael A, Moroder L, Wünsch E, Ruhenstroth-Bauer G (1981) Fast intracellular pH determination in single cells. Naturwissenschaften 68:265–266

Valet G, Rüssmann L, Wirsching R (1984) Automated flow-cytometric identification of colo-rectal tumour cells by simultaneous DNA, CEA-antibody and cell volume measurements. J Clin Chem Clin Biochem 22:935–942

Valet G, Kahle H, Wirsching R, Liewald F, Demmel N, Rübe Ch, Warnecke HH (1986) Die automatische Identifizierung und biochemische Charakterisierung menschlicher Tumorzellen mit Hilfe der Durchflußcytometrie. In: Engelhardt D, Mann K (eds) Endokrin-aktive Tumoren. Springer, Berlin Heidelberg New York

Vere White R de, Olsson CA, Deitch AD (1986) Flow cytometry: role in monitoring transitional cell carcinoma of bladder. Urology 28(1):15–20

Immunohistochemical and Functional Investigations of Gap Junctions in Human Bladder Carcinoma Cell Lines

K. Wilgenbus, R. Knüchel, F. Brümmer, O. Traub, and F. Hofstädter[1]

Introduction

Gap junctions are membrane channels connecting the cytoplasmic compartments of adjacent cells. They are described as bipartite arrays of units, so-called connectons, which receive equal structural contributions from each partner of the cell pair (Unwinn and Zampighi 1980). The connexon consists of six identical proteins that span the lipid bilayer of the junctional membranes. Metabolites of a molecular weight < 900 daltons and ions can pass through these intercellular channels (Flagg-Newton et al. 1979). Several substances are known to alter the permeability of gap junctions (Ramon 1985). The functional role of gap junctions is not completely understood, but intercellular communication may be required for (Lowenstein 1981): metabolic coupling, differentiation, growth control, regulation of enzyme systems.

Many quantitative and qualitative abnormalities have been described in cancer (Weinstein and Pauli 1986). These abnormalities may contribute to the physical properties and functional characteristics of tumors. Differential responses of cancer cells to irradiation were observed among communication-competent and communication-incompetent cells. Communication-competent cells are more radioresistant than communication-incompetent cells. This phenomenon has been termed the "contact-effect" (Dertinger et al. 1982). Studies of gap junctions have depended upon either morphological analysis (freeze-fracture) or physiological measurement of junctional communication. Hence isolation of gap junctions was undertaken to generate antibody probes specific to their protein component (Traub et al. 1982). A 21K and a 26K protein have been described. Immunochemical analysis indicates that the gap junction protein is highly homologous among vertrebrate organisms (Willecke et al. 1985). For this study we used two different tissue-culture models, the conventional monolayer and multicellular tumor spheroids (MCTS). MCTS is a model of tumor cell aggregates, showing a three-dimensional growth pattern (Mueller-Klieser 1987; Sutherland and Durand 1984). Differences in junctional communication rates among monolayer and spheroids were described (Dertinger and Hülser 1984). These differences may provide for different sensitivity rates between monolayers and spheroids to chemotherapy (Knüchel et al. 1988). The rabbit 26K mouse liver gap junction protein-specific antibody (Prof. Willecke, Bonn) was used for immunohistochemical investigations in human bladder carcinoma cell lines.

Material and Methods

Tissue Culture. The established transitional carcinoma cell lines J82 and MGH-U1 were used throughout all experiments. J82 and MGH-U1 were grown as monolayers

[1] Department of Pathology, RWTH-Aachen, Neues Klinikum, Pauwelsstraße, 5100 Aachen, FRG

Investigative Urology 3
Edited by H. Rübben et al.

in 10% fetal calf serum (FCS, Boehringer) containing Dulbecco's modified eagle medium (DMEM, Gibco) and penicillin/streptomycin (100 IU/ml; 100 mg/ml; Sigma) in tissue culture flasks (Falcon). To culture J82/MGH-U1 spheroids cells were plated on agarose-coated 96-multiwell test plates (Nunc, Falcon) in a concentration of 4000 cells/200 ml DMEM. Within 4 days of incubation at 37°C in humid air containing 5% CO_2, cells formed tight aggregates and increased in size until reaching a plateau phase after 2 weeks. Culture medium was changed every 2nd day.

Immunohistochemistry. For immunohistochemical studies we used a method described by Dermietzel et al. (1984). In short, after fixation the sections were incubated with 35–40 µl 26K-specific antibody (10 µg/ml PBS) for at least 30 min. The secondary antiserum (sheep rabbit-specific IgG), conjugated to fluorescein-isocyanate was used as 10 µl in 100 µl PBS per section.

Measurement of Intercellular Communication. Junctional permeability was probed with the fluorescent dye Lucifer yellow (Sigma). The dye was injected iontophoretically into the cells with the aid of a micropipette. For measurement of the junctional communication the spread of Lucifer-yellow fluorescence to the cell neighbors was viewed in the microscope darkfield. The frequency of dye transfer to neighboring cells (communication frequency) was determined within 2 minutes. We injected 25 superficial cells of 7 different spheroids and 20 cells growing as monolayer (both J82-derived and 7 days old).

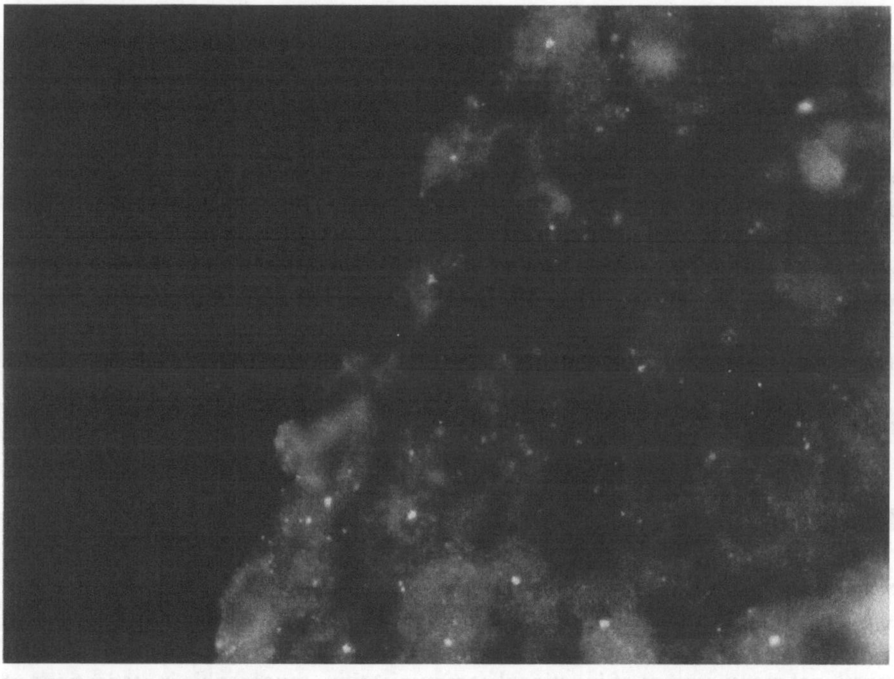

Fig. 1. Outer part of a spheroid (J82-derived and 7 days old). Fluorescent spots of about 1.0–2.0 µm in diameter are seen (2.0 cm = 20 µm)

Fig. 2. No fluorescent spots are seen in the negative control. The 26K-specific antibody was replaced by normal rabbit serum (1:100 PBS)

Results

We were able to show that the 26K-specific antibody also binds specifically to gap-junction proteins in human bladder carcinoma cell lines. In spheroids fluorescent spots were detected on apposed plasma membranes. The spots were shown to have a size of about 0.5–1.0 μm in diameter (Figs. 1, 2). Very few or no fluorescent spots were observed in the necrosis zone of spheroids. No differences in staining pattern were observed among J82- and MGH-U1-derived cell lines. Monolayers did not show any specific immunoreactivity. No spread of Lucifer yellow was observed in spheroids (communication frequency = 0%). The 20 injected cells growing as a monolayer showed spread of fluorescent dye to 60 neighboring cells ($n = 112$; communication frequency = 54%).

Discussion

Spheroidal aggregates of malignant cells serve as in vitro models imitating an early, avascular stage of tumor growth. Immunological studies with spheroids have shown many similarities between the original tumor and the respective spheroid. Besides functional measurement of junctional communication, topographic investigations of gap junctions in three-dimensional structures reveal valuable results. In this way, the use of antibody probes directed against the gap junction protein has opened new approaches to characterize gap junctions. Interestingly, our study has shown a discrepancy between the results obtained by immunohistochemistry and functional measurement of junctional communications. While Lucifer-yellow transfer is a relevant parameter of junctional communication the immunohistochemical demonstration of gap junction proteins does not prove functional gap junction channels. It was shown that in contrast to monolayers which have stable coupling rates, opening and closing of gap junction channels is a widespread phenomenon among spheroids (Hülser and Brümmer 1982). This may correspond with in vivo conditions. Furthermore it must be emphasized that it was only possible to inject Lucifer yellow into the superficial cells of spheroids and no statement is allowed about the coupling rate of cells in the inner parts of spheroids. The fact that gap junction proteins were not immunohistochemically detectable in monolayer may reflect a level of differentiation that cannot occur in monolayers (Pauli and Weinstein 1981).

Summary

The abnormalities of gap junctions in cancer may contribute to physical and functional characteristics of tumors. Using the anti-26K gap junction protein antibody, specific fluorescent spots were seen by indirect immunofluorescence in spheroids derived from human bladder carcinoma cell lines. No specific immunoreactivity was observed in these cell lines growing as monolayer. Vice versa, gap junctions were not detected in spheroids by measurement of the junctional communication, whereas monolayer showed high communication rates.

References

Dermietzel R, Leibstein A, Frixen U, Janssen-Timmen U, Traub O, Willecke K (1984) Gap junctions in several tissues share antigenic determinants with liver gap junctions. EMBO 3:2261–2270

Dertinger H, Hülser DF (1984) Intercellular communication in spheroids. Recent Results Cancer Res 95:67–85

Dertinger H, Hinz G, Jacobs KH (1982) Intercellular communication, three-dimensional cell contact and radiosensitivity. Biophys Struct Mech 9:89–93

Flagg-Newton JL, Simpson I, Loewenstein WR (1979) Permeability of the cell-to-cell membrane channels in mammalian cell junction. Science 205:404–407

Hülser DF, Brümmer F (1982) Closing and opening of gap junction pores between two- and three-dimensionally cultured tumor cells. Biophys Struct Mech 9:83–88

Knüchel R, Hofstädter F, Jenkins W, Masters JRW (1988) Sensitivities of monolayer and spheroids of the human bladder-cancer-cell-line MGH-U1 to drugs used for intravesical chemotherapy. Cancer Res (in press)

Loewenstein WR (1981) Junctional intercellular communication: the cell-to-cell channel. Physiol Rev 61:829–913

Mueller-Klieser W (1987) Multicellular spheroids: a review on cellular aggregates in cancer research. J Cancer Res Clin Oncol 113:101–122

Pauli BU, Weinstein RS (1981) Structure of gap junctions in cultures of normal and neoplastic bladder epithelial cells. Experientia 37:248–250

Ramon F, Zampighi GA, Rivera A (1985) Control of junctional permeability. In: Bennett MV, Spray DC (eds) Gap junctions. Cold Spring Harbor Laboratory, Cold Spring Harbor, New York, pp 155–166

Sutherland RM, Durand RE (1984) Growth and cellular characteristics of multicell spheroids. Recent Results Cancer Res 95:24–49

Traub O, Janssen-Timmen U, Drüge PM, Dermietzel R, Willecke K (1982) Immunological properties of gap junction protein from mouse liver. J Cell Biochem 19:27–44

Unwinn PNT, Zampighi G (1980) Structure of the junction between communicating cells. Nature 283:545–549

Weinstein RS, Pauli BU (1986) Cell junctions and the biological behaviour of cancer. In: Bock G, Clark S (eds) Junctional complexes of epithelial cells. John Wiley and Sons, Chichester, pp 241–250

Willecke K, Traub O, Janssen-Timmen U, Dermietzel R, Leibstein A, Paul D, Rabes H (1985) Immunochemical investigations of gap junction protein in different mammalian tissues. In: Bennett WV, Spray DC (eds) Gap junctions. Cold Spring Harbor Laboratory, New York, pp 67–77

Investigations for a Point Mutation in the c-Ha-*ras* 1 Oncogene in the Genome of Bladder Carcinomas by Southern Blot Analysis

S. HANDT[1], R. BÜTTNER, R. KNÜCHEL, H. RÜBBEN, F. HOFSTÄDTER, and C. WAGENER

Introduction

During the investigations of transforming retroviruses, DNA sequences were isolated which have been shown to play an important role in cell transformation of infected cells (Bishop 1986); these DNA sequences have been called viral oncogenes (v-*onc*). Further experiments revealed that similar or even identical DNA sequences can be found regularly integrated in animal or human cells. These oncogene sequences code for proteins which have important functions in cell growth and proliferation (Tomasi 1986). To distinguish these inherent oncogenes from the viral oncogenes they are called protooncogenes or cellular oncogenes (c-*onc*). It is believed that the cellular oncogenes have developed earlier in ontogeny and that the integration of oncogene sequences in viral genomes occurred later. The reintegration of the oncogenes by retroviral infections may be followed by an uncontrolled production of the sometimes slightly modified oncogene product, and this way may induce malignant cell transformation (Bishop 1986; Tomasi 1986). Under certain conditions the cellular oncogenes may become activated and can, independent from viral infections, lead to cellular transformation (Land et al. 1983; Chan and McGee 1987). Mechanisms which have been found to result in an activation of cellular oncogenes may be (Tomasi 1986): point mutations, translocations, and amplifications.

The c-Ha-*ras* 1 oncogene of the bladder carcinoma cell line EJ/T24 was found to differ from the normal oncogene in one nucleotide within the 12th codon, resulting in an amino acid change (Capon et al. 1983; Muschel et al. 1983; Parada et al. 1982; Taparowsky et al. 1982). The amino acid change influenced the function of the *ras*-coded p21 protein (Tabin et al. 1982; Reddy et al. 1982; Santos et al. 1982) which was made responsible for the cell transformation (Lacal et al. 1986; Chang et al. 1982; Gilbert and Harris 1988). This protein seems to have a G-protein-like function, activating the cellular adenylate cyclase (Toda et al. 1985). The GTPase activity, which regulates the duration of the proliferatory stimulus, seems to be decreased within the point-mutated ras p21 protein, thus leading to a prolonged stimulation (Bishop 1986).

A well-known example of a translocation of an oncogene leading to malignancy is the translocation of c-*myc* from chromosome 8 to chromosomes 14, 2, or 22 in the Burkitt lymphoma (Taub et al. 1982). On chromosomes 14, 2, and 22 the genes for immunoglobulin heavy and light chains are located which are transcribed in a high number. The translocation of c-*myc* near the highly transcribed immunoglobulin genes results in the production of an equally high number of c-*myc* copies, which are

[1] Department of Pathology, RWTH Aachen, Neues Klinikum, Pauwelsstraße, 5100 Aachen, FRG

Investigative Urology 3
Edited by H. Rübben et al.

no longer under the control of the growth-regulating elements of the cell (Croce and Nowell 1986; Yunis 1983).

Amplification of an oncogene may result in an unusually high transcription rate as well, thus leading to an overproduction of the oncogene-coded protein.

In this study we want to investigate whether the point mutation of the c-Ha-*ras* 1 oncogene in codon 12 is a frequent event in bladder carcinomas and whether it may serve as a suitable marker to estimate tumor progression.

Materials and Methods

To show the point mutation of the c-Ha-*ras* 1 oncogene Southern blot analysis (SBA) was used. DNA from different bladder cell carcinomas of different histological grading was extracted by standard methods (Maniatis 1982) and digested with restriction endonucleases (REs). REs recognize sequences of 4–6 nucleotides and cut double-stranded DNA at these sites. After digestion the DNA segments are separated on an agarose gel according to their length. Bathing the gel in sodium hydroxide makes the DNA segments single-stranded. Afterwards the DNA segments must be transferred from the gel to a solid support (e.g., nitrocellulose filter) for the following hybridization. The transfer method used is the Southern blot (Southern 1975); a high salt buffer is soaked from a towel of wicks placed above the nitrocellulose filter lying directly on the gel, thus transferring the DNA segments out of the gel to the filter. After the blotting the filter is baked for some hours at 80°C to obtain better binding of the single-stranded DNA segments to the nitrocellulose. The filter is then hybridized within a seal bag containing the radioactively labelled c-Ha-*ras* 1 probe, SDS, SSC, and some other ingredients depending on the protocol used (Maniatis 1983). After hybridization the unspecifically bound radioactivity is washed away, and the dry filter is exposed to an X-ray film for some days. The developed film then shows distinct bands of DNA fragments containing the *ras*-coding nucleotide sequences; the localization of the bands depends on the length of the restriction enzyme fragment. Thus the SBA enables one to detect restriction fragment length polymorphisms (RFLPs). Used for the detection of the c-Ha-*ras* 1 oncogene, the bladder carcinoma DNA is digested with the REs *Msp*I and *Hpa*II. These enzymes recognize the nucleotide sequences CCGG that can be found within the 11th and 12th codons of the normal c-Ha-*ras* 1 oncogene (GCC-GGC). Therefore the DNA is cut at this site, the resulting restriction fragment being 355 base pairs (bp) in length. An oncogene with the point mutation at codon 12 has a different nucleotide sequence at codons 11 and 12: GCC-GTC. The REs do not cut this sequence, the resulting restriction fragment not being 355 bp but 412 bp in length. This RFLP can be detected by SBA analysis using an agarose gel concentration of 3% and electrophoresis conditions of 70 V for at least 4 h.

Results

Twelve bladder carcinomas were analyzed for the presence of the point-mutated c-Ha-*ras* 1 oncogene. The tumor tissue was obtained by transurethral resection of bladder tumors at low stages; in most cases the histologic pattern was G2 (six cases), five were G1, and one tumor G3. Only one case showed a restriction fragment of 412 bp in length by SBA and therefore revealed the presence of the point mutated c-Ha-*ras* 1 oncogene. The other bladder carcinomas had restriction fragments of 355 bp and therefore contained the normal c-Ha-*ras* 1 oncogene.

Discussion

The results of our study imply that only in a few cases do bladder carcinomas show the point mutation of the 12th codon in the c-Ha-*ras* 1 oncogene. Only 1 of 12 bladder carcinomas investigated in this study show this point mutation. Similar results have been reported elsewhere (Fujita et al. 1985). It can be concluded that the determination of the point-mutated *ras* by SBA is not very suitable to yield information about tumor progress. Other methods of DNA recombinational techniques may provide more relevant information about the biology of the tumor: Northern blot analysis for determining the expression of oncogenes influencing tumor behavior and progression can be used as well as other techniques that can perhaps reveal important DNA sequences inducing malignancy (Büttner et al. 1988; Fenoglio-Preiser and Willman 1987).

Summary

12 early stage bladder carcinomas of different grading were analyzed for the presence of a point mutation within the 12th codon of the c-Ha-*ras* 1 oncogene. This point mutation, found within the bladder carcinoma cell line EJ/T24, is believed to play an important role in the development of malignancy. Only one bladder carcinoma of the tumors investigated in this study showed the point mutation within the 12th codon; therefore this seldom event does not seem to be a suitable marker in the evaluation of the progression of early stage bladder cell carcinomas.

References

Bishop JM (1986) Viral oncogenes. Cell 42:23–38

Büttner R, Knüchel R, Rübben H, Hofstädter F, Westphal KH (1988) Genetische Faktoren in der Entstehung von Urothelkarzinomen. Verhdlg dte Ges Pathol (in press)

Capon JC, et al (1983) Complete nucleotide sequences of the T24 human bladder carcinoma oncogene and its normal homologue. Nature 302:33–37

Chan V, McGee J (1987) Cellular oncogenes in neoplasia. J Clin Pathol 40:1055–1063

Chang E, et al (1982) Tumorigenic transformation of mammalian cells induced by a normal human gene homologous to the oncogene of Harvey murine sarcoma virus. Nature 297:479–483

Croce CM, Nowell PC (1986) Molecular genetics of human B cell neoplasia. Adv Immunol 38:245–274

Fenoglio-Preiser CM, Willman CL (1987) Molecular biology and the pathologist. Arch Pathol Lab Med 111:601–619

Fujita J, et al (1985) Frequency of molecular alterations affecting *ras* protooncogenes in human urinary tract tumors. Proc Natl Acad Sci USA 82:3849–3853

Gilbert P, Harris H (1988) The role of the *ras* oncogene in the formation of tumors. J Cell Sci 90: 433–446

Goldfarb M, et al (1982) Isolation and preliminary characterization of a human transforming gene from T24 bladder carcinoma cells. Nature 296:404–409

Lacal JC, et al (1986) Ras p21 proteins with high or low GTPase activity can efficiently transform NIH/3T3 cells. Cell 44:609–617
Land H, et al (1983) Cellular oncogenes and multistep carcinogenesis. Science 222:771–778
Maniatis T (1982) Molecular cloning – a laboratory manual. Cold Spring Harbor Laboratory, New York
Muschel RJ, et al (1983) The human c-*ras* 1H oncogene: a mutation in normal and neoplastic tissue from the same patient. Science 219:853–885
Parada LF, et al (1982) Human EJ bladder carcinoma oncogene is homologue of Harvey sarcoma virus *ras* gene. Nature 297:474–478
Reddy EP, et al (1982) A point mutation is responsible for the acquisition of transforming properties by the T24 human bladder carcinoma oncogene. Nature 300:149–152
Santos E, et al (1982) T24 human bladder carcinoma oncogene is an activated form of the normal human homologue of BALB- and Harvey-MSV transforming genes. Nature 298:343–347
Southern EM (1975) Detection of specific sequences among DNA fragments separated by gel electrophoresis. J Mol Biol 98:503–517
Spandidos DA, Wilkie NM (1984) Malignant transformation of early passage rodent cells by single mutated human oncogene. Nature 310:469–475
Tabin C, et al (1982) Mechanism of activation of a human oncogene. Nature 300:143–149
Taparowsky E, et al (1982) Activation of the T24 bladder carcinoma transforming gene is linked to a single amino acid change. Nature 300:762–765
Taub R, et al (1982) Translocation of the c-*myc* gene into the immunoglobulin heavy chain locus in human Burkitt lymphoma and murine plasmacytoma cells. Proc Natl Acad Sci USA 79:7837–7841
Toda T, et al (1985) In yeast, ras proteins are controlling elements of adenylate cyclase. Cell 40: 27–36
Tomasi T (1986) Oncogenes and cancer. In: Fenoglio-Preiser CM, Weinstein RS, Kaufmann N (eds) New concepts in neoplasia as applied to diagnostic pathology. Williams & Wilkins, Baltimore, pp 59–90
Yunis J (1983) The chromosomal basis of human neoplasia. Science 221:227–235

Prevention of Hyperchloremic Acidosis Following Ureterosigmoidostomy: The Functional Rectal Bladder

K. Miller, U. Matsui, and R. Hautmann[1]

Introduction

In recent years, some authors (Segura and Kelalis 1975; Zincke and Segura 1975; Hendren 1983; Spirnak and Caldamone 1986) have claimed that ureterosigmoidostomy is due for a renaissance. The long-term outcome of this technique parallels that of the ileal conduit (Miller 1987), which is still the method of urinary diversion most widely used. The advantage of ureterosigmoidostomy is that no stoma is required; on the other hand there is a high incidence of hyperchloremic acidosis and an increased risk of colonic cancer after an interval of 15–20 years (Stewart et al. 1981). The latter complication may not be a problem in elderly patients requiring urinary diversion after cystectomy for bladder cancer.

Hyperchloremic acidosis has so far been mainly attacked with drugs (Koch and McDougal 1985); modifications of the operative technique have rarely been attempted to solve this problem. We therefore initiated an experimental study, to find out whether intussusception of the sigmoid colon can be employed without disturbance of the fecal stream and whether this modification results in an improved metabolic situation.

Material and Methods

Foxhound dogs, weighing 25–35 kg each, were used for this study. All operations were carried out under general anesthesia. The abdominal cavity was entered by a midline incision. Following isolation of the urinary bladder from the urethra, the sigmoid colon was freed from its meso over a length of 6–7 cm. A 5-cm sigmoidotomy was then carried out and the colon intussuscepted in order to create a 3–4 cm long nipple. The intussusception was stabilized by preceeding sero-muscular scarification and absorbable sutures at the nipple base. The bladder was then opened at its dorsal surface and anastomosed to the sigma.

This vesico-sigmoidostomy provides a nonobstructive diversion without the need for ureteral stenting, as the ureteral orifices remained undisturbed. No drains or catheters were required; the anastomosis between the bladder and the sigmoid colon was sutured watertight. The wound was closed in layers. During the postoperative period the animals were kept on oral antibiotics for 7 days and were allowed water and food ad libitum.

To assess the effect of the sigmoidal intussusception on the metabolic situation, the dogs were randomly divided into two groups: Group 1 received the functional

[1] University of Ulm, Division of Urology, Prittwitzstraße 43, 7900 Ulm, FRG

Investigative Urology 3
Edited by H. Rübben et al.

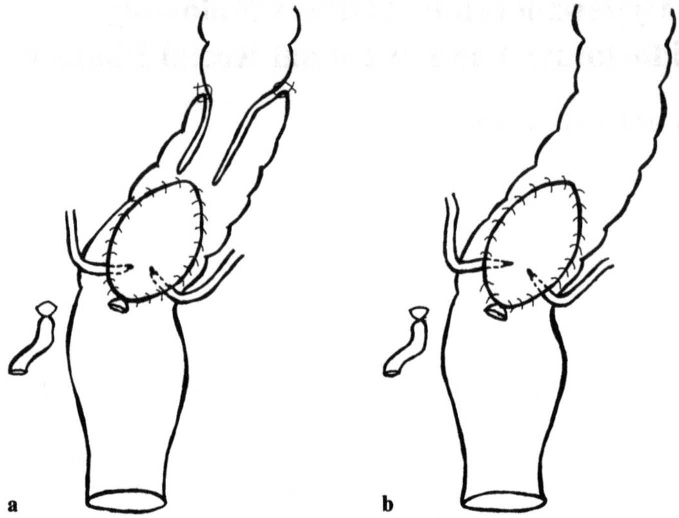

Fig. 1a, b. Schematic drawing of the operative techniques. **a** Vesico-sigmoidostomy with isoperistaltic intussusception of the sigmoid colon (functional rectal bladder, group 1); **b** vesico-sigmoidostomy without intussusception (group 2)

rectal bladder (i.e., vesico-sigmoidostomy with an intussuscepted sigmoid colon); group 2 had the same vesico-sigmoidostomy without intussusception (Fig. 1).

Blood samples were drawn twice weekly over a maximal period of 4 months postoperatively, and the following parameters were evaluated: creatinine, base excess, bicarbonate, pH. The normal range for these parameters was determined by two preoperative blood samples from each animal.

The metabolic results of the two groups were statistically compared using the Wilcoxon test.

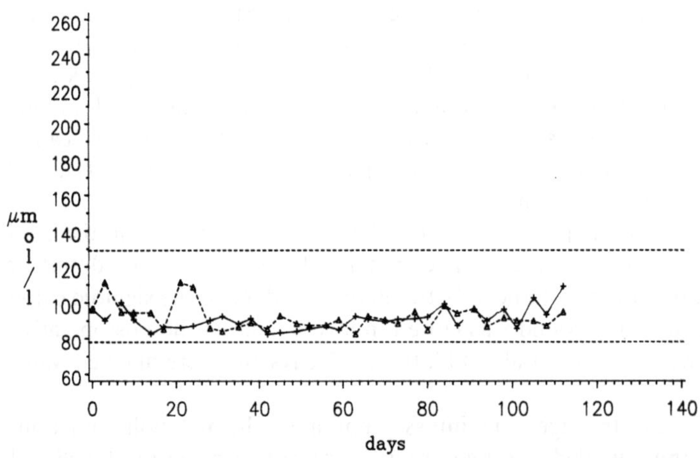

Fig. 2. Postoperative course of average creatinine values (each point represents the average of 3–7 values of a day). Group 1, *continuous line;* group 2, *dashed line;* normal range between the *two dotted horizontal lines*

The function of the colonic intussusception was assessed by a contrast filling of the rectal bladder under fluoroscopic control. An IVP was taken 6–8 weeks postoperatively to evaluate the upper urinary tract.

Results

In group 1, two dogs died of postoperative complications, one from hemorrhage, the other from a leak at the vesico-sigmoid anastomosis. Thus five dogs with 10 reno-

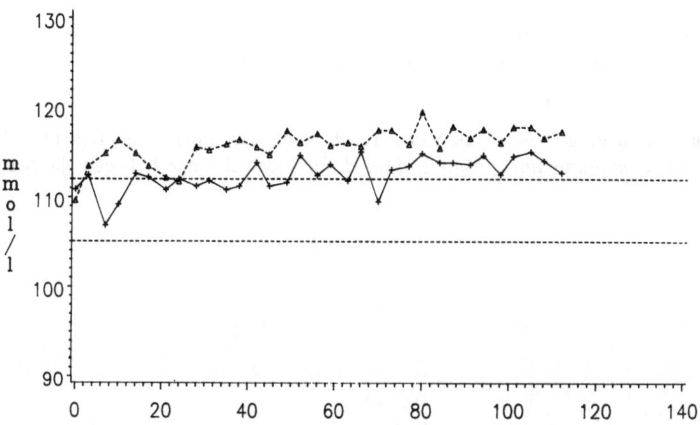

Fig. 3. Postoperative course of average chloride values (each point represents the average of 3–7 values of a day). Group 1, *continuous line;* group 2, *dashed line;* normal range between the *two dotted horizontal lines*

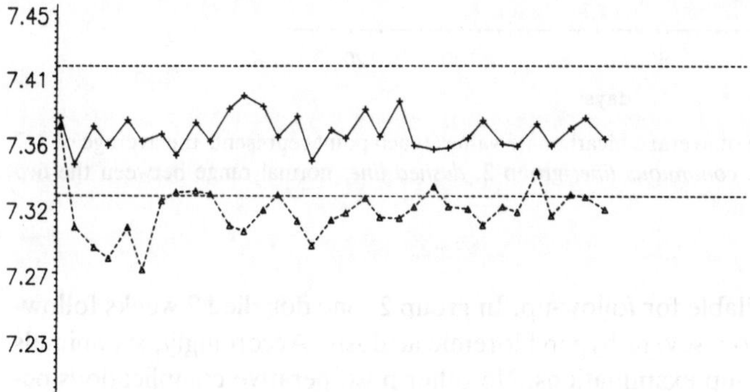

Fig. 4. Postoperative course of average pH values (each point represents the average of 3–7 values of a day). Group 1, *continuous line;* group 2, *dashed line;* normal range between the *two dotted horizontal lines*

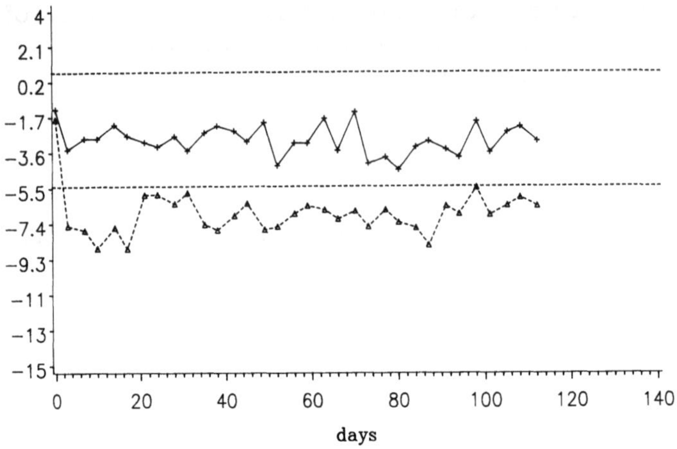

Fig. 5. Postoperative course of average base excess values (each point represents the average of 3–7 values of a day). Group 1, *continuous line;* group 2, *dashed line;* normal range between the *two dotted horizontal lines*

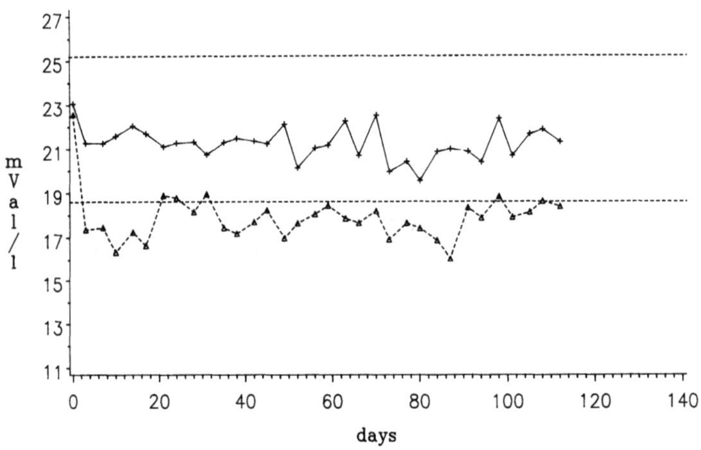

Fig. 6. Postoperative course of average bicarbonate values (each point represents the average of 3–7 values of a day). Group 1, *continuous line;* group 2, *dashed line;* normal range between the *two dotted horizontal lines*

ureteral units were available for follow-up. In group 2, one dog died 2 weeks following the operation due to a severe hyperchloremic acidosis. Accordingly, six animals were left for the follow-up examinations. No other postoperative complications occurred; in particular no signs of an obstructed fecal stream were found in the intussuscepted group. In this group, dye filling of the rectal bladder revealed one reflux up the colon due to a shortening of the nipple and one ureteric reflux. The IVPs showed normal upper urinary tracts throughout both groups.

Evaluation of the blood samples showed no difference for creatinine (Fig. 2); the animals of both groups had normal values throughout the follow-up period. Thus, equivalent, undisturbed, renal function was confirmed. Chlorid was elevated in both groups and was significantly higher in the non-intussuscepted group (Fig. 3). All acid-base parameters (pH, base excess, bicarbonate) were significantly better in group 1 (Figs. 4–6).

Discussion

Hyperchloremic acidosis in the postoperative course of ureterosigmoidostomy occurs in 50%–80% of the patients (Ferris and Odel 1950). These patients require permanent alkalinization of the urine to control the side effects of this metabolic disturbance. The most important pathophysiologic force for the induction of acidosis is the absorption of chloride ions (Koch and McDougal 1985); the amount of this absorption is influenced by the size of the exposed bowel surface. It has been shown that in patients with ureterosigmoidostomy the entire colon up to the ileocecal valve is rinsed with urine. Confinement of the reservoir therefore was expected to result in an improvement of hyperchloremic acidosis. Accordingly, patients with an isolated rectal bladder (when the rectum is completely isolated from the fecal stream and a colostomy provides fecal diversion) show little or no problems with metabolic disturbances (Pyrah 1963; Ghoneim and Ashamallah 1974). Our results, constructing a functional rectal bladder in dogs by intussusception of the sigmoid colon confirm these clinical observations: during a 4-month follow-up of the important metabolic parameters (chloride, pH, base excess, bicarbonate), the functional rectal bladder yielded significantly better results than a control group with the same form of urinary diversion but without intussusception of the colon. Amazingly, this intussusception did not cause any obstruction of the fecal stream as known from accidental intussusception of the bowel: this phenomenon may be explained by the fact that only accidental intussusception leads to edema and necrosis of the intussuscepted part which in turn causes the obstruction (Perrin and Lindsay 1921).

As the gut of dogs resembles the human intestine with regard to absorption and motility (Adler et al. 1941), a similar outcome as shown in our study can be expected in a clinical setting. Therefore, this technique may be a valid alternative in patients in whom other forms of continent urinary diversion cannot be applied.

References

Adler HF, Atkinson AJ, Ivy AC (1941) A study of the motility of the human colon: an explanation of dysynergia of the colon, or the "unstable colon". Am J Dig Dis 8:197

Ferris DO, Odel JM (1950) Electrolyte pattern of the blood after bilateral ureterosigmoidostomy. JAMA 142:634

Ghoneim MA, Ashamallah A (1974) Further experience with the rectosigmoid bladder. Br J Urol 46:511

Hendren WH (1983) Ureterocolic diversion of urine: management of some difficult problems. J Urol 129:719

Koch MO, McDougal WS (1985) The pathophysiology of hyperchloremic acidosis after urinary diversion through intestinal segments. Surgery 98:561

Miller K (1987) The continent functional rectal-bladder: an experimental study on dogs. Thesis, University of Ulm, Medical School

Perrin WS, Lindsay EC (1921) Intussusception. Br J Surg 9:46
Pyrah LM (1963) The rectosigmoid bladder as a method of urinary diversion. J Urol 90:189
Segura JW, Kelalis PP (1975) Long term results of ureterosigmoidostomy in children with bladder exstrophy. J Urol 114:138
Spirnak JP, Caldamone AA (1986) Ureterosigmoidostomy. Urol Clin North Am 13:285
Stewart M, et al (1981) The role of *N*-nitrosamine in carcinogenesis at the ureterocolic anastomosis. Br J Urol 53:115
Zincke H, Segura JW (1975) Ureterosigmoidostomy: a critical review of 173 cases. J Urol 113:324

Tumors Experimentally Produced in a Rat Model for Carcinogenesis in Ureterosigmoidostomy

W.-D. MIERSCH[1] and J. VOGEL[2]

Introduction

The first description of ureterosigmoidostomy by Simon in 1852 caused euphoria concerning an operative technique that preserved continence and did not bother the patient with another stoma. Yet soon the state of euphoria was subdued by three complications that followed the operation. Ascending pyelonephritides and hyperchloremic acidoses oppressed the patient. Furthermore, after a medium latency period of about 20 years adenocarcinoma of the colon, which were induced by the operation, occurred in the region of the anastomosis. Up to now 103 malignant tumors near the anastomosis of the ureterosigmoidostomy have been described. In addition especially in recent times 70 benign polyps were found in the course of postoperative endoscopic examinations performed by many clinics as routine. Most of these polyps are adenomas, often showing clear atypias.

Even with use of different bowel segments for the urinary diversion, development of adenocarcinomas is described. Here the colon conduit as well as the ileum conduit are to be mentioned. In the meantime case reports have been published which describe adenocarcinomas in the bowel segment of bladders being augmented by the small and large intestine (Harzmann et al. 1986).

Different experimental studies postulate different theories concerning the genesis of these tumors. Aaronson (Aaronson and Sinclair-Smith 1984; Aaronson et al. 1987) supposes an irritation of the transitional cell epithelium caused by the feces, and therefore interprets the tumors to be primary adenocarcinomas of the transitional cell epithelium. Crissey (Crissey et al. 1979, 1980; Gittes 1986) emphasizes the importance of carcinogens developing in the mixture of urine and faeces for the carcinogenesis at the site of the anastomosis.

Materials and Methods

In the model we inaugurated with Han:WISTAR rats we first of all wanted to eliminate the possible influence of the metabolic process on carcinogenesis through the development of a hyperchloremic acidosis. Furthermore, we simulated the operation performed on humans by a strict use of microsurgical techniques. Therefore, the left ureter was antirefluxively implanted into the sigma after the method of Goodwin/Hohenfellner. The right ureter was left in situ. The anastomoses were microsurgically performed and checked about 6 weeks after the operation by urogram. As a control

[1] Urologische Universitätsklinik Bonn
[2] Pathologisches Institut der Universität Bonn, FRG

Investigative Urology 3
Edited by H. Rübben et al.

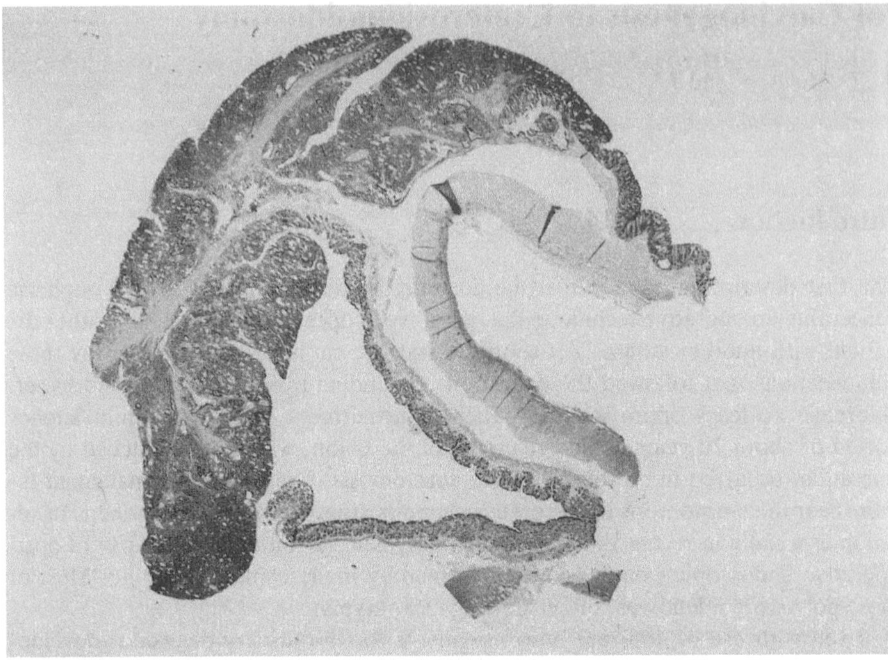

Fig. 1. Adenocarcinoma of the intestinal type at the site of the anastomosis

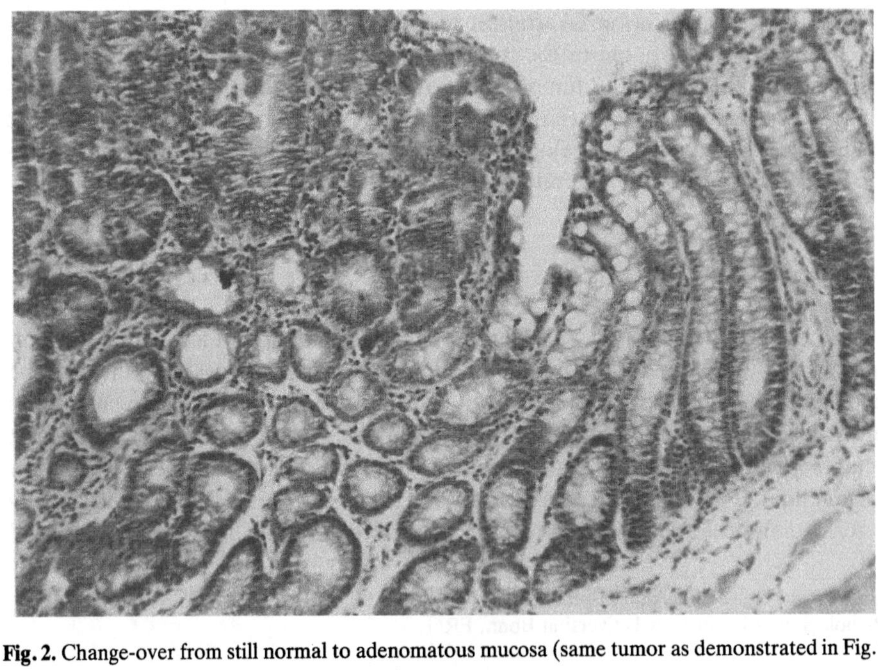

Fig. 2. Change-over from still normal to adenomatous mucosa (same tumor as demonstrated in Fig. 1)

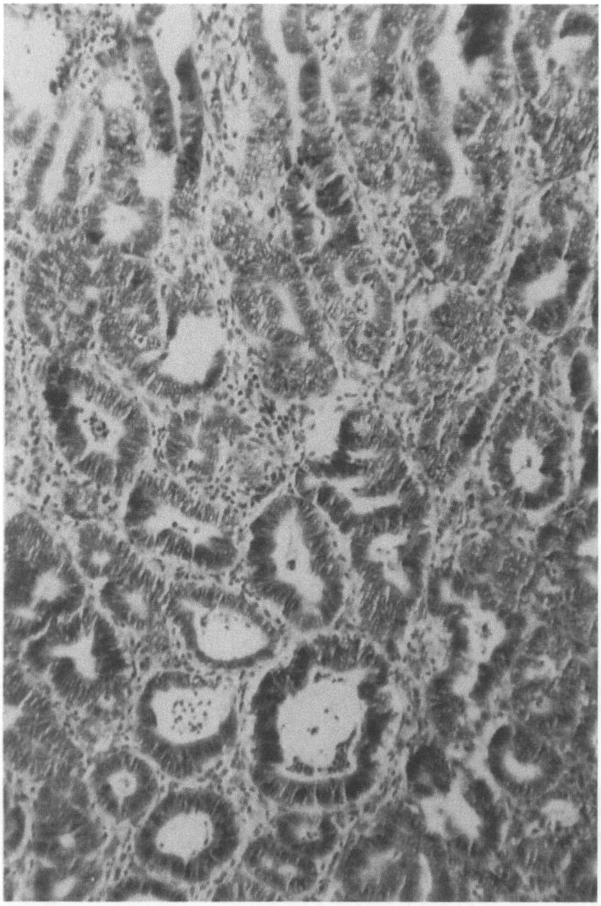

Fig. 3. The central part of the tumor demonstrated in Fig. 1 shows the adenocarcinoma

group rats were sigmoidostomated. Opposed to the sigmoidostomy a mucosal tunnel and a defect in the mucous membrane were performed, just as though the ureter would be implanted. Of course the implantation itself was not performed in the control group. The bowel was opened by a longitudinal section and closed transversely by Schmieden's continuous suture (Miersch 1988, 1989).

After the section the animals were examined macroscopically and with the help of magnifying lenses. If tumor formation was seen, the region of the ureterocolic anastomosis was taken by a longitudinal section. It was embedded in paraffin and later on worked up by many different sections. The histological examination was performed with routinely stained sections.

Results

In 22 of 50 animals operated after this model a clear tumor formation was found. As a result of the histological examination 12 tumors were found to be real neoplasia.

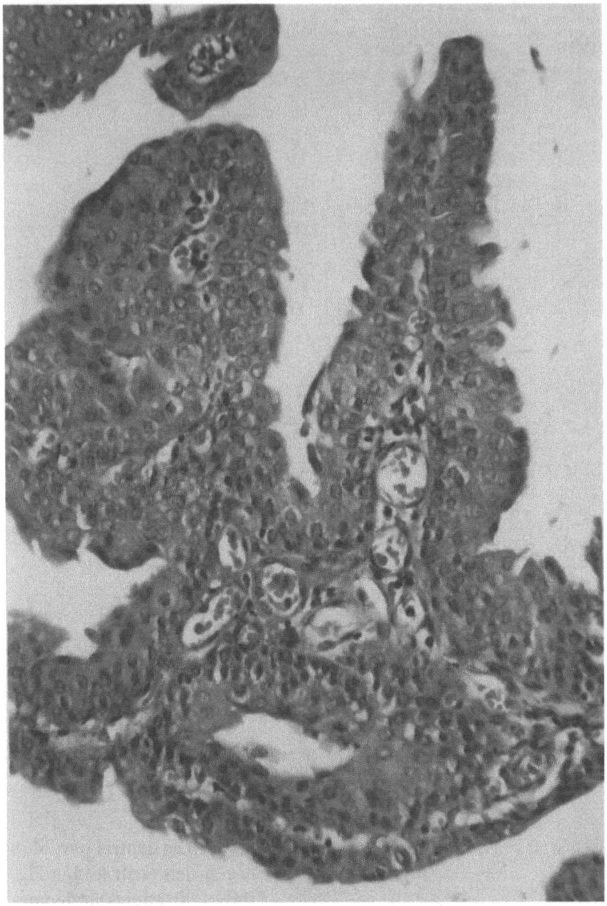

Fig. 4. Urothelial papilloma at the site of the anastomosis

These 12 tumors could be divided into the following groups: an adenoma of the colon with a central ulcus; four adenocarcinomas of the intestinal type which partly have been developed in the region of a previous adenoma (Fig. 1). One of them was combined with a squamous cell carcinoma, another one with a urothelial papilloma and an anaplastic tumor. The enlargement shows the change-over from still normal to adenomatous mucosa (Fig. 2). In the central part of the same tumor the carcinoma is proved (Fig. 3).

Five urothelial papillomas were found altogether, yet just once was it discovered as an isolated form.

Histological enlargement presents the proliferating transitional cell epithelium (Fig. 4). At the top of some of the tumors we also found goblet cells and cylindrical epithelium. This strange intermixture of intestinal mucosa and transitional cell epithelium often struck us when examining these tumors, but we also found this in anastomoses which have not changed neoplastically (Fig. 5).

In the other four cases the urothelial papilloma was associated with different tumors at the site of the anastomosis, in the proximal and distal ureter, and in the renal

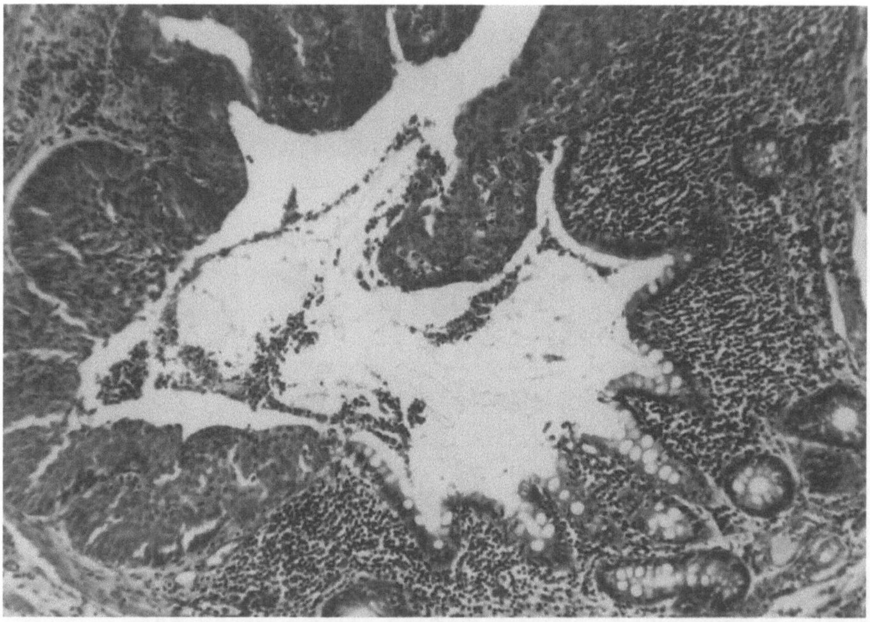

Fig. 5. Strange intermixture of intestinal mucosa and transitional cell epithelium in an implanted ureter which is not neoplastically changed

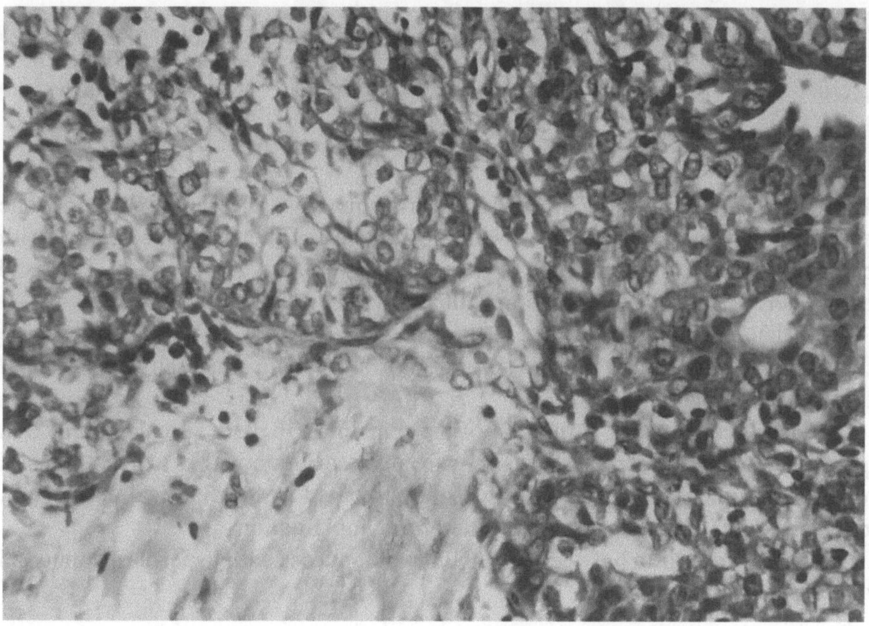

Fig. 6. Solid urothelial carcinoma developed at the site of the anastomosis

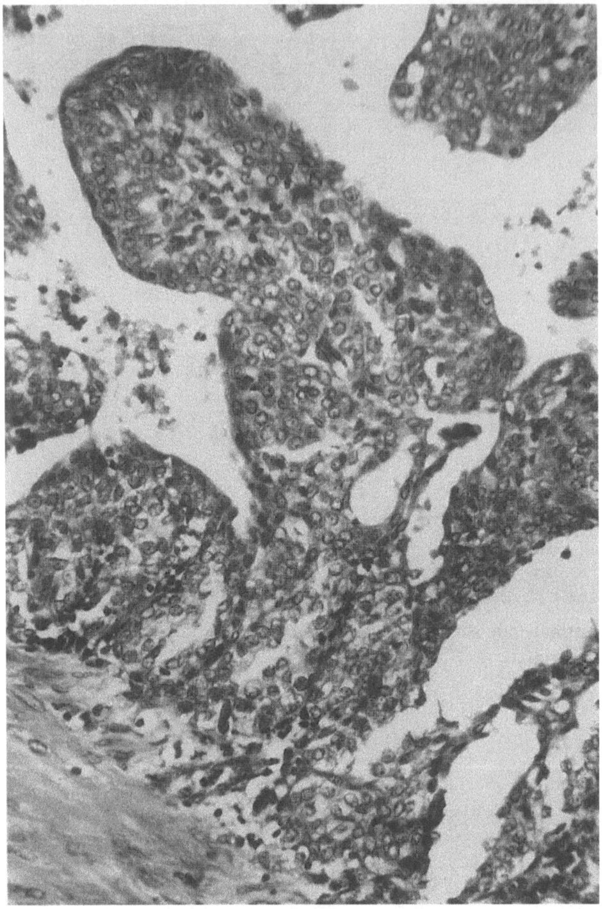

Fig. 7. Papillary urothelial carcinoma of the distal part of the implanted ureter

pelvis. Once we found the combination with a squamous cell carcinoma, once the urothelial papilloma was associated with a carcinoma of the renal pelvis, once with a carcinoma of the intestinal type and an undifferentiated carcinoma of the distal ureter. There was also a combination with a polypous mucosal hyperplasia.

Urothelial carcinomas occurred in three cases (Figs. 6, 7). In all cases they were associated with a polypous mucosal prolapse or a polypous mucosal hyperplasia at the site of the implantation.

The macroscopic tumor formation of the remaining 10 cases revealed a mucosal hyperplasia or mucosal prolapse in six, twice an association with a scarred mucosal fold, once with an intramural, submucosal cyst coated with cylindrical epithelium, and once with an ulcus situated at the site of the implantation.

The abrupt transition between urothelium and mucosa with hyperplastic mucosal changes was striking (Fig. 5).

Discussion

The medium observation period was 20 months for the group with the implantation of the left ureter. The tumor which developed in the shortest time was a urothelial carcinoma and was found after only 9 months. In the sham-operated control group with 30 evaluated animals and a medium observation period of 17.4 months no tumor could be discovered either in the kidney, renal pelvis, ureter, bladder, or large intestine.

To sum up the results, we can say that in the group of rats which has been examined and evaluated so far, 12 animals developed adenocarcinomas, transitional cell carcinomas, squamous cell carcinomas, or mixed forms as well as still benign adenomas and urothelial papillomas exclusively on the operated side. According to Deerberg who examined the spontaneous incidence of tumors in Han:WISTAR rats, papillomas of the bladder did not develop before the 3rd or 4th year. Transitional cell carcinomas of the renal pelvis or the ureter did not occur in 609 evaluated rats. The spontaneous incidence rate of adenocarcinomas of the colon is 0.3% up to the 2nd year and increases to 1.3% by the 4th year. Benign adenomas could not be discovered in male rats. As to female rats Deerberg found one adenoma of the colon in 305 observed rats after 3 years (Deerberg et al. 1980).

So with a well-balanced metabolism the tumor rate is in no way as high as described in other models. Yet a clear increase of the tumor rate is still seen with our operating technique. We attribute the increased rate to the unstable and highly sensitive, artificially produced borderline between transitional cell epithelium and the mucosa of the colon, which is exposed to different stimuli, namely the mechanical irritation of the feces or also perhaps carcinogens being developed by the mixture of urine and feces (Aaronson and Sinclair-Smith 1984; Aaronson et al. 1987; Crissey et al. 1979, 1980; Gittes 1986; Stewart et al. 1981). As a result surplus repairs develop, processes on both mucosae; the transitional cell mucosa tries to protrude into the lumen of the bowel as far as possible and the mucosa of the colon seems to try to coat the lumen of the ureter. In the course of these processes atypias occur, and finally carcinomas develop.

References

Aaronson IA, Sinclair-Smith CC (1984) Dysplasia of ureteric epithelium: a source of adenocarcinoma in ureterosigmoidostomy? Z Kinderchir 39:364–367

Aaronson IA, Constantinides CC, Sallie LP, Sinclair-Smith CC (1987) Pathogenesis of adenocarcinoma complicating ureterosigmoidostomy. Experimental observations. Urology 29:538–543

Crissey MM, Steele GD Jr, Gittes RF (1979) Carcinoma in colonic urinary diversion in rats. Surgical Forum 30:554–555

Crissey MM, Steele GD, Gittes RF (1980) Rat model for carcinogenesis in ureterosigmoidostomy. Science 207:1079–1080

Deerberg F, Rapp KG, Pittermann W, Rehm S (1980) Zum Tumorspektrum der Han:WIST-Ratte. Z Versuchstierk 22:267–280

Gittes RF (1986) Carcinogenesis in ureterosigmoidostomy. Urol Clin North Am 13:201–205

Harzmann R, Kopper B, Carl P (1986) Karzinominduktion durch Harnab- oder -umleitung über Darmabschnitte? Urologe A 25:198–203

Miersch W-D (1988) Mikrochirurgisches Modell zur Untersuchung der Karzinominduktion durch Harnableitung über Darmabschnitte an der Ratte – Erste Ergebnisse. In: Verhandlungsbericht der Deutschen Gesellschaft für Urologie, 39, Stuttgart 1987, Springer, Berlin Heidelberg New York, pp 329–330

Miersch W-D (1988) A new microsurgical model for the study of carcinogenesis in colonic urinary diversion in rats. Urol Int 43:269–271

Simon C (1852) Ektopia vesicae. Lancet 2:568–570

Stewart M, Hill MJ, Pugh RCB, Williams JP (1981) The role of N-nitrosamine in carcinogenesis at the ureterocolic anastomosis. Br J Urol 53:115–118

Efficacy of Systemic Chemotherapy in Metastatic Murine Bladder Cancer

W. Kropp, M.-L. Mlynek, G. Cevc, and R. Hartung[1]

Introduction

So far, the efficiency of chemotherapy has been tested on FANFT-induced tumors of the bladder in mice and in rats, as well as on transplanted carcinoma of the bladder in immunocompetent mice and nude mice (Huland et al. 1985; Soloway 1977; Soloway and Masters 1980). Animal models for the study of cancer metastasis have been developed for a number of tumors and have been used for the study of the mechanisms of metastasis (Nicolson 1982).

Using a specially designed experimental bladder tumor model, the measurable effects of both mono- and polychemotherapy regarding the survival rate, absence of tumor, rate of tumor growth, and rate of metastasis were assessed on an invasive, in situ growing tumor. In the present study, this model was utilized to evaluate the effectiveness of the chemotherapeutic agents *cis*-platinum (CDDP), methotrexate (MTX), adriamycin (ADM), cyclophosphamide (CYC), and vinblastine (VLB) commonly used in the treatment of advanced bladder cancer.

Material and Methods

Animals. Female C3H/He-Han mice (weight: 22–24 g) were kept five to a cage. They were fed and given water ad libitum.

Tumor. MBT-2 is a poorly differentiated cell line derived from a FANFT-induced murine bladder carcinoma. The tumor has been maintained by serial transplantation in syngeneic C3H/He-Han mice. The cells obtained from a tumor-bearing C3H/He-Han mouse were cultivated in petri dishes and extracted with the help of trypsin during the exponential growth phase before being applied as single-cell suspensions in 0.1 ml medium (RPMI 1640 + 10% CS).

Procedure. For the experiments, the animals were anesthetized and catheterized (PE-10 polyethylene tube). After mechanical lesion of the bladder urothelium (by scraping with a silver wire) 1×10^5 MBT-2 cells were instilled. A 1-h cerclage ensured that the suspension remained in the bladder. Experiments were terminated at day 28 or 35.

Histology. Postmortem tissue analysis involved the urinary bladder, liver, lungs, and kidneys in serial slides.

[1] Urologische Klinik und Poliklinik der Technischen Universität München, Klinikum Rechts der Isar, Ismaninger Str. 22, 8000 München 80, FRG

Investigative Urology 3
Edited by H. Rübben et al.

Chemotherapy. Intraperitoneal chemotherapy was performed either on day 14, 21, and 28 (group A) or 7, 14, and 21 (groups B, C). Intraperitoneal drug dosages were: CDDP (7.2 mg/kg), MTX (4.8 mg/kg), ADM (1.2 mg/kg), CYC (0.6 mg/kg), and VLB (0.6 mg/kg).

Group C differed from group B in so far as the dosages of the chemotherapeutic agents were reduced. Control animals (C) were given intraperitoneal injections of saline solution.

Results and Conclusions

Group A. Only 2/30 animals (6.6%) in the CISCA group were still alive at the end of the experiment on day 35. In all animals tumor growth could be demonstrated. None of the therapies could halt tumor expansion (Table 1).

The rate of metastasis was lower in those animals which underwent chemotherapeutic treatment than in the control group. The lack of efficacy of the chemotherapy can be associated with the large tumor mass at the onset of therapy and the following rapid progression.

Table 1. Effect of chemotherapy on the survival rate (SR), the absence of tumor (AoT), and the rate of metastasis (RoM) in relation to initiation of therapy (14th day after tumor implantation). Control animals (C) were treated with a puffer solution

Expt. groups	SR	(%)	AoT	(%)	RoM	(%)
C	0/16	(0)	0/16	(0)	7/16	(43)
CDDP	0/31	(0)	0/31	(0)	11/31	(35)
MTX	0/22	(0)	0/22	(0)	9/22	(40)
CDDP + MTX	0/30	(0)	0/30	(0)	9/30	(30)
MVAC	0/27	(0)	0/27	(0)	8/27	(29)
CISCA	2/30	(6)	0/30	(0)	8/30	(26)

Table 2. Effect of chemotherapy on the survival rate (SR), the absence of tumor (AoT), and the rate of metastasis (RoM) in relation to initiation of therapy (7th day after tumor implantation)

Expt. groups	SR	(%)	AoT	(%)	RoM	(%)
C	7/30	(23)	1/30	(3)	13/30	(43)
CDDP	15/40	(37)	7/40	(17)	5/40	(12)
MTX	14/40	(35)	3/40	(7)	15/40	(37)
ADM	7/20	(35)	0/20	(0)	2/20	(10)
CDDP + MTX	2/20	(10)	4/20	(20)	4/20	(20)
CDDP + ADM	4/20	(20)	1/20	(5)	3/20	(15)
MVAC	2/20	(10)	9/20	(45)	0/20	(0)
CISCA	4/22	(18)	18/22	(82)	0/22	(0)

Table 3. Effect of reduced dosage chemotherapy on the survival rate (SR), the absence of tumor (AoT), and the rate of metastasis (RoM) in relation to initiation of therapy (7th day after tumor implantation)

Expt. groups	SR	(%)	AoT	(%)	RoM	(%)
C	7/30	(23)	1/30	(3)	13/30	(43)
CDDP + MTX	3/21	(14)	0/21	(0)	3/21	(14)
CDDP + ADM	4/20	(20)	1/20	(5)	4/20	(20)
MVAC	5/19	(26)	1/19	(5)	5/19	(26)
CISCA	12/19	(63)	2/19	(11)	6/19	(31)

Group B. Early initiation of chemotherapy, on day 7 after tumor instillation, led to an improvement in the survival rate (Table 2). This effect was more prominent when monochemotherapy with CDDP, MTX, or ADM was applied. On the other hand, animals treated with combination chemotherapy were to a large degree free of tumor and metastasis. These results underline the greater efficacy of polychemotherapy, especially of the MVAC and CISCA schemes. The lower survival rate of animals treated with polychemotherapy may well have been caused by the toxicity of the therapeutic agents used in combination.

Group C. Reduction of the dosage of single substances used in combination chemotherapy led to a marked improvement of the survival rates in both the MVAC and the CISCA groups, whereas fewer animals survived in the CDDP + MTX and CDDP + ADM groups (Table 3). Improvement of the survival rate can only be achieved at the cost of a lower rate of tumor absence and a greater rate of metastasis.

Summary

This bladder carcinoma model allows evaluation of the effectiveness of chemotherapy protocols and regimens.

The later chemotherapy is initiated, the lesser are the chances of successful tumor destruction, reduction of metastasis, and improvement of the survival rates, due to the continuous increase in tumor size.

Reduced dosages in the polychemotherapy protocols led to reduction of toxicity (increase of the survival rate), but also to an increase in the rate of metastasis. Polychemotherapy did not prove superior to monochemotherapy.

References

Huland H, Otto U, Paleske AV (1985) Chemotherapy and human bladder carcinoma transplanted into NMRI NU/NU mice. J Urol 184:601

Nicolson G (1982) Cancer metastasis. Organ colonization and the cell-surface properties of malignant cells. Biochim Biophys Acta 695:113

Soloway MS (1977) Intravesical and systemic chemotherapy of murine bladder cancer. Cancer Res 37:2918

Soloway MS, Masters S (1980) Urothelial susceptibility to tumor cell implantation. Cancer 46:1158

Selective Arterial Chemoembolization of the Urinary Bladder with Reabsorbable *cis*-Platinum Microcapsules in the Dog Using a Double Balloon Embolization Catheter

C. Bornhof[1], E. Vecera[1], and B. Mosier[2]

Introduction

The side effects of new active cytostatic drug combinations for the treatment of transitional cell carcinomas are remarkable. The nephrotoxicity of *cis*-diammine-dichloroplatinum (DDP) represents a specific problem for the chemotherapy of bladder cancer. Of the patients with tumors staged T_3 and T_4 35% suffer from renal insufficiency due to obstruction of the kidneys (Greiner et al. 1983) and are not candidates for chemotherapy.

Targeted drug delivery, therefore, resulting in high tissue levels within the bladder wall and low systemic toxicity, could be of particular interest for multidrug chemotherapy as well as for integrated radiochemotherapy of bladder cancer. The present study deals with the selective arterial chemoembolization of the superior vesical artery of the dog using new, reabsorbable, DDP microcapsules.

Materials and Methods

An embolization catheter was placed by open surgery in the iliac internal artery at the origin of the superior vesical artery in 18 male Beagle dogs (Fig. 1). The double balloon was blocked and the position of the catheter controlled scintigraphically using ^{99}Technetium-albumin microspheres.

In the control dogs (group 1, $n = 3$) DDP (1.6 mg/kg body weight) was injected intravenously. There were five groups of dogs (each $n = 3$) receiving different preparations of DDP microcapsules (diameter 125 µm) (preparation by B. Mosier, Institute for Research, Houston, Texas, USA):

Group 2: Phosphoglyceride-phospholipid, DDP 0.8 mg/kg bw, concentration of DDP 17.2%
Group 3: Polyglyceride-protein, DDP 0.63 mg/kg bw, 14.2%
Group 4: Polyglyceride-cellulose, DDP 0.62 mg/kg bw, 14.2%
Group 5: Polyglyceride-phospholipid-cellulose, DDP 0.55 mg/kg bw, 12.4%
Group 6: Polyglyceride-phospholipid-protein, DDP 0.53 mg/kg bw, 12.0%
Group 7: Placebo microcapsules devoid of DDP, $n = 3$

All dogs received a forced diuresis. Platinum in the tissues and serum was measured with atomic absorption. The animals were killed after 10 days. Tissue samples

[1] Department of Urology, University of Erlangen, 8520 Erlangen, FRG
[2] Institute for Research, Houston, Texas, USA

Investigative Urology 3
Edited by H. Rübben et al.

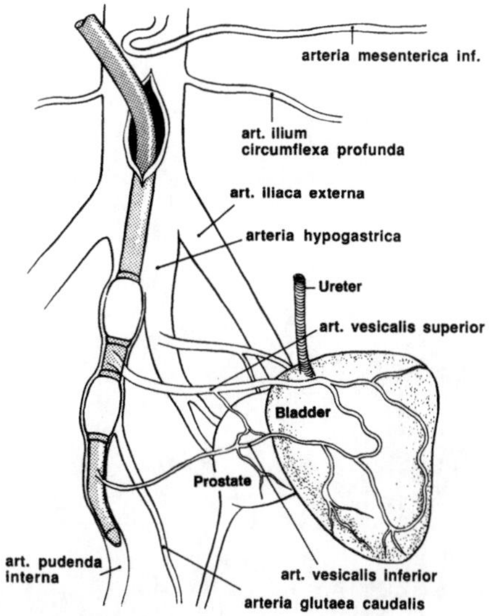

Fig. 1. Experimental design for the selective chemoembolization of the right superior vesical artery. The embolization catheter is placed in the right hypogastric artery with its tip in the internal pudendal artery

a 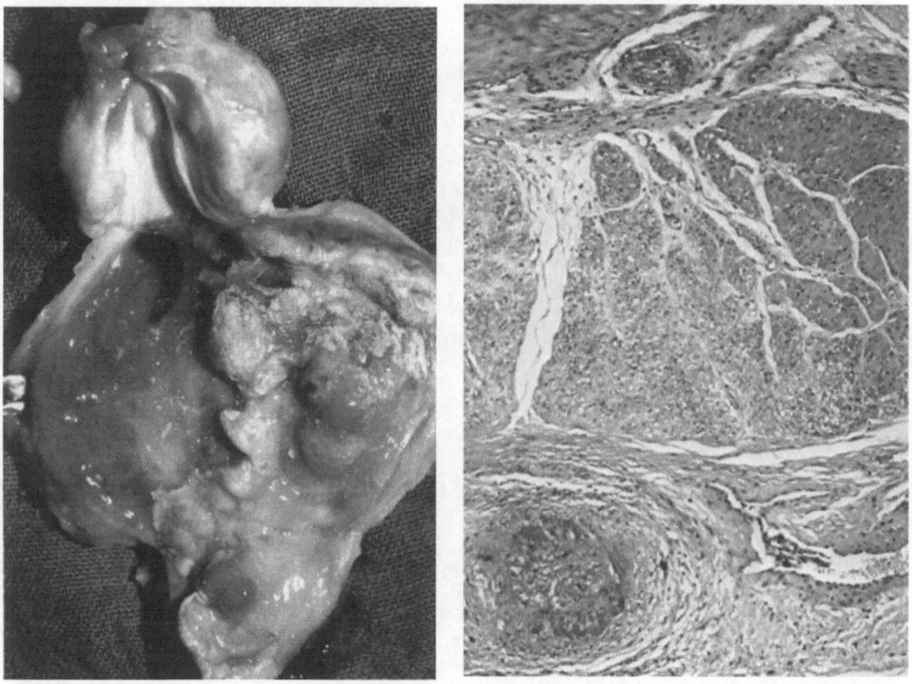 b

Fig. 2. a Macroscopic aspect of the inner surface of the bladder wall 10 days after chemoembolization. **b** Regressive muscle fibers in the muscularis propria of the bladder. In the *lower portion* a subserous artery with an organized thrombus; in the *upper portion* a small artery with a thrombus. Group 6, H & E stain, × 69

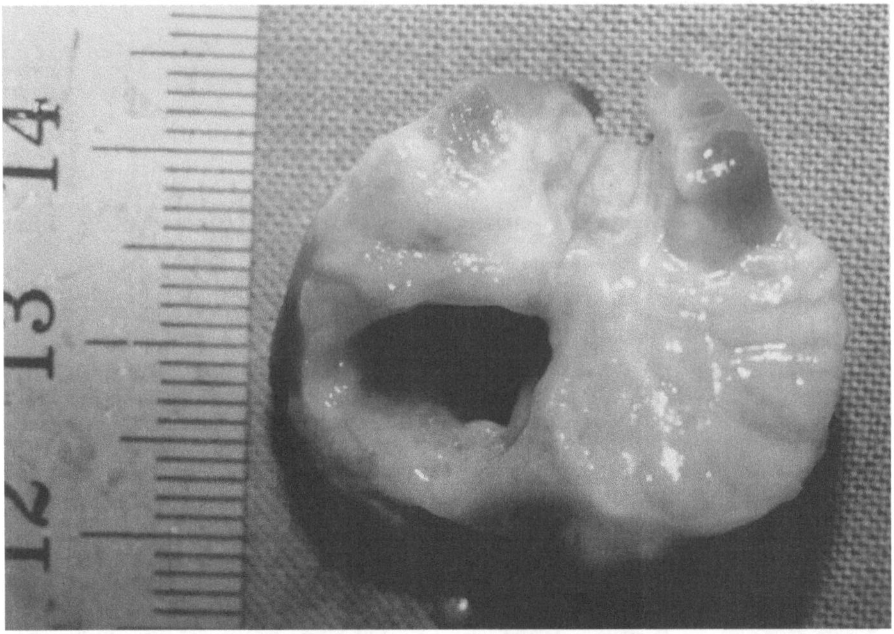

a

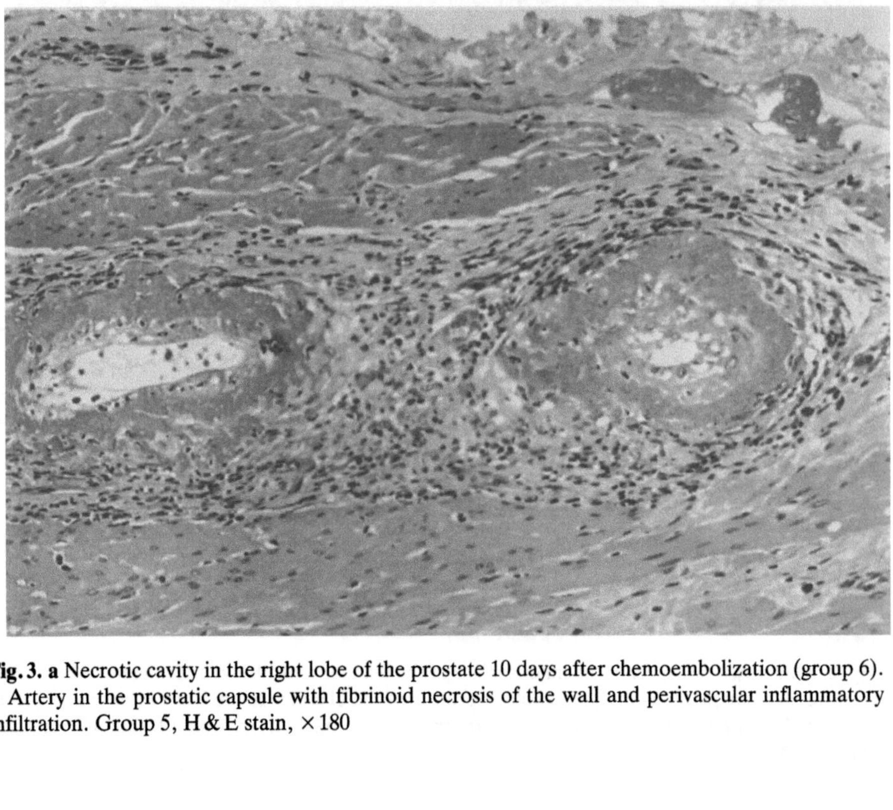

b

Fig. 3. a Necrotic cavity in the right lobe of the prostate 10 days after chemoembolization (group 6). **b** Artery in the prostatic capsule with fibrinoid necrosis of the wall and perivascular inflammatory infiltration. Group 5, H & E stain, × 180 were taken for histology and for measurement of platinum levels separately from the right and left side of the bladder wall and prostate and from the respective regional lymph nodes, as well as from the kidneys, liver, lungs, skeletal muscle, and brain.

Statistics were performed using the nonparametric H-Test according to Kruskal and Wallis for interindividual and the Wilcoxon Test for intraindividual comparisons with $P < 0.05$ as level of significance.

Results

Scintigraphy revealed a selective injection of the microcapsules into the superior vesical artery, resulting in a well-defined accumulation of activity in the bladder wall and the prostate in all dogs. Histology showed thrombotic occlusions of the intramural vessels with fibrosis of the bladder wall (Fig. 2). Necroses penetrating the whole of the wall were never seen. The ipsilateral lobe of the prostate was replaced centrally by a necrotic cavity (Fig. 3) surrounded with atrophy of the glands and scarring of the tissue.

Table 1. Tissue levels of platinum (ng/g tissue) 10 days after DDP injection

Organ	Intravenously (1.6 mg/kg bw)	Intraarterially[a] (0.53 mg/kg body weight)	
		Side of injection	Opposite side
Bladder	160 ± 30	1687 ± 1291	496 ± 262
Prostate	297 ± 43	2538 ± 1181	660 ± 257
Lymph nodes	320 ± 93	222 ± 147	106 ± 89

DDP, *cis*-diammine-dichloro-platinum

[a] Microcapsules: DDP 12%; polyglyceride-phospholipid-protein

Table 2. Tissue levels of platinum (ng/g tissue) 10 days after DDP injection

Organ	Intravenously (1.6 mg/kg bw)	Intraarterially[a] (0.53 mg/kg bw)
Kidney	985 ± 44	172 ± 55
Liver	860 ± 283	136 ± 58
Lung	390 ± 52	< 20
Skeletal muscle	90 ± 43	< 20
Brain	23 ± 7	< 20

DDP, *cis*-diammine-dichloro-platinum

[a] Microcapsules: DDP 12%, polyglyceride-phospholipid-protein

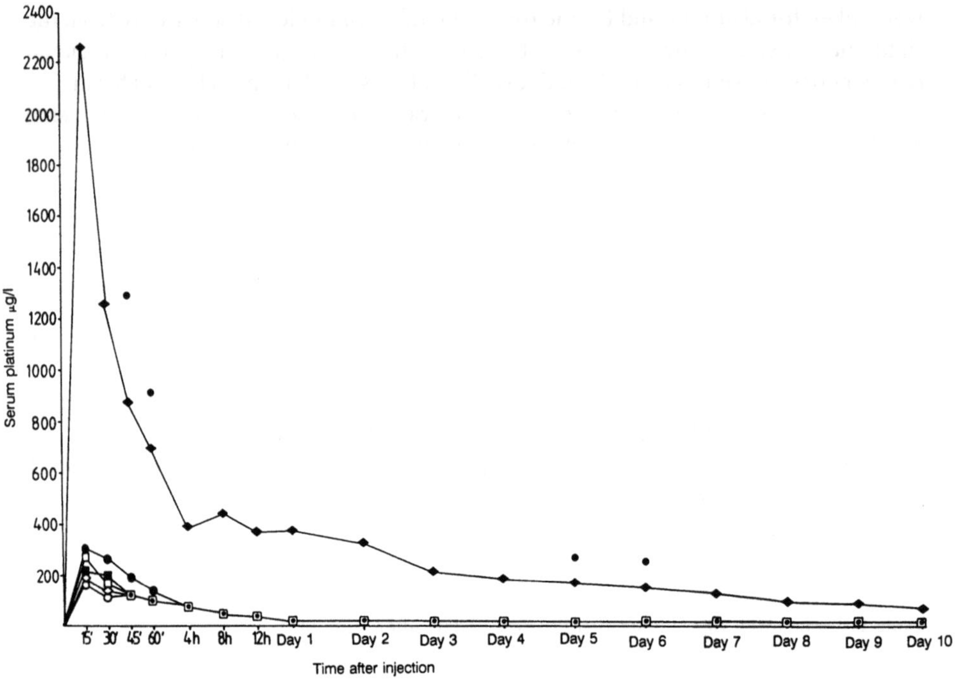

Fig. 4. Serum platinum levels in the six experimental groups. ◆, Group 1; ● group 2; □ group 3; ■ group 4; ○, group 5; ◇, group 6; •, denotes significant differences between group 1 and groups 2–6. Each dot represents the mean value of three experiments

Table 3. Half-life times ($t_{1/2}$) of serum platinum concentrations

Group	$t_{1/2}\ \alpha$ (min)	$t_{1/2}\ \beta$ (h)
1	29	96
2	39	104
3	39	79
4	38	99
5	–	105
6	56	97

The platinum levels (Table 1) were elevated in the bladder wall ($P<0.05$) and in the prostate ($P=0.05$) and lower in the lymph nodes in the chemoembolized groups compared with the controls. The platinum levels were significantly higher on the side of the injection as compared with the opposite side. The platinum levels in the kidneys, liver, lungs, and skeletal muscle were significantly lower in the dogs treated with chemoembolization than in the control group (Table 2).

The serum platinum levels (Fig. 4) reached a peak 15 min after injection and were markedly lower after chemoembolization for 10 days compared with the control dogs. In either group the serum platinum falls in a biphasic pattern ($t_{1/2}\ \alpha = 29–56$ min; $t_{1/2}\ \beta = 79–105$ h; Table 3). The urinary excretion of platinum was significantly lower in the groups receiving DDP microcapsules than in the control dogs for 6 days, reaching a peak on day 1 of the experiment (161 ± 38 μg/h vs 4535 ± 1180 μg/h).

The most pronounced increase of platinum in the bladder wall and the prostate is achieved by the injection of the DDP microcapsules in the groups 4, 5, 6.

Discussion

Arterial chemoembolization for the treatment of bladder cancer was investigated experimentally and clinically by Kato (Nemoto and Kato 1984), but has not gained wide acceptance outside Japan for several reasons: first, mitomycin-C, used by Kato, does not belong to the first line cytostatic drugs for urothelial tumors; secondly, ethylcellulose used as the shell material is not degradable and, therefore, its toxicologic and immunogenic effects are not predictable. Moreover, painful and extensive necroses of the skin and gluteus muscle due to the occlusion of the superior gluteal artery were described in 37% of the patients (Kato et al. 1981).

In the present study for the first time biologically degradable microcapsules, containing DDP, were used. Other cytostatic drugs, like methotrexate, vinblastine, or adriamycin can be microencapsulated with the same technique (Mosier 1985). The DDP microcapsules can easily be dispersed in a dextran solution and injected through conventional plastic syringes. Due to their small size, they reach the peripheral intramural vessels of the bladder wall, which is the desired target site. Injection of placebo microcapsules, devoid of DDP, also results in pronounced cytotoxic effects, which, however, are further enhanced by the incorporation of DDP. The results of our study clearly show that a highly selective chemoembolization of the vesical artery can be performed with high platinum levels at the target site and low systemic toxicity. Most importantly, the nephrotoxicity of DDP is significantly diminished due to the low accumulation of platinum within the kidneys.

Hence, also patients with a mild to moderate renal insufficiency can be treated with DDP-containing drug regimens or, in patients with normal renal function, a lower dosage of DDP is sufficient to reach therapeutic drug levels.

Far advanced bladder cancer, frequently, is a systemic disease with a tendency to distant spread. If, therefore, cytotoxic systemic drug levels are to be achieved, a preparation of microcapsules can be chosen with an enhanced release of DDP. Thus, locoregional therapy does not rule out effective systemic treatment, but permits a fine adjustment of the dosage for the individual patient. Currently, studies are under way to investigate the selective chemoembolization of bladder cancer in humans using a transfemoral approach for angiographically guided insertion of the embolization catheter without open operation.

The high platinum levels in the prostate indicate that the method described could be useful, too, in patients with advanced prostatic carcinoma, resistant to the antiandrogen therapy, in whom the side effects of a conventional systemic chemotherapy cannot be tolerated.

References

Greiner R, Studer U, Bleher S (1983) Zur Indikation der Strahlentherapie des Blasenkarzinoms. In: Schmiedt E, Bauer HW (eds) Blasenkarzinom-Entscheidungshilfen bei der Therapie. Zuckschwerdt, München, pp 176–189

Kato T, Nemoto R, Mori H, Takahashi M, Tamakawa Y, Harada M (1981) Arterial chemoembolization with microencapsulated anticancer drug. JAMA 245:1123–1127

Mosier B (1985) Method of preparing microspheres for intravascular delivery. United States Patent Number 4.492,720

Nemoto R, Kato T (1984) Microencapsulation of anticancer drug for intraarterial infusion and its application. In: Davis SS, Illum L, McVie JG, Tomlinson E (eds) Microspheres and drug therapy, pharmaceutical, immunological and medical aspects. Elsevier, Amsterdam, pp 229–243

Tissue Concentration of Chloraluminum-Phthalocyanine in Xenotransplanted Human Bladder Cancer

K. Miller[1], B. Bartos[1], A. Rück[2], E. Schmidt[1], R. Steiner[2], and R. Hautmann[1]

Introduction

In recent years, photodynamic therapy (PDT) for the treatment of various malignant tissues has gained increasing attention. PDT is based on the more or less selective retention of a systemically administered photosensitizer in malignant tissues. Irradiation of the tissue with light of an appropriate wavelength causes cell death by activation of the photosensitizing drug.

In the beginning most in vitro and in vivo studies focussed on hematoporphyrin derivative (HPD) as sensitizer. More recent experimental work has been done in order to develop new and better sensitizers. This search for alternative sensitizing agents has been accelerated by the fact that HPD is far from being an ideal photosensitizer: HPD contains a mixture of different components, making a chemical definition difficult. The absorption peak in the desirable red portion of the visible light spectrum, which would provide the best tissue penetration, is weak. Moreover, as it has a strong absorption in the ultraviolet, exposure of the skin to sunlight causes photosensitization with severe side effects.

Metallophthalocyanines, a group of tetra-azo-tetra-benzoporphyrin dyes fulfill some of the aforementioned needs for an ideal sensitizer: they have a clearly defined chemical composition and are therefore easily synthesized. Water solubility can be achieved by sulfonation (Moan et al. 1987), and the resulting substances are chemically stable (Bown et al. 1986). Moreover, they have a strong absorption peak in the red part of the spectrum (at 675 nm).

Phototoxicity of phthalocyanines (PC) has been demonstrated in vitro and in vivo by several authors (Ben Hur and Rosenthal 1985; Brasseur et al. 1988; Moan et al. 1987; Selman et al. 1986). To assess the potential of PC for the treatment of bladder cancer, we have studied the uptake of sulfonated chloraluminium-phthalocyanines, using nude mice with xenotransplanted human bladder tumors as the experimental model.

Material and Methods

Tumor Model. The tumor used for this study was cut from a high-grade human bladder tumor removed during a radical cystectomy. The solid tumor tissue was divided into pieces of approximately 0.5 g and stored at −20°C. Nude mice, 4–6 weeks old, with an average weight of 25 g were used as hosts for the human tumor tissue. For transplantation, the thawed tumor pieces were inserted into both flanks of the mice

[1] Division of Urology, University of Ulm, 7900 Ulm, FRG
[2] Institute for Laser Technologies in Medicine, Ulm, 7900 Ulm, FRG

Investigative Urology 3
Edited by H. Rübben et al.

via a 5-mm dorsal skin incision. For this procedure, the animals were anesthetized with ether. Postoperatively, they were given food and water ad libitum. The tumor took 4–5 weeks to grow to a size of 6–10 mm in diameter. Tumors older and larger than this showed signs of liquefied necrosis and were therefore not suitable for concentration measurements. For our studies we used 4–5-week-old tumors showing minimal or no necrosis.

Photosensitizer. Chloraluminum-phthalocyanine (ClAlPc), averaging 3–4 sulphonic acid groups per molecule, supplied by BASF was used. It was dissolved in Hank's solution and administered by intraperitoneal injection at a dosage of 5 mg/kg. The sensitized animals were kept in the dark.

Measurement of Tissue Concentrations. The concentration of ClAlPc was measured in tumor, skin, muscle, liver, and bladder at 8, 16, 24, 48, and 72 h post sensitization in five animals at each interval. Mice were killed by carbon dioxide and approximately 0.5 g of tumor, muscle, skin, liver, and the whole bladder were removed and stored at −20°C in the dark until extraction. Tissue samples were prepared as described by Bown et al. (1986) with minor modifications; the samples were weighed and homogenized in 7 ml 0.1 *M* NaOH, then centrifuged at 20000 rpm for 20 min at 4°C. The supernatant was separated and the fluorescence read at 675 nm, excitation at 600 nm, with a fluorescence spectrometer (Kontron 25 SPF). The results obtained were calibrated against fluorescence standard curves of known concentrations of ClAlPc in unsensitized tissue. The samples of unsensitized tissue were prepared as described above and concentrations expressed in ng ClAlPc/g tissue.

Results

The quantity of ClAlPc measured in the different tissues as a function of time is shown in Fig. 1. The ClAlPc concentration was lowest in tumor tissue followed by bladder and skin. The highest concentration was found in the liver and muscle.

Discussion

Urothelial cancer of the bladder continues to be a therapeutic challenge as the treatment modalities on hand do not yet provide satisfactory results. As bladder tumors

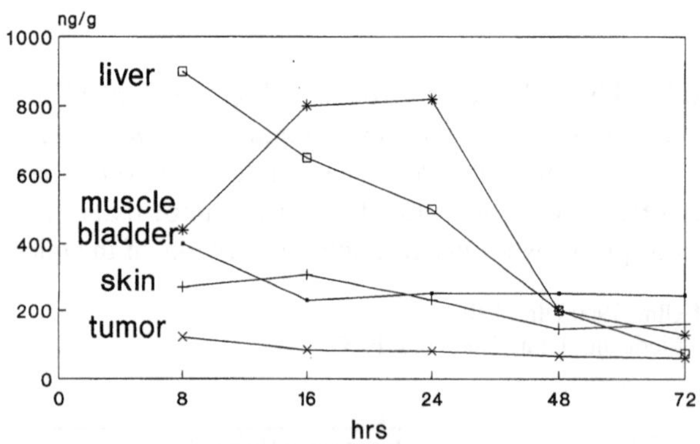

Fig. 1. Distribution of ClAlPc in various tissues during the 72 h after intraperitoneal application of the sensitizer

are easily accessible for endoscopic treatment, conventional laser therapy, using the Neodym-Yac-Laser (Hofstetter et al. 1985) and photodynamic therapy (Benson 1985) have been attempted as an alternative. Those attempts have so far failed to yield a significantly superior result when compared with conventional endoscopic therapy (electroresection). Development of integral photodynamic therapy for bladder cancer (Jocham et al. 1984) was a promising advancement with regard to the experimental results. The idea of integrated PDT is to destroy selectively even invisible tumor cells within the bladder by a diffuse radiation of the whole bladder wall, following photosensitation. It is easy to understand that this treatment would be an ideal therapy for bladder cancer, with its potentially multifocal growth, especially for carcinoma in situ. To minimize side effects caused by phototoxic damage of the normal bladder wall, this treatment modality would require a highly tumor-selective photosensitizer. It is therefore of particular interest to compare tissue concentrations of the sensitizers in various organs and cell types at different intervals following application, to find the optimal time for irradiation. Using a high-grade urothelial bladder cancer we failed to demonstrate a tumor-selective uptake or retention of ClAlPc during up to 72 h after application. Other groups, using different tumor models, found better ratios: Moan et al. could show the concentration of ClAlPc in CHHH-mouse mammary carcinomas being double when compared with skin concentration.

Tralau et al., using a rat fibrosarcoma, found the highest concentration in the skin, following the systemical administration of 5 mg/kg ClAlPc. Tumor concentration was twice as high as muscle concentration 48 h after sensitisation.

At present, it is difficult to analyze the reasons for the different results obtained with different tumor models. More studies, using different bladder carcinomas and other transplantation sites (mouse bladder), are necessary to evaluate definitely the tumor-selective uptake and retention of phthalocyanines.

References

Ben Hur E, Rosenthal I (1986) Photosensitized inactivation of Chinese hamster cells by phthalocyanines. Photochem Photobiol 42:145

Benson RC (1985) Hematoporphyrin photosensitization and the Argon-dye laser. In: Smith JA (ed) Lasers in urologic surgery. Year Book, Chicago, pp 103–119

Bown SG, Tralau CJ, Coleridge-Smith PD, Akdemir D, Wilman TJ (1986) Photodynamic therapy with porphyrin and phthalocyanine sensitisation: quantitative studies in normal rat liver. Br J Cancer 54:43–52

Brasseur N, Hasrat A, Rejan L (1988) Biological activities of phthalocyanines-IX photosensitisation of V-79 Chinese hamster cells and EMT-6 mouse mammary tumor by selectively sulfonated zinc phthalocyanines. Photochem Photobiol 47:705–711

Hofstetter AG (1985) Laser treatment of the bladder: experimental and clinical results. In: Smith JA (ed) Lasers in urologic surgery. Year Book, Chicago, pp 63–81

Jocham D, Chaussy C, Staehler G, Löhrs U, Unsöld E (1984) Integrale Photoradiotherapie des Blasenkarzinoms nach tumorselektiver Photosensibilisierung mit Hämatoporphyrin-Derivat (HpD). Akt Urol 15:109–115

Moan J, Peng L, Evensen JF, Berg K, Western A, Rimingington C (1987) Photosensitizing efficiencies, tumor and cellular uptake of different photosensitizing drugs relevant for photodynamic therapy of cancer. Photochem Photobiol 46:713–721

Selman S, Kreimer-Brinbaum M, Audhuri C, Gargo GM (1986) Photodynamic treatment of transplantable bladder tumors in rodents after pretreatment with chloroaluminum tetrasulfophthalocyanine. J Urol 136:141–145

Tralau CJ, MacRobert AJ, Coleridge-Smith PD, Barr H, Bown SG (1987) Photodynamic therapy with phthalocyanine sensitisation: quantitative studies in a transplantable rat fibrosarcoma. Br J Cancer: 389–394

Biological Effects of Recombinant Human Tumor Necrosis Factor on Human Bladder Cancer Cells

W. Heckl, B. Klossner, and B. Halliger[1]

Introduction

The tumor necrosis factor (TNF) was detected by Carswell et al. (1975) in the serum of animals injected sequentially with bacillus Calmette-Guerin or *Corynebacterium parvum* and endotoxin. This treatment induces proliferation of macrophages, which are stimulated to secrete TNF by endotoxin (Beutler et al. 1986). TNF causes hemorrhagic necrosis of certain transplantable mouse and human tumors with no apparent effect on the host (Haranata et al. 1984). Partially purified preparations of human TNF as well as recombinant TNF have been shown to exhibit selective cytotoxic effects in vitro against several tumor cell lines with no cytotoxic effect on normal fibroblasts (Wang et al. 1985; Sugarman et al. 1985) but growth-enhancing effects on normal diploid skin (Detroit 551), lung (WI38), and foreskin (FS-4) fibroblastic cultures (Viket et al. 1986). Although the mechanism of selective toxicity of TNF to tumor cells is unknown, the selectivity is supposed to be at the TNF-receptor level.

The in vitro cytotoxicity of TNF to tumor cells can be enhanced by the addition of actinomycin D (Flick and Gifford 1984) as well as by other chemotherapeutic drugs (Alexander et al. 1987a). This observation and the increasing interest of using immunomodifiers in the therapy of bladder cancer focused our interest on the examination of the effect of the recombinant human tumor necrosis factor in combination with chemotherapeutic drugs on human bladder cancer cell lines.

Materials and Methods

Chemotherapeutic Agents. The recombinant human tumor necrosis factor (rHuTNF) was provided by Knoll AG, Ludwigshafen, FRG (specific activity 6.63×10^6 U/mg protein using standard L929 assay). Actinomycin D and adriamcycin were purchased from Sigma.

TNF Assay. The human transitional cell carcinoma (TCC) cell lines EJ, BT-1, SD, HT-1376, J-82, 5637, 639V, RT-112, RT-4, and T-24 were seeded at a density of 1×10^5 cells/microtiter well in 96 well microtiter plates. After 24-h incubation in the appropiate culture medium (RPMI-1640 or DMEM) the supernatant was replaced by 0.2 ml/well of a new medium containing increasing concentrations (5–1400 U/ml) of recombinant human TNF. In a second experiment these tumor cells were treated with 0.1 µg/ml actinomycin D or 1 ng/ml adriamycin, as single agents or along with

[1]Department of Urology, University of Würzburg, Medical School, Josef-Schneider-Str. 2, 8700 Würzburg, FRG

Investigative Urology 3
Edited by H. Rübben et al.

increasing concentrations of rHuTNF (up to 200 U/ml). After a further 24-h incubation the cytotoxicity was calculated using crystal violet as a staining dye (absorption at 540 nm). All samples were corrected for standardization with a correction factor estimated by running a standard curve with L 929 (50 ng/ml rHuTNF). Percentage cytotoxicity was calculated by comparing treated monolayers with untreated.

The response of the human bladder cancer cell lines to the treatment with various drugs was determined as follows: no response, <20% dead cells; moderate response, 20%–50% dead cells; response, >50% dead cells.

Results

With increasing concentrations of rHuTNF there was an increase of cytotoxicity to the human bladder cancer cell lines tested. However, there was a discrepancy in the TNF sensitivity. Whereas the cell lines T-24 and RT-4 were quite resistant to the TNF, 639V and RT-112 showed a high sensitivity to this drug, i.e., out of these two cell lines between 50% and 70% of the tumor cells were killed using 300 U/ml and between 60% and 70% with the highest concentration (1400 U/ml of TNF used. The other six cell lines (EJ, BT-1, HT-1376, SD, 5637, J-82) had only a moderate TNF sensitivity. Even with the highest TNF concentration (1400 U/ml) no more than 24%–35% of these cells were killed (Fig. 1). However, in the presence of actinomycin D (1 μg/ml), a striking cytotoxic effect on the human bladder cancer cell lines

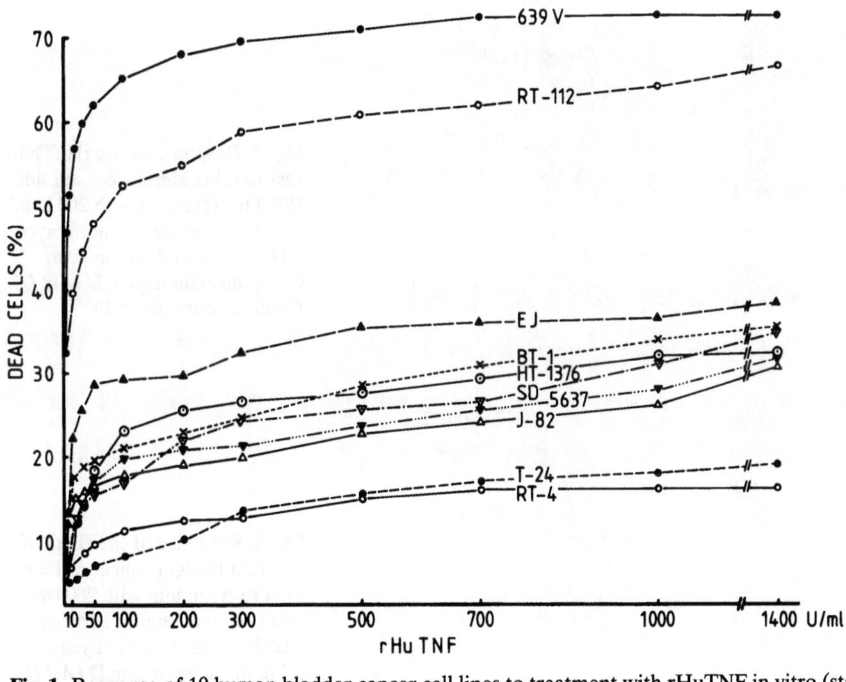

Fig. 1. Response of 10 human bladder cancer cell lines to treatment with rHuTNF in vitro (standard error means ≤5%)

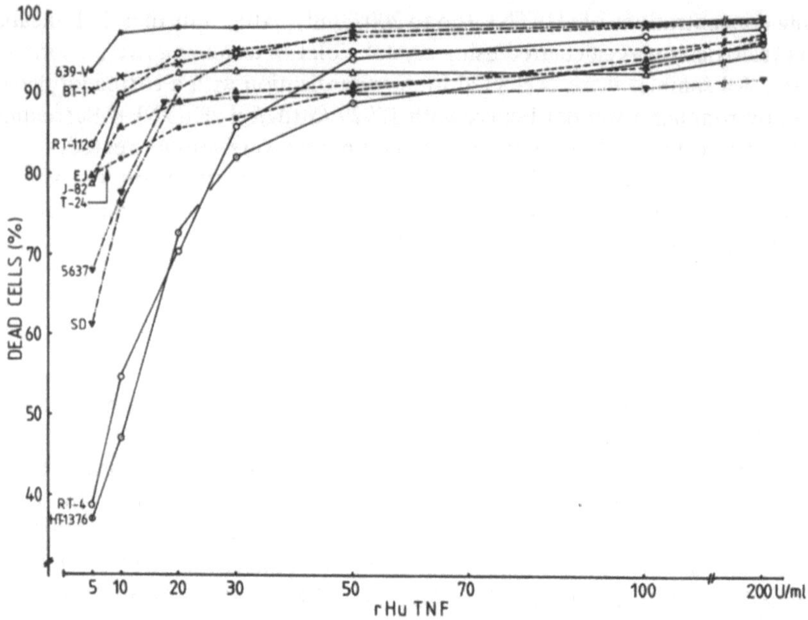

Fig. 2. Response of 10 human bladder cancer cell lines to treatment with rHuTNF (5–200 U/ml) and actinomycin D (0.1 µg/ml) (standard error means ≤5%)

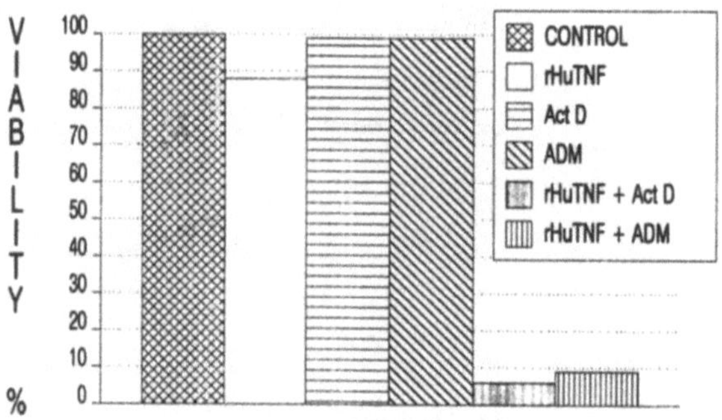

Fig. 3. Response of the rHuTNF-resistant bladder cancer cell line RT-4 to treatment with 200 U/ml *rHuTNF* and 1 ng/ml adriamycin *(ADM)*, 1 ng/ml adriamycin, 0.1 µg/ml actinomycin D *(Act D)*. *Control,* untreated cells

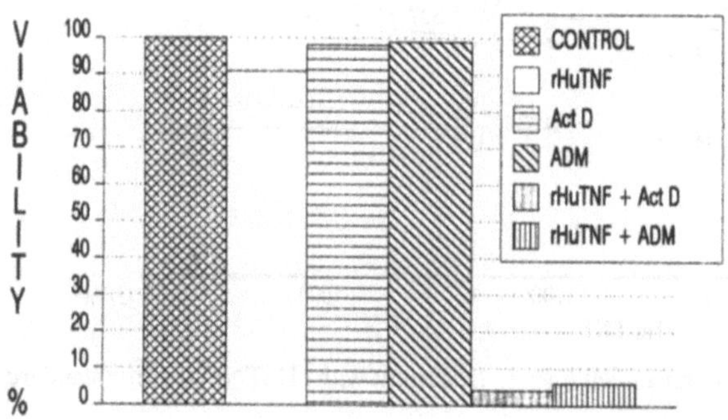

Fig. 4. Response of the rHuTNF-resistant bladder cancer cell line T-24 to treatment with 200 U/ml *rHuTNF* and 1 ng/ml adriamycin *(ADM)*, 1 ng/ml adriamycin, 0.1 µg/ml actinomycin D *(Act D)*. *Control,* untreated cells

from rHuTNF was seen. The combination of both agents resulted in a dose-dependent synergy of cytotoxicity, detected as an upward deflection of the dose-response curve in the presence of actinomycin D (Fig. 2). This deflection of the response curve was obvious in the combination of 1 µg/ml actinomycin D and 30 U/ml rHuTNF, a concentration with apparently no effect on the tumor cells, when given as a single agent. Hence, any effect of actinomycin D alone upon the cells was not detected.

We found similar results with adriamycin and rHuTNF. The TNF-resistant cell lines T-24 and RT-4 showed a synergistic enhanced cytotoxicity upon addition of both agents. The maximum effect was apparent with an rHuTNF concentration of 200 U/ml and 1 ng/ml of adriamycin. As already demonstrated with actinomycin D, adriamycin as a single agent has a negligible effect on these tumor cells, using the same concentrations as in the combination experiment (Figs. 3, 4).

Discussion

Optimal dosing and scheduling of treatment seems critical in determining the magnitude of cytotoxicity by rHuTNF. Whereas a 24-h continuous exposure of high doses of rHuTNF demonstrated a moderate response of most of the bladder cancer cell lines tested, cells exposed to lower concentrations of TNF and for shorter times recover (data not shown). Heterogeneity in the cell response to rHuTNF within the human bladder cancer cells may offer one explanation for this moderate response of the tumor cells. Another explanation may be that rHuTNF cytotoxicity is a multihit phenomenon, i.e., excess amounts of rHuTNF are constantly necessary to cause cell killing.

It is tempting to hypothesize that these tumor cells, like some normal cells, tend to be resistant to TNF-mediated cell killing because either they produce low levels of TNF or these cells have high levels of an endogeneous protective activity that renders them resistant to the rHuTNF action.

The increase in cytotoxicity of the human bladder cancer cells after addition of actinomycin D or adriamycin to rHuTNF has already been demonstrated in other cell systems (Ruff and Gifford 1981; Ostrove and Gifford 1979). The actinomycin D inhibits the RNA synthesis and interacts with the DNA topoisomerase II (Tewey et al. 1984), an enzyme which is able to catalyze the formation of various changed forms of DNA (Liu 1983). The topoisomerase targeted drugs like actinomycin D or adriamycin accumulate the changed DNA by stabilizing the usually transient reaction intermediate. As mentioned by Alexander and coworkers (1987a) the synergistic action of rHuTNF and topoisomerase-targeted drugs is closely related to the DNA damage caused. However, the exact mechanism of this action is still unknown.

The usefulness of rHuTNF as a single agent in the treatment of human bladder cancer remains to be determined; in vivo experiments with the murine bladder cancer cell line MBT-2 have been done (Lee et al. 1987). However, reports of rHuTNF as a single agent in other tumors are not very encouraging.

Our results are in agreement with the findings of others (Alexander et al. 1987b) and provide a good basis for future experiments regarding the combined treatment of bladder cancer with rHuTNF and topoisomerase-targeted chemotherapeutic drugs like adriamycin.

References

Alexander RB, Nelson WG, Coffey DS (1987a) Synergistic enhancement by tumor necrosis factor of in vitro cytotoxicity from chemotherapeutic drugs targeted at DNA topoisomerase II. Cancer Res 47:2403–2406

Alexander RB, Isaacs JT, Coffey DS (1987b) Tumor necrosis factor enhances the in vitro and in vivo efficacy of chemotherapeutic drugs targeted at DNA topoisomerase II in the treatment of murine bladder cancer. J Urol 138:427–429

Beutler B, Krochin N, Milsark IW, Luedke C, Cerami A (1986) Control of cachectin (tumor necrosis factor) synthesis: mechanisms of endotoxin resistance. Science 232:977–980

Carswell EA, Old LJ, Kassel RL, Green S, Fiore N, Williamson B (1975) An endotoxin-induced serum factor that causes necrosis of tumors. Proc Natl Acad Sci USA 72:3666–3670

Flick DA, Gifford GE (1984) Comparison of in vitro cell cytotoxic assays for tumor necrosis factor. J Immunol Methods 68:167–175

Haranaka K, Satomi N, Sakurai A (1984) Antitumor activity of murine tumor necrosis factor (TNF) against transplantable murine tumors and heterotransplanted human tumors in nude mice. Int J Cancer 34:263–267

Lee K-E, O'Donnell RW, Schoen S, Cockett ATK (1987) Effect of intravesical administration of tumor necrosis serum and human recombinant tumor necrosis factor on a murine bladder tumor. J Urol 138:430–432

Liu LF (1983) DNA topoisomerases – enzymes that catalyze the breaking and rejoining of DNA. CRC Crit Rev Biochem 15:1–24

Ostrove JM, Gifford GE (1979) Stimulation of RNA synthesis in L929 cells by rabbit tumor necrosis factor. Proc Soc Exp Med 160:354–358

Ruff MR, Gifford GE (1981) Tumor necrosis factor. In: Pick E (ed) Lymphokines, vol 2. Academic, New York, pp 235–272

Sugarman BJ, Aggarwal BB, Hass PE, Figari IS, Palladino MA, Shepard HM (1985) Recombinant tumor necrosis factor-α: effects on proliferation of normal and transformed cells in vitro. Science 230:943–945

Tewey KM, Rowe TC, Yang L, Halligan BD, Liu LF (1984) Adriamycin-induced DNA damage mediated by mammalian DNA topoisomerase II. Science 226:466–468

Vilcek J, Palombella V, Henriksen-Destefano D, Swenson C, Feinman R, Hirai M, Tsujimoto M (1986) Fibroblast growth enhancing activity of tumor necrosis factor and its relationship to other polypeptide growth factors. J Exp Med 163:632–643

Wang AM, Creasey AA, Ladner MB, Lin LS, Strickler J, van Arsdell JN, Yamamoto R, Mark DF (1985) Molecular cloning of the complementary DNA for human tumor necrosis factor. Science 228:149–154

Influence of Immunomodulation on Chemically Induced Bladder Tumors

F. Recker[1], S. Markos-Pustai[2], W. Küpper[3], and H. Rübben[4]

Introduction

The immunosurveillance theory describes that one of the factors responsible for the development of cancer is the extent of the immunoresponse (Klein 1975). Modulation of the immune system is possible by suppression or stimulation. Cyclosporine A is a powerful immunosuppressive drug which is used for the prevention of allograft rejection in organ transplant patients (Morris 1981). It is relatively specific for T lymphocytes and is thought to act by inhibiting the expression of antigen-induced signals from T cells necessary for the subsequent recruitment, proliferation, and maturation of the T-cell-dependent immune response (Lafferty and Borel 1983). In contrast, keyhole-limpet hemocyanin (KLH) is known to produce a nonspecific immune stimulation. Klippel et al. (1977) injected this agent submucosally into the bladder wall of sensitized and nonsensitized rats. A marked inflammatory reaction was noted with a typical mononuclear cell infiltration without ulceration. A measurable antitumor effect in transplantable murine bladder tumors (MBT2) by KLH was reported by Lamm et al. (1982). In contrast, Walsh et al. (1983) could not find any effect of KLH in a chemically induced (FANFT) murine bladder tumor model. We used a well-established model of bladder carcinoma, chemically initiated by *N*-butyl-*N*(4 hydroxybutyl) nitrosamin (BBN). The following project was performed to evaluate the influence of two contrary immunoregimens on chemically induced bladder cancer.

Materials and Methods

Immunosuppression. In a first series, 175 Wistar rats with an average weight of 200 g were randomized into five groups (Fig. 1). The carcinogen BBN was administered as a 0.05% solution in the drinking water over a period of 8 weeks. CsA was dissolved in olive oil and ethyl alcohol and administered orally to experimental animals at doses ranging from 5 mg/kg per day (group II) to 12.5 mg/kg per day (group III) over a period of 11 weeks. Group I received only BBN; groups IV and V were treated exclusively with CsA. Details of the different experiments carried out in the five groups are shown in Fig. 1. CsA blood levels were sampled in half of each group using radioimmuno assay (RIA). Sample checks were made on creatine and ureate

[1] Dept. of Urology, University Hospital, Zürich, Switzerland
[2] Dept. of Med. Immunology, RWTH Aachen, 5100 Aachen, FRG
[3] Dept. of Veterinary Medicine, RWTH Aachen, 5100 Aachen, FRG
[4] Dept. of Urology, Knappschaftskrankenhaus Bardenberg, FRG

Investigative Urology 3
Edited by H. Rübben et al.

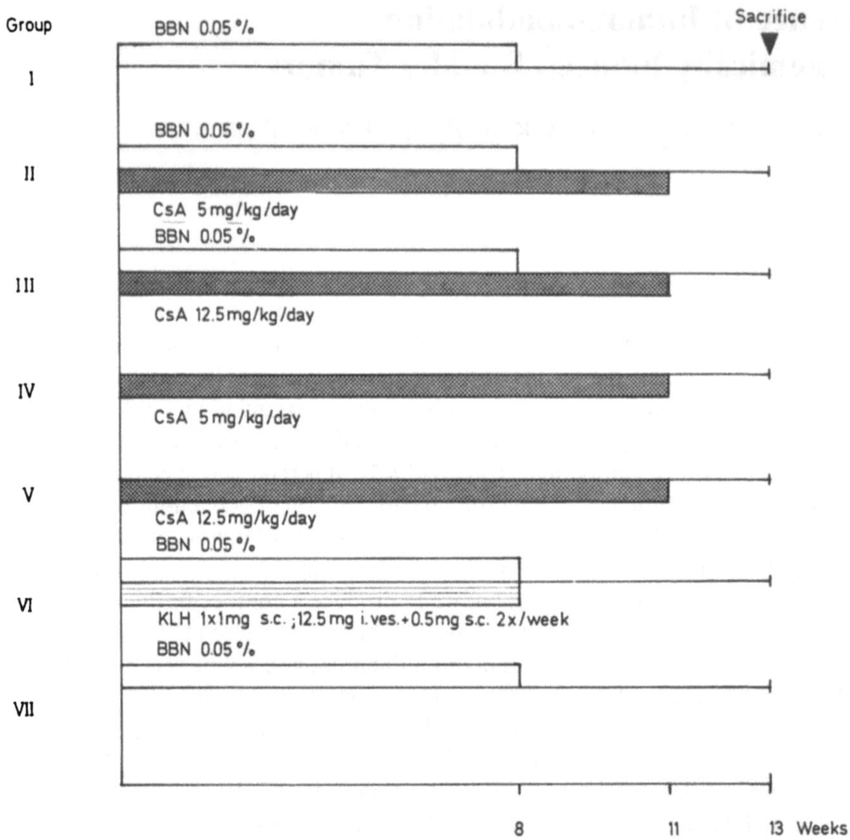

Fig. 1. Schematic presentation of the protocol used for the induction of bladder carcinoma in Wistar rats with 0.05% BBN in the drinking water. Immunosuppression by CsA, immunostimulation by KLH

levels in the blood specimen, and the blood count was analyzed. All animals were killed at the end of the 13th week using ether.

Immunostimulation. In the second experiment, 40 male Wistar rats (group VI) were treated after being sensitized with 1 × 1 mg KLH into the foot pad two times a week with 12.5 mg KLH intravesical and 0.5 mg KLH subcutaneously over a period of 8 weeks (Fig. 1). Simultaneously, the carcinogen BBN was administered as a 0.05% solution in the drinking water over the same period. The control group consisted also of 40 male Wistar rats receiving only BBN in the same way as group VI. Interleukin 2 was determined in half of each group. At the end of the 13th week the animals were killed. The histological examinations of bladder, ureter, kidney, liver, lung, and thymus were fixed in 8% formalin, embedded in paraffin, and stained for microscopic study with hematoxylin and eosin. The bladder was dissected into four rings, each divided into sixteen segments. A percentage tumor expansion and invasion for each segment was determined according to a point system. Statistical analysis was performed using the Student's *t* distribution. Results were considered to differ significantly if the probability of error was less than 0.05%.

Results

Immunosuppression. Exophytic tumors displayed extensive epithelial proliferation with a tendency to formation of papillomas. Cellular irregularity was slight to moderate, and a few mitotic figures were detected in the proliferative areas of the bladder epithelium. Infiltrative tumors crossed the lamina propria and were more irregular in appearance than exophytic bladder tumors. Using the previously described point system, the proportion of the bladder affected by tumors was determined. Group 1, receiving solely 0.05% BBN, had a proportion of 4.2 ± 0.4% exophytic and 0.7% ± 0.08% infiltrative tumors in the bladder. In contrast, rats treated with BBN and low dose CsA (group II) developed a twofold higher incidence of exophytic urothelial tumors than group I and a threefold higher incidence of infiltrative transitional cell tumors (Table 1). Tumor enhancement was greatest in group III: 11.6 ± 1.4% of the bladder surface was covered by exophytic urothelial tumors, three times more than group I. The proportion of infiltrative tumors in group III amounted to 3.31 ± 0.4%, a four and a half-fold increase over group I.

Statistical significance for the exophytic tumors was $P < 0.004$, for the infiltrative urothelial carcinoma $P < 0.001$. Neither bladder tumors nor hyperplasia were detected in groups IV and V. None of the animals displayed any metastasis. The intakes of 0.05% BBN in groups I, II, and III were similar throughout the experimental period. CsA serum levels ranged from low values of 251 ± 106 ng/ml (group II) and 203 ± 93 ng/ml (group IV) to toxic values of 1238 ± 505 ng/ml (group III) and 1340 ± 580 ng/ml (group V).

Immunostimulation. In group VI (KLH stimulated) the proportion of exophytic tumors amounted to 9.8 ± 2.7% in contrast to group VII (only BBN) in which the percentage of papillary tumors was 14.2 ± 2.8%. Infiltrative tumors were also lower in group VI compared with the unstimulated group VII ($P < 0.05$). The BBN intake was similar in both groups in spite of more being given than in groups I, II, and III, which is responsible for the higher tumor induction in control group VII compared with group I. The interleukin 2 levels in the KLH-treated rats were higher (7.2 U/ml) than in the BBN control rats (3.2 U/ml) and untreated rats (3.0 U/ml).

Table 1. Percentage of bladder tumor expansion. A CsA dose-dependent enhancement (II, III) of bladder tumor induction was observed. Under immunostimulation with KLH (VI) bladder tumor induction was reduced compared with controls (VII)

	I	II	III	IV	V	VI	VII
Exophytic	4.2 ± 0.4%	8.0 ± 0.9%	11.6 ± 1.4%	∅	∅	9.8 ± 2.7%	14.2 ± 2.8%
Infiltrative	0.7 ± 0.08%	2.5 ± 0.3%	3.3 ± 0.4%	∅	∅	2.7 ± 1.6%	4.6 ± 1.3%

Discussion

The results of our experiments demonstrate that modulation of the immunosystem has a marked effect on BBN-induced bladder tumors. BBN fulfills the criteria for a classic tumor initiator. It is known to produce bladder tumors selectively in great numbers after a short induction period (Druckrey et al. 1964). Besides the initiation, the promotion is one step in the process of carcinogenesis. The promoting agent CsA alone had no tumorigenic effect (groups IV, V); thus the immunosuppression must contribute a tumor-promoting environment. The decrease in immunosurveillance can be mediated by a lower activation of T helper cells through inhibition of interleukin 1 secretion and diminished interleukin 2 production (Bunjes et al. 1984) in T helper cells. A subsequent reduced activation of cytotoxic T cells and an NK-cell deficiency under CsA may be postulated as the reason for the observed enhanced tumor induction. In contrast, the results after nonspecific immunostimulation with KLH represent a marked reducing effect on chemically induced bladder carcinoma. The enhanced interleukin 2 levels after KLH administration confirmed the stimulation effect. Findings are similar to those reported by Lamm et al. (1981); he showed that intralesional KLH in presensitized mice resulted in a significant reduction of tumor growth with prolongation of animal survival. In contrast, Walsh et al. (1983) failed in preventing the subcutaneous or intravesical growth of FANFT-induced bladder tumors by immunostimulation with KLH. In spite of this, our results after immunostimulation support recent clinical reports about prevention of recurrent superficial bladder cancer by KLH (Jurinic et al. 1988) and confirm the concept of immunotherapy in bladder cancer.

Summary

The effects of immunomodulation on the induction of bladder carcinoma were investigated in Wistar rats using *N*-butyl-*N*(4 hydroxybutyl) nitrosamine (BBN) as a known initiator of bladder carcinoma. In a first series the immunosystem was suppressed by Cyclosporine A (CsA). Rats treated with 0.05% BBN + CsA 5 mg/kg/day or CsA 12.5 mg/kg/day orally developed a CsA dose dependent (2–4 fold) enhancement of bladder tumor expansion as compared to 0.05% BBN application alone. In contrast immunomodulation by stimulation with Keyhole-Limpet Haemocyanin (KLH) 12.5 mg i.ves. + 0.5 mg s.c./2×/week after being sensitized with 1 mg KLH s.c., resulted in a reduction of BBN induced bladder tumors. The results confirm the immunosurveillance theory that effective expression of immune response may be important in the control of tumor development. The effective immunostimulation by KLH support the concept of immunotherapy in bladder cancer.

References

Bunjes D, Hardt C, Röllinhoff M (1984) Cyclosporine A mediates immunosuppression of primary cytotoxic T cell responses by imparing the release of interleukin 1 and interleukin 2. Eur J Immunol II:657

Druckrey H, Preussmann R, Ivankovic S, Schmidt C, Stahl K (1964) Selective Erzeugung von Blasenkrebs an Ratten durch Dibutyl and *N*-Butyl-*n*-butanol (4) nitrosamin. Z Krebsforschung 66: 280

Jurinic CG, Engelmann U, Gasch J, Klippel K (1988) Immunotherapy in bladder cancer with keyhole-limpet haemocyanin: a randomized study. J Urol 139: 723

Klein G (1975) Immunological surveillance against neoplasia. Harvey Lectures 69: 71

Klippel KF, Paulini G, Hutschenreiter G (1977) The effect of keyhole-limpet haemocyanin (KLH) on the rat bladder. Cancer Immunol Immunother 3: 65

Lafferty K, Borel JF (1983) Hypothesis about the mechanism of action of Cyclosporine A. Proc 1st Inter Congr Cyclosporine, Houston, TX

Lamm DL, Reyna JA, Reichert DF (1981) Keyhole-limpet haemocyanin and immune ribonucleic acid immunotherapy of murine transitional cell carcinoma. Urol Res 9: 227

Lamm DL, Reichert DF, Harris SC, Lucio RM (1982) Immunotherapy of murine transitional cell carcinoma. J Urol 128: 1104

Morris PJ (1981) Cyclosporine A. Transplantation 38: 349

Walsh WG, Tomashefsky P, Olsson CA, de Vere White R (1983) Keyhole-limpet haemocyanin (KLH) immunotherapy of murine transitional cell carcinoma. Urol Res 11: 263

Effects of High Energy Shock Waves on BBN-Induced Bladder Tumors in Rats

N. Fischer, F.-J. Deutz, N. Meyers, and H. Rübben[1]

Introduction

At the time of introduction of extracorporal shock wave lithotripsy (ESWL) into the clinical treatment of urinary calculi, it was regarded as completely harmless and non-traumatizing to biological tissues (Chaussy et al. 1986c). First experiments on leukocyte cultures revealed no influence of high energy shock waves on the proliferative activity of human cells.

With the spread of the method, more and more groups were concerned with its side effects on kidney parenchyma, and it had been noticed that ESWL causes tissue damage of marked extent (Muschter et al. 1987). Interstitial edema and multiple hemorrhages were observed, mainly due to glomerular and tubular lesions and ruptures of small vessels at the corticomedullar junction (Recker et al. 1988). Cavitation effects turned out to be the most probable cause of these tissue injuries (Fischer et al. 1988).

Previously, working groups of Chaussy and Fair reported on some effects of shock waves on malignant cells in vitro and in vivo and postulated a partially selective antiproliferative activity of shock wave exposition (Chaussy et al. 1986a, b; Fair et al. 1986; Russo et al. 1986). The aim of our investigations was to evaluate the effects of high energy shock waves in a chemically induced carcinoma. Tumor induction was performed with *N*-butyl-N-(4-hydroxybutyl)-nitrosamine in female Wistar rats. This bladder tumor model is well-established in our institution and has been used for several experiments before.

A pilot test with cress semen (Müller and Fischer, personal communication, 1987) showed a delay of sprout and a reduction of growth after shock wave exposure as a hint to the antiproliferative effect and encouraged us to perform animal experiments.

Methods

Epithelial bladder tumors were induced in female Wistar rats by 0.05% BBN in the drinking water for 12 weeks. Beginning in the 9th week, 6×250 high energy shock waves (HESW) of 14 kV were applied either alone or in combination with intravesical instillation of 2.0 mg/ml *cis*-platinum (DDP) over a period of 4 weeks. Control groups were instillated only with *cis*-platinum or saline solution. One week after the last treatment cycle, the animals were killed. The extent of superficial and infiltrative tumor growth was estimated by light microscopy. Due to the disappointing results of this first series of investigations, the experimental setup was modified in a second series. Therapy was not started until termination of tumor induction in the 12th week, shock wave energy was increased to 24 kV, shock wave treatment was com-

[1] Dept. of Urology, Klinikum der RWTH, Aachen, 5100 Aachen, FRG

Investigative Urology 3
Edited by H. Rübben et al.

bined with a systemic chemotherapy with 1 mg/kg *cis*-platinum, and the intervals between the treatment courses were shortened to 6 treatments in 2 weeks.

This resulted in the following experimental setup:

1. Series of experiments
Group A.1: 6 × 250 HESW + DDP intravesical ($n = 29$)
Group A.2: 6 × 250 HESW ($n = 22$)
Group A.3: DDP intravesical ($n = 21$)
Group A.4: control group ($n = 21$)
2. Series of experiments
Group B.1: 6 × 250 HESW + DDP intravenous ($n = 30$)
Group B.2: 6 × 250 HESW ($n = 25$)
Group B.3: DDP intravenous ($n = 25$)
Group B.4: control group ($n = 20$)

Results

Superficial necrosis and edema of the bladder wall were observed as typical effects of shock wave application. Hemorrhages were only found in group B.1 with a combination of HESW and systemic administration of *cis*-platinum. Organs with near relation to the bladder, especially the intestine, showed no pathological changes.

With a combination of shock wave treatment and intravesical chemotherapy, a slight reduction of superficial tumor growth could be achieved in the first experi-

Table 1. First series of experiments (12 weeks tumor induction, 6 × 250 HESW 14 kV 9th–12th week)

	Infiltrative tumor	Exophytic tumor	Lethality
HESW + DDP i.ves.	4.0%	12.0%	27.6%
HESW	5.2%	18.1%	4.5%
DDP i.ves.	3.8%	15.8%	–
Control	3.4%	17.6%	–
Kruskal-Wallis test	$P = 0.41$	$P = 0.11$	

Table 2. Second series of experiments (12 weeks tumor induction, 6 × 250 HESW 24 kV 13th–14th week)

	Infiltrative tumor	Exophytic tumor	Lethality
HESW + DDP i.ves.	4.1%	15.3%	20.0%
HESW	4.3%	14.3%	12.0%
DDP i.ves.	1.3%	10.9%	12.0%
Control	7.8%	23.4%	12.0%
Kruskal-Wallis test	$P = 0.0001$	$P = 0.0034$	

ment, whereas infiltrative tumor growth was not influenced. The second series of experiments showed a statistical significant suppression of both superficial and infiltrative tumor growth either by systemic *cis*-platinum therapy or by shock wave application. There was no additional effect, when both therapies were combined (Tables 1, 2).

Discussion

In our experiments, we could demonstrate that both high energy shock waves and systemic therapy with *cis*-platinum can reduce the growing of BBN-induced bladder tumors in rats. As there is no synergism between these two therapies, we conclude that the effect of high energy shock waves on the tumor tissue is unspecific and energy-dependent. There is no hint as to a selective antiproliferative mechanism of shock waves in neoplastic cells.

Nevertheless, our results indicate that the spatial configuration of tumors can be influenced by shock wave exposure. This is probably due to the tissue damage caused by cavitation effects.

Therefore, in opposition to the aims of development in shock wave lithotripsy, cavitation has to be maximized when used in tumor treatment. First experiments have been performed by Hahn and Riedlinger (Hahn et al. 1988) using high energy pulsed ultrasound to produce strong cavitation in subcutaneous transplanted tumors in nude mice. The same morphological findings as in our investigation were observed. Further investigations are needed to see whether these effects can be enhanced by using weak reflectors to produce tensile waves instead of regular shock waves.

References

Chaussy C, Randazzo R, Fuchs G (1986a) The effects of extracorporeal shock waves on FANFT bladder tumours in C3H/He mice. J Urol 135:739

Chaussy C, Randazzo R, Fuchs G (1986b) The effects of extracorporeal shock waves on human renal carcinoma cells and normal embryonic kidney cells. J Urol 135:864

Chaussy C, Schmiedt E, Jocham D, Fuchs G, Brendel W (1986c) Extracorporeal shock wave lithotripsy: technical concept, experimental research, and clinical application. Karger, Basel

Fair W, Yang C, Russo P (1986) The effect of high energy shock waves on the G2 and M phases of the cell cycle as determined by flow cytometry and clonogenic assay. J Urol 135:867

Fischer N, Müller H, Gülhan A, Sohn M, Deutz F, Rübben H, Lutzeyer W (1988) Cavitation effects. J Endourol 2:215

Hahn E, Riedlinger R, Mattern J, Überle W, Bak M, Peschke P, Lorenz A, Zuna I, Gerlach L, Volm M, van Kaick G, Lorenz W (1988) High energy pulsed ultrasound: cytotoxic effects on rodent tumors. Biomed Technik 33/2:141

Muschter R, Schmeller N, Kutscher K, Reimers I, Hofstetter A, Löhrs U (1987) Morphologische Nierenveränderungen durch die Anwendung der extracorporalen Stoßwellenlithotripsie und ihr klinisches Korrelat. In: Verhandlungsbericht der Deutschen Gesellschaft für Urologie, 39. Springer, Berlin Heidelberg New York

Recker F, Fischer N, Rübben H, Deutz F (1988) Rasterelektronen- und lichtmikroskopische Veränderungen der Nieren unter dem neuen Stoßgenerator des Lithotriptors HM3. In: Verhandlungsbericht der Deutschen Gesellschaft für Urologie. Springer, Berlin Heidelberg New York

Russo P, Stephenson R, Mies C, Huryk R, Heston W, Melamed M, Fair W (1986) High energy shock waves suppress tumor growth in vitro and in vivo. J Urol 135:626

V. Urodynamics

Papaverine in Human Bladder Muscle

L. Hertle[1] and H. Nawrath[2]

Introduction

It is generally assumed that drugs which induce relaxation of smooth muscles may be of clinical importance in some urological disorders; such drugs are indeed widely used, for example, in the therapy of unstable bladders or to facilitate the passage of ureteral stones. Recently, papaverine has been shown to be very effective, e.g., in relaxing smooth muscles of the corpus cavernosum penis, thereby inducing erections in many impotent men (Virag 1982). The purpose of this study is to determine the relaxing properties of papaverine in isolated muscle strips from the human detrusor and to evaluate its potential clinical importance.

Materials and Methods

Detrusor specimens from the dome of the bladder were taken from seven patients (six male, one female) with a mean age of 58 years (range 49–68), who were undergoing radical cystectomy because of bladder carcinoma. None of these patients had received radiation therapy or chemotherapy prior to operation, and all patients had sterile urine cultures. All tissue specimens were taken from a macroscopically normal part of the detrusor. Immediately after removal of the bladder, the tissue specimen (1 or 2 from each patient) were immersed in cold (4°C) Tyrode solution. The serosal and mucosal layers were carefully dissected away, and up to 16 muscle pieces, approximately 10 by 3–4 mm and weighing 50–100 mg, were excised from each specimen. Some of the preparations were used within 2–4 h after the operation, while some were stored at 4°C for up to 24 h. No qualitative or quantitative differences in response were found between muscle strips which were used within 4 h after cystectomy and those which were used 24 h later.

Contractions. By tying both ends with fine silk sutures (5 × 0) the preparations were suspended in 10-ml organ baths containing Tyrode solution at 37°C gassed with 95% O_2 and 5% CO_2. The tension was measured under isometric conditions with inductive force displacement transducers and recorded on paper. The preload tension was adjusted to 10 m*N*. An interval of at least an hour was allowed for equilibration, after which the experiments were performed.

Solutions. The Tyrode solution used was prepared with distilled, deionized water and had the following composition (in mmol/l): NaCl 136.9, KCl 5.4, $MgCl_2$ 1.05,

[1] Department of Urology, University of Bochum, 4630 Bochum, FRG
[2] Department of Pharmacology, University of Mainz, 6500 Mainz, FRG

Investigative Urology 3
Edited by H. Rübben et al.

NaH_2PO_4 0.42, $NaHCO_3$ 11.9, $CaCl_2$ 5.4, and glucose 5.5. The pH of the solution was 7.2. The Tyrode solution used for potassium-induced contractions contained KCl 85 mmol/l and NaCl 57.3 mmol/l; the other ingredients remained the same as above. The stock solutions of norepinephrine, phenylephrine, serotonin, histamine, carbachol, and papaverine were prepared in distilled water. From these stock solutions, desired concentrations of the drugs were prepared in Tyrode solution and added in appropriate volume into the muscle bath to give the desired final concentrations. The pH was maintained at 7.2 ± 0.1. The experimental arrangement permitted a rapid exchange (1–2 s) of solutions.

Drugs. The following drugs were used: carbamoyl choline hydrochloride (carbachol, Merck), histamine 2-hydrochloride (Serva), L-norepinephrine bitartrate (Serva), L-phenylephrine hydrochloride (Boehringer), serotonin creatinine sulfate (Merck), and papaverine hydrochloride (Serva).

At the end of each experiment the preparations were blotted with filter paper for 90 s under constant pressure (280 g) and weighed. Concentrations given are the final concentrations of drugs in the organ bath in moles/liter. The EC_{50} value of papaverine was determined graphically, taking into account 2 points on the steep portion of each individual concentration-response curve, and geometric mean values were calculated. Results are expressed as means ± standard error of the means (SEM).

Results

Norepinephrine, phenylephrine, and serotonin in concentrations of 10^{-4} mol/l had only very small effects on the tension of isolated human bladder dome preparations. In contrast, histamine (10^{-4} mol/l), carbachol (10^{-4} mol/l), and high extracellular potassium concentrations (85 mmol/l) produced strong increases in tension, carbachol being the strongest stimulatory agent. Therefore, carbachol and high potassium were used as stimulants to study the relaxing properties of papaverine.

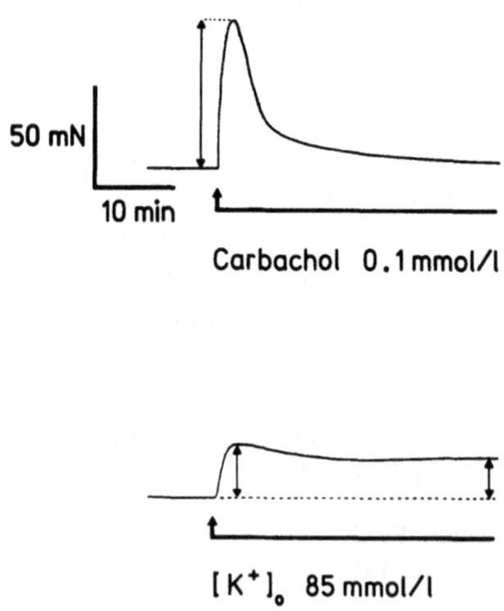

Fig. 1. Original recording of effects of carbachol 10^{-4} mol/l and extracellular potassium concentration (85 mmol/l) on tension of muscle strips of human bladder dome ($CaCl_2$: 1.8 mmol/l). Carbachol-induced contractions were transient in nature, whereas stimulation by high potassium produced a stable plateau following an initial tension peak

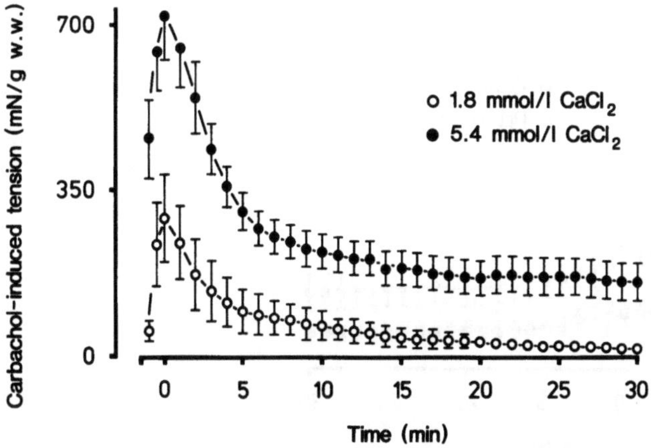

Fig. 2. Time course of effects of carbachol 10^{-4} mol/l on tension of isolated human bladder muscle at two different extracellular calcium concentrations. *Open circles,* 1.8 mmol/l $CaCl_2$ ($n = 4$, two patients); *closed circles,* 5.4 mmol/l $CaCl_2$ ($n = 20$, seven patients). Means ± SEM; *w.w.*, wet weight

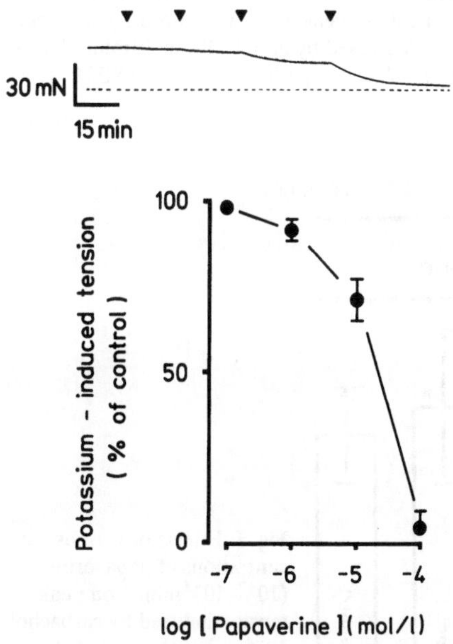

Fig. 3. Effects of papaverine on residual (plateau) tension induced by extracellular potassium 85 mmol/l. Original recording and concentration-response curve. Means ± SEM ($n = 12$, three patients)

The response to carbachol was biphasic and transient in nature (original recording is shown in Fig. 1). After an initial rapid increase in tension, which peaked, tension continuously decreased in a second phase. The decrease in tension returned to baseline level within 20 min, when the extracellular calcium concentration was 1.8 mmol/l (Fig. 2). At a calcium concentration of 5.4 mmol/l carbachol produced a significantly higher increase in peak tension and a more sustained plateau in the fading phase (Fig. 2).

Depolarization of the detrusor muscle strips with an extracellular potassium concentration of 85 mmol/l induced a rapid increase in tension, which peaked and was followed by partial relaxation and sustained contraction (original recording is shown in Fig. 1).

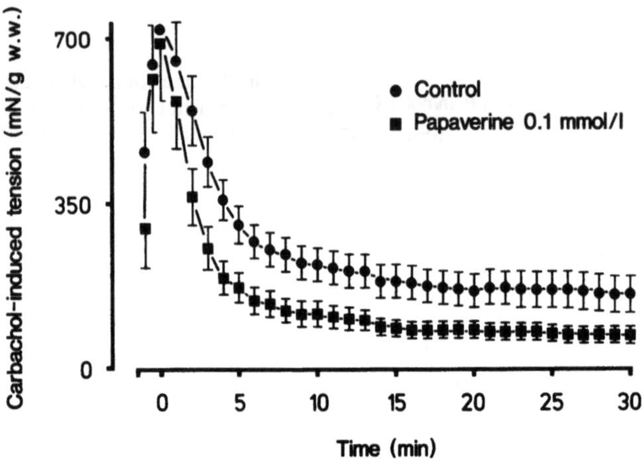

Fig. 4. Time course of effects of papaverine 100 μmol/l on carbachol-induced tension of isolated human bladder muscle. Papaverine had virtually no effect on peak tension induced by carbachol 10^{-4} mol/l. Fading was accelerated and steady state was depressed by about 54% at 30 min. *Circles,* control ($n = 20$, seven patients); *squares,* papaverine ($n = 7$, seven patients). Means ± SEM; *w.w.,* wet weight

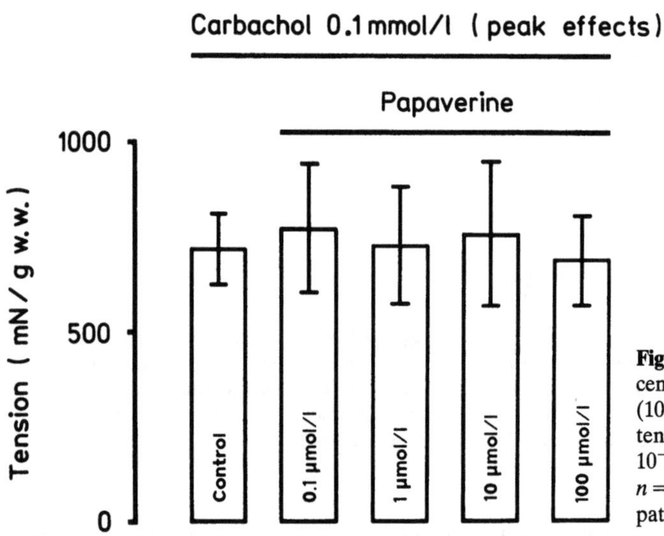

Fig. 5. Effects of various concentrations of papaverine (10^{-7}–10^{-4} mol/l) on peak tension induced by carbachol 10^{-4} mol/l. Means ± SEM; $n = 7$ in each group, seven patients; *w.w.,* wet weight

Figure 3 displays the relaxing effects of papaverine in high potassium-induced contractions. The muscle strips were activated with an extracellular potassium concentration of 85 mmol/l at a calcium concentration of 5.4 mmol/l. After the contraction had stabilized papaverine was added cumulatively, allowing time between additions for stabilization of relaxation. The inhibition of depolarization-induced contraction was measured as a function of drug concentration. The values are given as percentages of inhibition of equilibrium contraction (control) after depolarization. A concentration of papaverine of 10^{-7} mol/l was the threshold for relaxing activity, and the potassium-induced activation was completely antagonized at a concentration of

10^{-4} mol/l. The concentration of papaverine producing half maximum relaxation was 2.1×10^{-5} mol/l.

The effects of papaverine on carbachol-induced contractions were also studied at extracellular calcium concentrations of 5.4 mmol/l. In the control group ($n = 20$, seven patients) muscle strips were activated with carbachol 10^{-4} mol/l. In the test group ($n = 7$, in each group, seven patients) the muscle strips were preincubated for 60 min with papaverine in concentrations of 10^{-7} to 10^{-4} mol/l. Peak tension and the time course of tension generation were evaluated under control and test conditions. Figure 4 presents the time course of the effects of papaverine 10^{-4} mol/l on carbachol-induced contractions. The concentration-response relationships of papaverine on peak tension of detrusor strips activated by carbachol are displayed in Fig. 5. Both figures clearly show that papaverine, even at high concentrations of 10^{-4} mol/l, had no significant effects on peak tension generation. However, the fading of the carbachol-induced peak response was accelerated by papaverine. The steady state tension at 30 min which amounted to 24% ± 5% of peak tension under control conditions was reduced by papaverine 10^{-4} mol/l by about 54%.

Discussion

In the present study we found that contractions induced by carbachol and high extracellular potassium in human isolated bladder muscle were differently affected by papaverine. In carbachol-induced contractions, papaverine, even in high concentrations of 10^{-4} mol/l, had virtually no effects on peak tension generation, whereas the fading was accelerated, and the steady state tension at 30 min was reduced by about 54%. In contrast, high potassium-induced contractions were relaxed by papaverine in a concentration-dependent way; a concentration of papaverine of 10^{-4} mol/l produced full relaxation.

In our experiments carbachol and high extracellular potassium proved to be the two most prominent means of activation of bladder smooth muscle. It is well-established that carbachol and high potassium differ in the way they induce contractions: carbachol acts by binding to its specific muscarinic receptors on the smooth muscle membrane, and high potassium acts by depolarization of the cell membrane, which is not related to any specific receptor activation (Bolton 1979).

Papaverine is a non-specific smooth muscle relaxant and is thought to act at a site distal to the cholinergic receptor site. However, the precise mode of its action is unknown. One possible mechanism is related to cyclic adenosine 3′5′-monophosphate (cAMP). Pöch et al. (1969) first reported an inhibition of cAMP breakdown in vitro by a number of spasmolytic drugs. An increase in cAMP is supposed to lead to an enhanced calcium binding to membrane and intracellular storage sites, thereby reducing influx and/or release of calcium. A rise in cAMP may be induced by an inhibition of phosphodiesterase, which degrades cAMP to 5′-adenosine monophosphate (5′AMP). Papaverine has been described as inhibiting cAMP phosphodiesterase activity of smooth muscle, causing a rise in cAMP levels (for review, see Bolton 1979).

An alternative mechanism of smooth muscle relaxation was proposed by Grün et al. (1969) and Fleckenstein et al. (1971) for verapamil and some other drugs with relaxing properties. Inhibition of transmembrane calcium influx, first observed with verapamil and D600 in the heart (Fleckenstein et al. 1968), was suggested to be their mechanism of action.

Many of papaverine's actions might possibly be explained if it is assumed that it blocks calcium ion channels in the cell membrane (Bolton 1979). In many smooth muscles papaverine reduces tension induced by high extracellular potassium concentrations and inhibits ^{45}Ca uptake from the preparations when stimulated by high potassium depolarization (for review, see Bolton 1979; Huddart et al. 1984). Contractions induced by high extracellular potassium concentrations are easily blocked by low concentrations of calcium channel blockers, suggesting that the continuing entry of calcium through the membrane is necessary to keep the contractile machinery activated (Högestätt and Andersson 1984). The data presented here confirm the earlier postulate that papaverine inhibits calcium influx (Bolton 1979; Huddart et al. 1984).

The mechanisms responsible for the peak tension generation in carbachol-induced contractions are obviously not affected by papaverine even in high concentrations. On the other hand, papaverine accelerates the fading and reduces the steady state tension of carbachol-induced contractions, suggesting some effects on the not yet defined calcium movements in that phase of the carbachol-induced contraction. However, so little is known about the cellular mechanism of papaverine's action that at present this study cannot add substantial information to the understanding of the calcium movements during carbachol-induced contractions.

In order to establish whether papaverine is useful clinically, double-blind studies should be performed. Although papaverine had little effects on carbachol-induced contractions it cannot be excluded that the drug is effective in diseases in which noncholinergic mechanisms are involved.

References

Bolton TB (1979) Mechanism of action of transmitters and other substances on smooth muscle. Physiol Rev 59:606–718

Fleckenstein A, Grün G, Tritthart H, Byon K, Harding P (1971) Uterus-Relaxation durch hochaktive Ca^{++}-antagonistische Hemmstoffe der elektromechanischen Koppelung wie Isoptin (Verapamil, Iproveratril), Substanz D600 und Segontin (Prenylamin). Klin Wochenschr 49: 32–41

Fleckenstein A, Döring HJ, Kammermeier H (1968) Einfluß von Beta-Rezeptorenblockern und verwandten Substanzen auf Erregung, Kontraktion und Energiestoffwechsel der Myokardfaser. Klin Wochenschr 46:343–351

Grün G, Fleckenstein A, Tritthart H (1969) Elektromechanische Entkoppelung durch muskulotrope Relaxantien der Uterusmuskulatur. Naunyn-Schmiedebergs Arch Pharmacol 264:239–240

Högestätt ED, Andersson KE (1984) Mechanism behind the biphasic contractile response to potassium depolarization in isolated rat cerebral arteries. J Pharm Exp Ther 228:187–195

Huddart H, Langton PD, Saad KHM (1984) Inhibition by papaverine of calcium movements and tension in the smooth muscles of rat vas deferens and urinary bladder. J Physiol 349:183–194

Pöch G, Juan H, Kukovetz WR (1969) Einfluß von herz- und gefäßwirksamen Substanzen auf die Aktivität der Phosphodiesterase. Naunyn-Schmiedebergs Arch Pharmacol 264:293–294

Virag R (1982) Intracavernous injection of papaverine for erectile failure. Lancet ii:983 (Letter to the Editor)

On the Locational Dependency and Diuresis Dependency of the Ureteral Dynamic: An Experimental Study in the Endoureteral Simultaneous Measurement of Pressure and Developed Force

J. POHL and U. DAMBACHER[1]

Introduction

The driving force of urine transport originates in the muscular contraction ring which, under normal conditions, closes the ureteral lumen and progresses towards the bladder. All previous methodical approaches to the in vivo investigation of the dynamics of urine transport have largely concentrated on secondary phenomena such as intraluminal pressure and urine flow, or on the electrical potentials which accompany the muscular contraction. We were able to show in a previous study that it is possible, using a catheter which we developed, to measure the forces occurring in the contraction ring (Pohl et al. 1986). With the present study we want to investigate on the one hand, how the contracting forces change over the whole course of the ureter and on the other hand, how they change with increased diuresis.

Methods

A ureteral catheter, specially developed for the simultaneous registration of force and pressure, was cystoscopically inserted into 12 pyeloureteral units from 8 mongrel dogs. Individual measurements of locational dependency were taken at defined positions in the ureter. Following intravenous administration of 0.5 mg/kg body weight of furosemide and consequently increased diuresis, measurements were taken in the central third of the ureter over a period of 120 min with the bladder empty.

The longitudinal section of the measuring probe (Fig. 1), which is mounted on a 5F vein catheter, shows the main element, the measuring window, into which the free end of the force-measuring cantilever protrudes. At the base of the cantilever are attached highly sensitive strain gauges which modulate electrical signals in analogue response to forces acting on the cantilever.

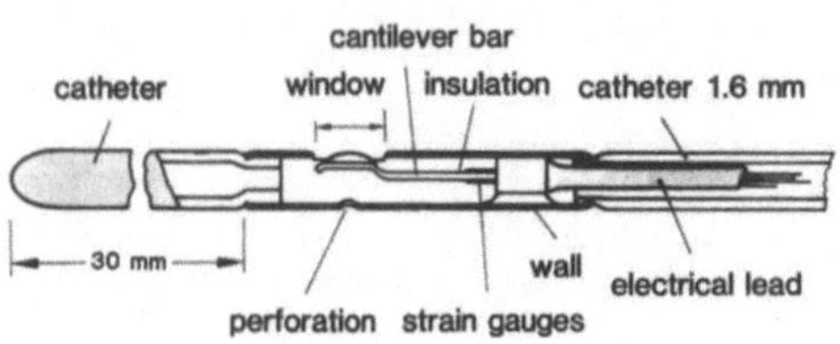

Fig. 1. Two-channel measuring catheter to register force and pressure. Longitudinal section of measuring probe

[1] Urologische Klinik und Poliklinik der Westf. Wilhelms-Universität, 4400 Münster, FRG

Investigative Urology 3
Edited by H. Rübben et al.

The measured value in m*N* is a measure of the force with which the ring-shaped contraction narrows or closes the luminal cross section. The intraluminal pressure is recorded simultaneously by means of a second channel.

Results

An example of the simultaneous registration of force (F) and of intraluminal pressure (P) is shown in Fig. 2. First of all the bolus pressure superimposes on the basal

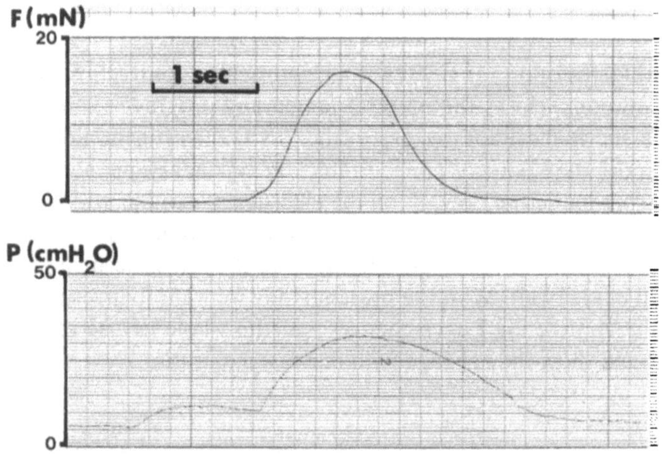

Fig. 2. Simultaneous registration of developed force *(F)* and pressure *(P)*

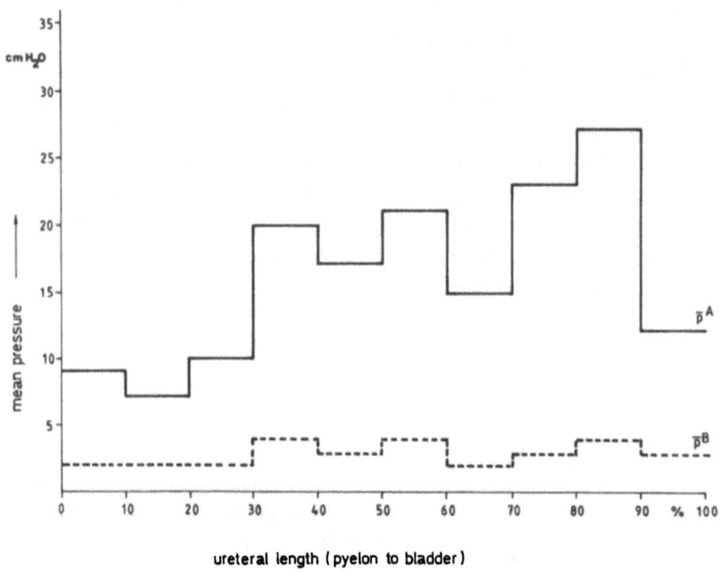

Fig. 3. Mean basal pressure *($\bar{p}B$)* and mean pressure amplitudes *($\bar{p}A$)* depending on point of measurement in the ureter

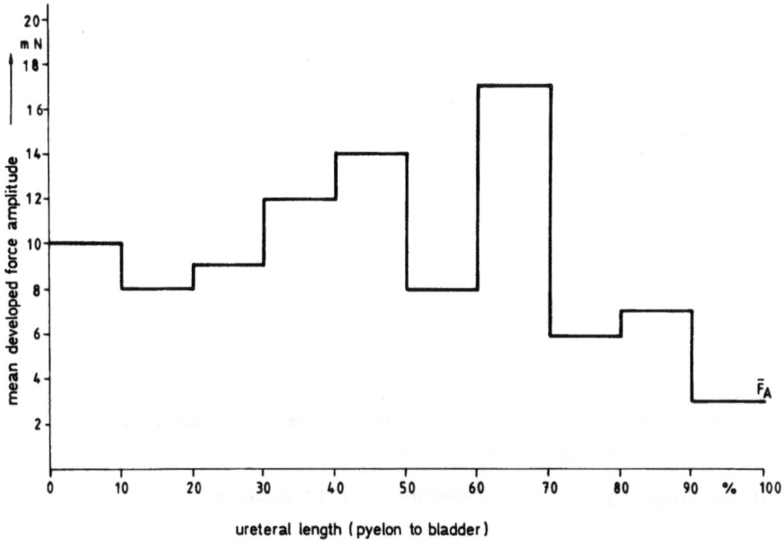

Fig. 4. Mean force amplitude *($\bar{F}_A$)* depending upon point of measurement in the ureter

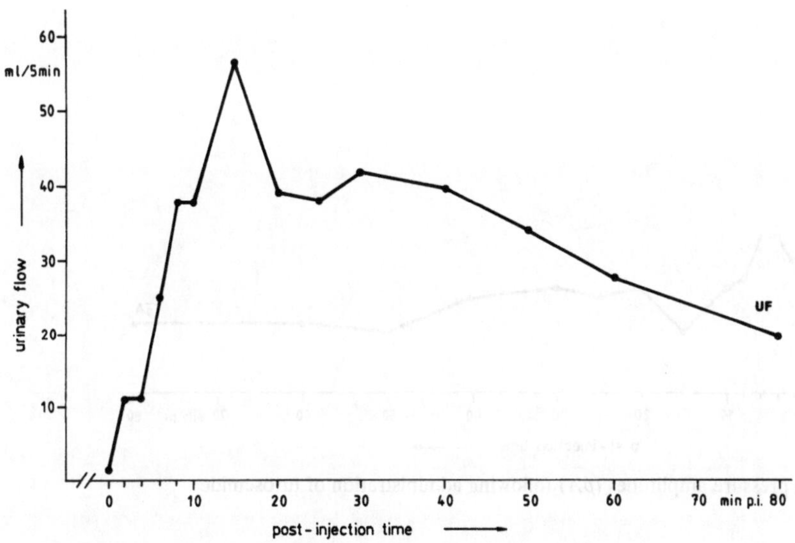

Fig. 5. Mean urine flow *(UF)* following administration of furosemide

pressure and so produces a preliminary wave. The muscular contraction process (F) is recorded quantitatively by the developed force probe. The typical pressure process occurs secondarily in the contraction ring.

Measurements over the whole extent of the ureter show that from the pyeloureteral junction to the bladder the average peristaltic frequency reduces from 13 to 8 per minute. The mean pressure amplitudes in the contraction ring are also dependent on

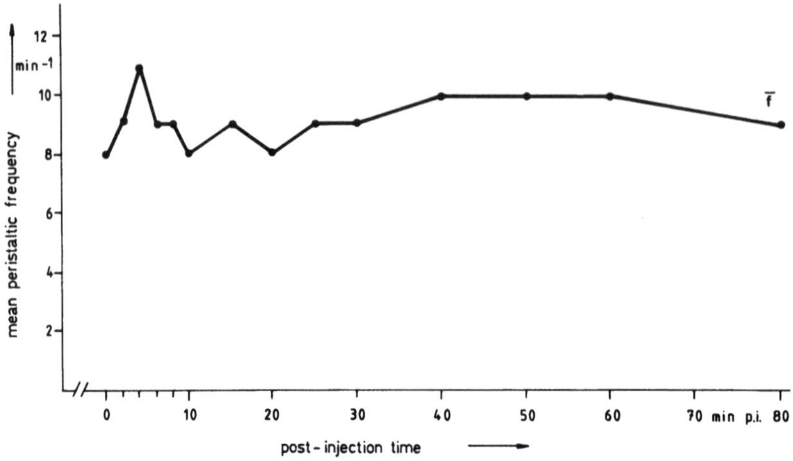

Fig. 6. Mean peristaltic frequency *($\bar{f}$)* following administration of furosemide

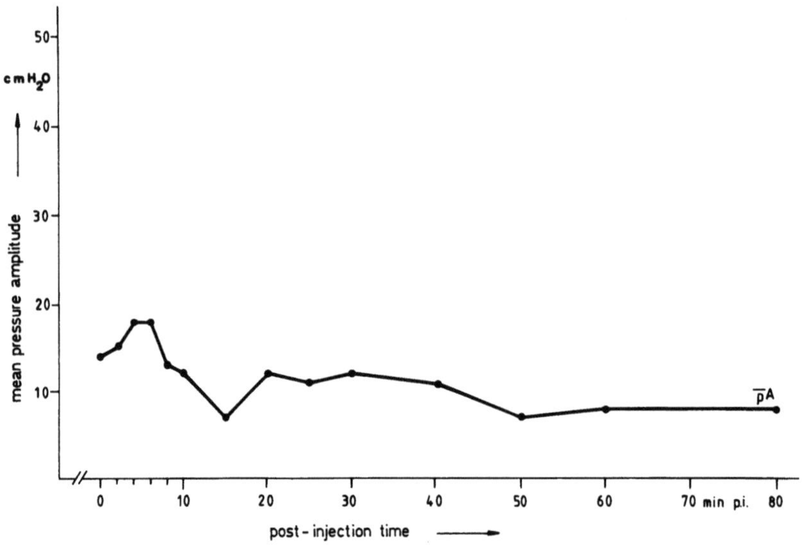

Fig. 7. Mean pressure amplitudes *($\bar{p}A$)* following administration of furosemide

location; showing a rising tendency, they fluctuate between 7 and 27 cmH_2O, with the highest values being registered prevesically. Compared with the surrounding area, the pressure values in the area of the iliac vessels (60%–70% of the length of the ureter) are noticeably low. Only the basal pressure shows no considerable variation over the whole extent of the ureter (Fig. 3).

The force distribution profile, ascertained over the whole length of the ureter (Fig. 4), differs clearly from the pressure distribution profile described above (Fig. 3) and shows, among other things, a noticeable minimum prior to the iliac vessels and a noticeable maximum within the area of the iliac vessels.

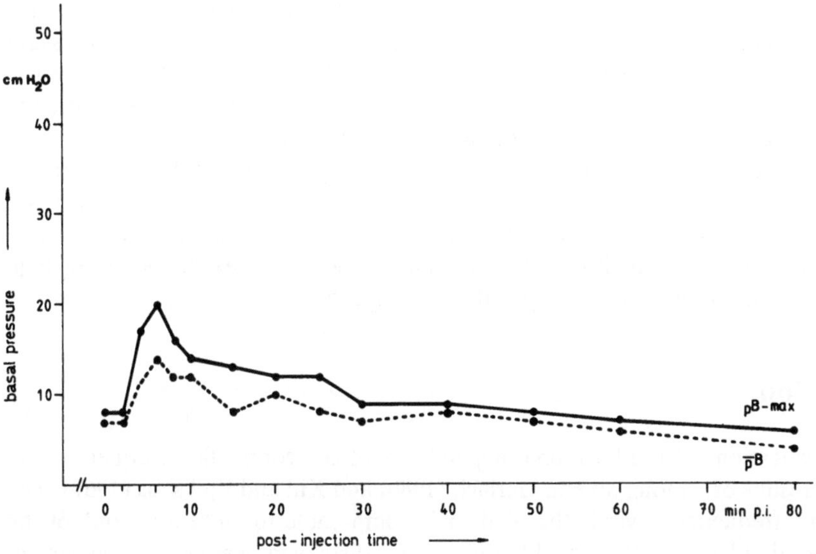

Fig. 8. Mean basal pressure *(pB)* and maximal basal pressure *($\bar{p}B$-max)* following administration of furosemide

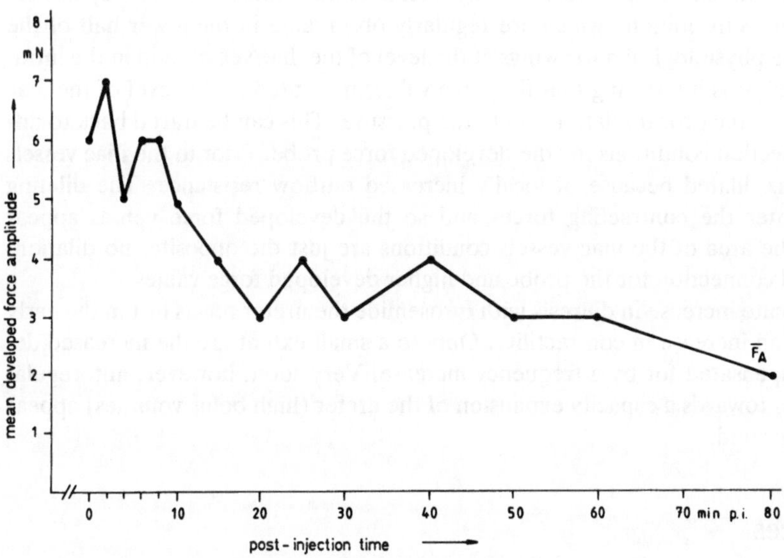

Fig. 9. Mean force amplitudes *($\bar{F}_A$)* following administration of furosemide

Following administration of furosemide there is first of all a rise in urine flow to up to 50 times the initial volume, the maximum being reached after 15 min (Fig. 5). The return of urine flow volume to the levels registered before administration of furosemide takes more than 120 min.

Under the changing diuresis conditions, the variation in peristaltic frequency was unexpectedly small (Fig. 6). In contrast to urine volume, which is highest after

15 min, the peristaltic frequency, pressure parameter, and developed force have already reached a maximum after 3–6 min (Figs. 6–9). The change in mean pressure amplitude also varies within relatively narrow limits (Fig. 7). By contrast, there is a clearer increase in basal pressure (Fig. 8), which first of all registers three times the initial value and then returns to the initial value over 60 min.

The development of the mean force amplitudes appears unexpected (Fig. 9): The muscular response to the increased diuresis is only a very fleeting and slight increase in the contraction forces. We then observed an at first rapid and later more gradual falling-off in the force amplitudes. In about half of the ureters examined during high diuresis, the developed force dropped down even as far as zero.

Discussion

Our investigations of the locational dependency of the contraction frequency confirm the results of, among others, Gerlach (1980) and Kiil and Kjekshus (1967). The decreasing frequency towards the bladder is comparable to an "extinction" of the myogenic stimulus. The cause could originate in a distally increasing stimulus threshold.

The likewise location-dependent contraction pressure was attributed by Gerlach (1980) to fluctuating wall strength or myoarchitecture. Rutishauser (1970) has related two pressure minima which are regularly observable in the lower half of the ureter to the physiological narrowings at the level of the iliac vessels and in the intramural ureter. It is interesting that the force values measured at the level of the iliac vessels show a reciprocal relationship to the pressure. This can be traced back to different connection conditions for the developed force probe. Prior to the iliac vessels the ureter is dilated because of locally increased outflow resistance. The dilating forces counter the contracting forces and so the developed force values appear lower. In the area of the iliac vessels conditions are just the opposite: no dilation, thus a good connection for the probe and higher developed force values.

To an acute increase in diuresis with furosemide the ureter reacts just in the early phase with an increase in contractility. Only to a small extent are the increased demands compensated for by a frequency increase. Very soon, however, autoregulative changes towards a capacity expansion of the ureter (high bolus volumes) appear in the foreground.

References

Gerlach R (1980) Harnleiterdynamik und Harnleiterersatz. Stippack, Aachen, pp 19–37

Kiil F, Kjekshus J (1967) The physiology of the ureter and renal pelvis. In: Proc 3rd Int Congr Nephrol, vol 2, Washington, 1966. Karger, Basel, pp 321–335

Pohl J, Stroh N, Marx G, Dambacher U (1986) In-vivo Kraftaufnahme im Harnleiter. 8. Sympos Exp Urol, Mainz, FRG

Rutishauser G (1970) Druck und Dynamik in den oberen Harnwegen. Fortschritte der Urologie und Nephrologie, vol 2. Steinkopff, Darmstadt, pp 22–31

Detrusor Contractility and Its Relationship to Different Degrees of Tension

D. Rohrmann[1], H.-A. Spormann[2], J. Hannappel[2], D. Albrecht[3], and W. Lutzeyer[2]

Introduction

Bladder function and its modulation have been the topic of much experimental work ever since Budge (1958) described the bladder innervation for the first time. Special contributions have been achieved by the use of neurohistochemical and pharmacological methods.

Up to now, Lipshultz's model concerning the vegetative innervation of the bladder, which was published in 1973 (Lipschultz et al. 1973), has remained undoubted: α-adrenergic, excitatory receptors are predominant in the bladder neck and the proximal urethra, whereas the detrusor is mostly influenced by cholinergic excitatory receptors. The adrenergic influence in the detrusor region is limited to a slight inhibitory effect mediated by β-adrenergic receptors. The physiological bladder function is coordinated by an alternate activation of different receptors: During the filling phase, the bladder is dominated by the sympathetic nervous system, which makes the bladder neck contract, while the detrusor remains quiet, due to the influence of inhibitory β-receptors. Voiding is mostly mediated by an activation of the parasympathetic nervous system resulting in a detrusor contraction while the bladder neck relaxes as the sympathetic nervous system is inhibited (Fig. 1).

In 1975, Benson et al. described another theory of bladder function modulation. In these experiments, detrusor muscle strips from guinea-pig bladder showed a changing reaction to drugs such as adrenaline according to their degree of tension. After a certain degree of lengthening detrusor muscle strips no longer showed an inhibitory sympathetic reaction, but they were, on the contrary, activated by adrenergic substances. Benson's experiments suggest a totally different view of micturition; that is why we started a series of experiments to prove the influence of adrenergic substances on bladder muscle strips with different degrees of tension.

Material and Methods

The autonomic innervation of the bladder can easily be shown in the organ bath (Fig. 2). Bladder muscle strips about 1 mm wide are brought into a special organ bath containing sufficient concentrations of oxygen and nutritive substances. The strips are connected to an isometric force transducer. As the muscle strips' tension can be changed from the outside, it is easy to investigate their reaction to drugs with reference to different degrees of tension.

[1] Dept. of Surgery, University of Karlsruhe, Moltkestr. 14, 7500 Karlsruhe, FRG
[2] Dept. of Urology der RWTH Aachen, Pauwelsstraße, 5100 Aachen, FRG

Investigative Urology 3
Edited by H. Rübben et al.

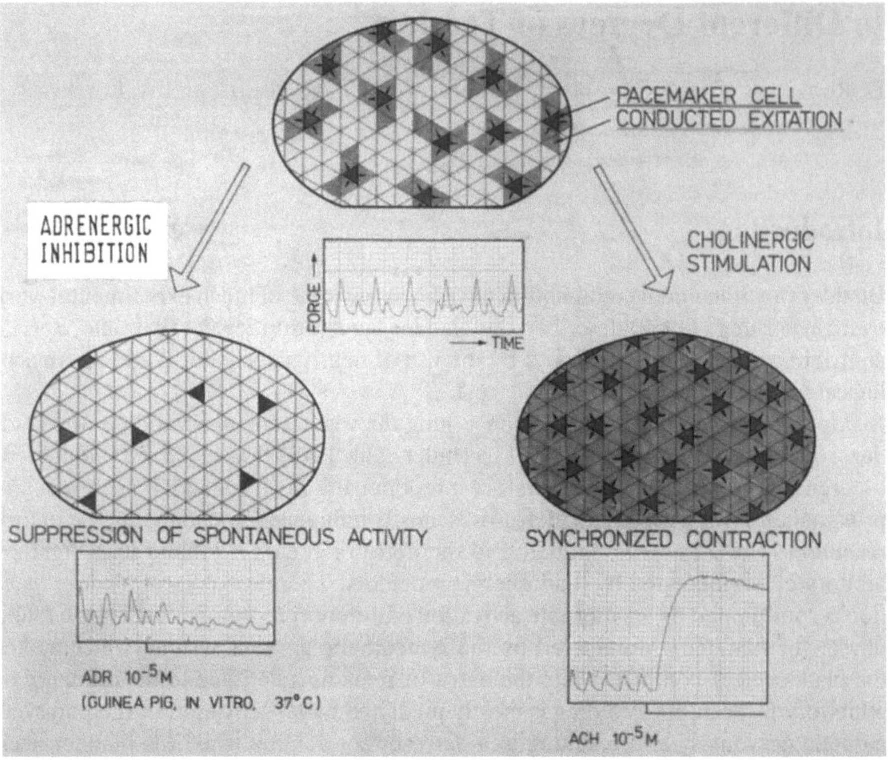

a

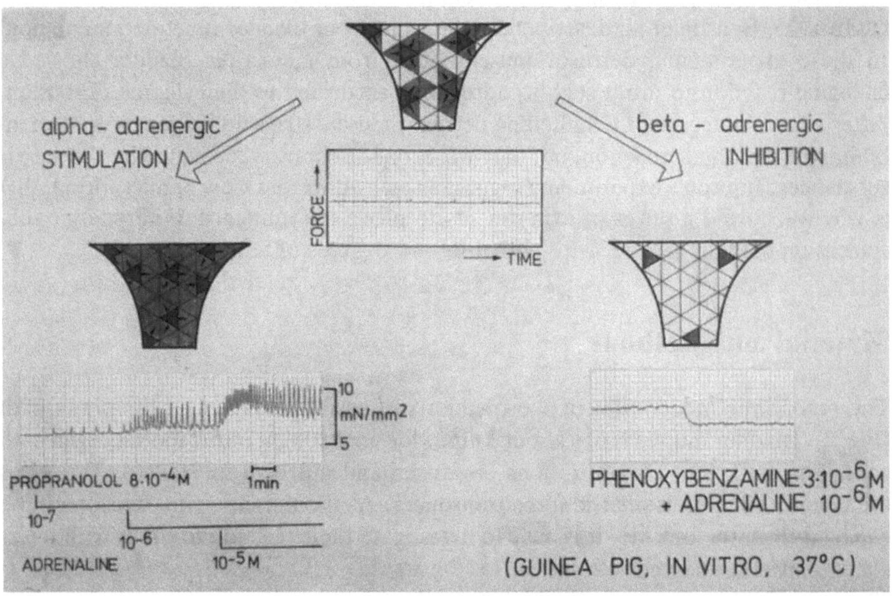

b

Fig. 1a, b. Vegetative control of the detrusor (**a**) and bladder neck (**b**). *ADR*, adrenaline; *ACH*, acetylcholine

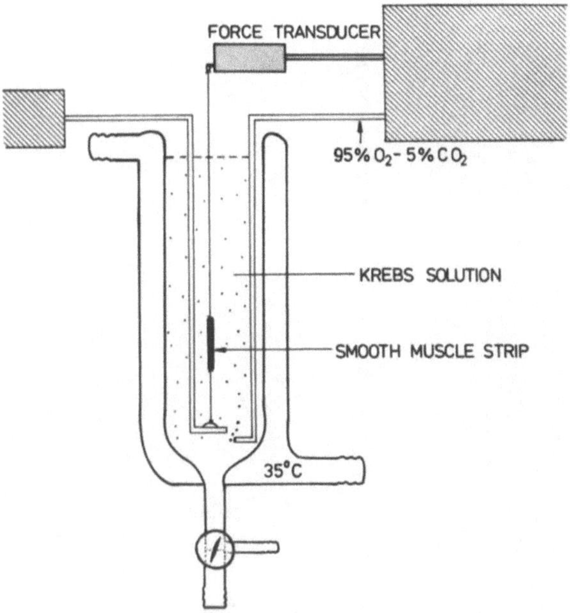

Fig. 2. Illustration of the organ bath

Results

Isolated muscle strips of the guinea-pig bladder normally show a typical pattern of spontaneous activity. Strips of the detrusor region do show spontaneous activity, whereas the bladder neck preparations remain quiet. If a certain degree of tension is applied to the strips, they show a change in length according to the degree of tension.

Detrusor and bladder neck strips show different reactions to the addition of adrenergic substances. Adrenaline (10^{-8} to 10^{-5} *M*/l) inhibits the spontaneous activ-

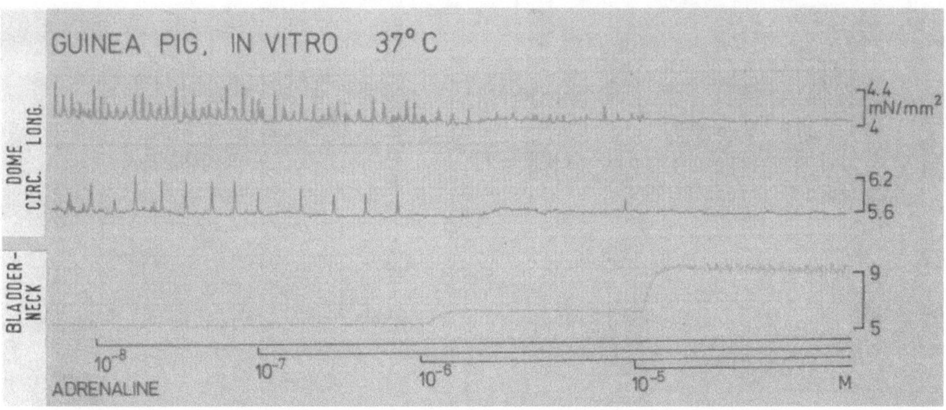

Fig. 3. Example of guinea-pig detrusor and bladder neck strips' reaction to adrenaline

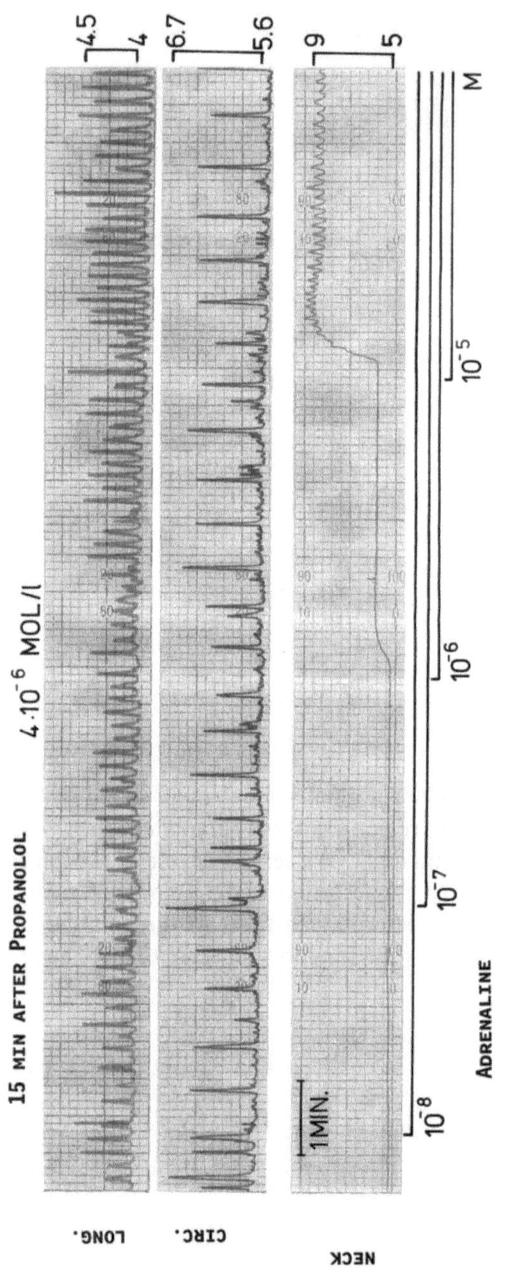

Fig. 4. Example of guinea-pig detrusor and bladder neck strips' reaction to adrenaline after application of the β-blocking agent propranolol

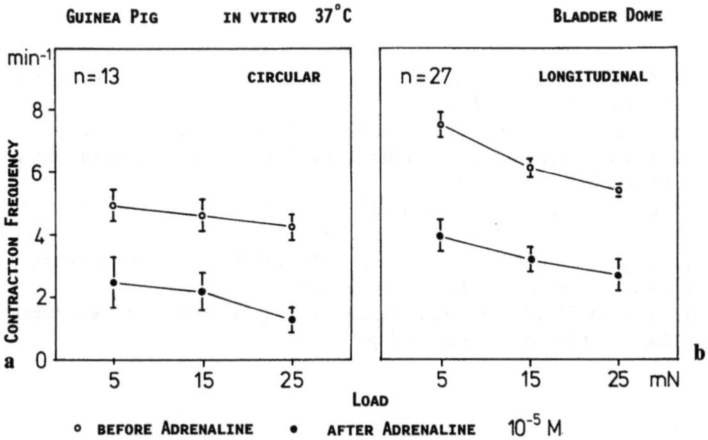

Fig. 5a, b. Contraction frequency of circular (**a**) and longitudinal (**b**) detrusor muscle strips related to different degrees of tension (here equated with load)

ity of detrusor strips, a phenomenon which is dose-dependent; the bladder neck strips are, on the contrary, activated by adrenaline and show a dose-dependent tonic contraction (Fig. 3). The inhibitory effect of adrenaline on detrusor strips is mediated by β-adrenoreceptors. This can easily be demonstrated by the addition of the β-blocking agent propranolol. Propranolol eliminates the depressing effect of adrenaline on detrusor strips, while the excitatory adrenergic reaction of bladder neck strips remains unchanged (Fig. 4).

Different degrees of tension applied to guinea-pig detrusor strips did not change the frequency of spontaneous activity (Fig. 5, upper row). If we looked at the adrenergic reaction of detrusor strips while increasing the degree of muscle strip tension, we always saw an inhibitory effect of adrenaline (Fig. 5, lower row). Bladder neck strips were always stimulated by adrenaline no matter at what level of muscle tension the experiment started.

Discussion

In our series of experiments, we could not confirm Benson's results of detrusor muscle changing its sensitivity to adrenergic substances according to its degree of tension. Though our experiments dealt with the same range of tension changes as Benson's did, we did not see an excitatory reaction to adrenaline with higher degrees of muscle strip tension. Several other authors, e.g., De Sy (1971) or Finkbeiner and Bissada (1980), could not confirm that either. Rohner et al. (1978), however, described an excitatory reaction of detrusor muscle strips to noradrenaline, but the experiments dealt with cases of bladder outlet obstruction, and this effect did not correlate to different degrees of muscle strip tension.

We think that it is not justified to doubt today's model of micturition in favor of a predominance of the sympathetic nervous system and its receptors changing sensitivity according to the degree of bladder volume, but voiding appears to remain mediated by the parasympathetic nervous system.

References

Benson GS, Raezer DM, Wein AJ, Corriere JN Jr (1975) Effect of muscle length on adrenergic stimulation of canine detrusor. Urology 5:769
Budge (1858) Über das Centrum genitospinale des N. sympathicus. Virchows Arch 15:115
De Sy W (1971) The reactivity of isolated urinary bladder strips of the guinea-pig toward electric stimulation. Arch Int Physiol Biochem 79:459
Finkbeiner AE, Bissada NK (1980) Effect of detrusor muscle length and tension and its response to pharmacologic and electrical stimulation. Part II. In vitro study. Urology 16:650
Lipshultz LI, Rohner TJ, Curry TH, Raezer DM, Schoenberg HW (1973) The effect of imipramine on in vitro dog bladder muscle contractility. Invest Urol 11:182
Rohner TJ, Hannigan JD, Sanford EJ (1978) Altered in vitro adrenergic responses of dog detrusor muscle after chronic bladder outlet obstruction. Urology 11:357

VI. Kidney Trauma, Pathophysiology, Urolithiasis

Renal Kinematics During Experimental Impact

R. A. ZINK[1], M. WEBER, M. WEISS, P. MÜSSELER, W. BRENDEL, and F. SCHUELER

Introduction

The aim of this study is to investigate the mechanism of renal trauma in detail. For this reason it is desirable to know how and to which extent the kidneys are accelerated, which movements they perform in relation to their hilar fixation and relative to the surrounding skeletal system, or which mechanism finally leads to the rupture of the organ. An experimental model should be developed to study this. Standardized free falls with the same impact characteristics as used by the automobile industry in their routinely performed car crash tests should allow a comparison with these tests (Kallieris and Mattern 1984; Nusholtz et al. 1980).

Piezoresistive microaccelerometers, implanted in the kidneys and in a reference point on the vertebral spine, were used for the first time in order to measure these parameters during standardized critical impact. Simultaneously taken high speed movies should allow the correlation of the electronically registered signals with optical information of the total body movements. Additionally performed measurements should allow in some of the experiments the registration of the pressures within the renal pelvis and the renal artery during the instance of impact.

Material and Methods

Animals. The 45 experiments were performed on pig cadavers since previous investigations showed that no significant difference could be demonstrated between the reactions of living versus dead animals in respect to the parameters of interest.

The animals were approximately 3 months old and had a body weight of 16.7 ± 3.2 kg. A premedication with 2 mg/kg azaperon i.m. was administered just before the experiments. They were then heparinized with 10000 IU i.v. and received a lethal dose i.v. of 20 ml pentobarbital-sodium. The anesthesized animals used in the experiments received metomidate-HCl (10 mg/kg of body weight). They were intubated, and the anesthesia was maintained with adequate amounts of this drug during the application of the probes and during the free fall.

Instrumentation. The two microaccelerometers (Endevco, type 7264) weighing 2 g and measuring ± 200 *g* were mounted to an adapter (10 × 10 × 13 mm) with orthogonal vector coordinates. The kidneys were exposed through a flank incision, and the probes implanted into the middle group of calices and fixed to the surrounding parenchyma. The cables were surrounded with silastic shrinking hose and lead through

[1] Department of Urology, LM-University, Marchioninistr. 15, 8000 München 70, FRG

Investigative Urology 3
Edited by H. Rübben et al.

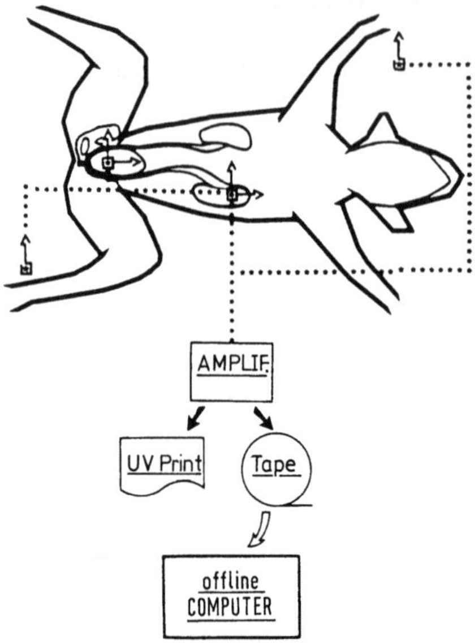

Fig. 1. Schematic drawing of the experimental design. ...., Cable for recording; □→, accelerometer; *AMPLIF,* multichannel amplifier; *UV-Print,* high-speed UV-printer; *Tape,* multichannel tape recorder

the skin by the use of a separate stab wound. The coaxial position of the probes was adjusted by fluoroscopy and marked on the body surface for the optical control.

The dorsal spine of the 2nd lumbar vertebra was removed and another accelerometer (Endevco, type 2261) weighing 16 g (16 × 25 mm), which was attached to a bonescrew, was put in place. Two accelerometers of the same type were used in the free fall frame in order to check its movements.

Micropressure transducers (Endevco, type 8507) weighing 1.1 g with a diameter of 1.6 mm were implanted in the renal artery or in the renal pelvis of the contralateral kidney in those experiments with simultaneous pressure measurements.

Equipment. A specially designed lift system with a guided frame allowed free falls from up to 20 m. The deceleration obtained by this system showed a nonoscillating, rectangular characteristic by the means of "breaking plates". They were attached to 65-cm long "breaking legs" which were pushed into plastic granulate during the impact. The depth of penetration equalled the deformation distance. The duration of the impact and its extent could be modified by the adjustment of the diameter of the breaking plates.

All signals from the probes were registered on multichannel UV-printer (Yokogawa, 291 S) and tape recorded (Bell + Howell, 236810/1) for further off-line computation (Fig. 1).

High-speed cameras (Stalex, WS-I) were placed on three different sides of the free fall frame, in those experiments with optical control. The movies were taken at 500 frames/s. A conventional 16-mm camera (Arriflex; 36 frames/s) was additionally used for the overall documentation of the experiments.

The animals were either placed in the prone position (with hanging legs) or onto their left flank with the accelerometers ipsi- or contralateral to the impact. The first position corresponded, e.g., to a frontal, the second one, to a side collision in a car.

Computation. A computer program for the analysis of car crash experiments, performed by the automobile industry, which was adjusted to the measuring equipment in use, allowed the following parameters to be computed:

1. Maximal ("touch down") speed (V_{max}):
   $V_{max} = \sqrt{2\,g\,h}$ [m/s]; *h*, free fall height; *g*, constant of gravity
2. Maximum differential acceleration (δA_{max}) e.g. kidney-skeleton:
   $\delta A_{max} = A_{max}\langle kid.\rangle - A_{max}\langle skel.\rangle$ [ms^{-2}]; *A*, acceleration
3. Stretch distance (L) kidney-skeleton at a given time (*Tn*):
   $L = \delta Vx \times Tn$ [m]; δVx, differential velocity at the time *Tn*
4. Maximum difference of stretch distances (δL_{max}):
   $\delta L_{max} = \int_{T_{end}}^{T_o} \times T_{end}$ T_o, time of "touch down", beginning of measurement; T_{end}, time of standstill
5. Renal oscillation (τ) (sine wave characteristic assumed):
   $\tau = 1/t$ [Hz]; *t*, distance between 2 maxima

Results

The frame system obtained after a free fall from 10 m a maximal speed of 14.0 m/s ≈ 50.4 km/h ≈ 31.2 mph and an acceleration of 23.8 ± 3.4 *g* at a deformation distance of 41.1 ± 2.9 cm.

Time Course. The first maximum of the acceleration (= 1st compression) was found ca. 70 ms after the beginning of the impact (T_o = touch down at the granulate). The second maximum occurred after 200–220 ms. Practically the same time course could be demonstrated by the high speed movies, analyzing the indicated spots at the cervical spine (C7), at the lumbar spine (L2), and at the sacral spine (S1).

Mean Acceleration. The kidneys and the skeleton probes showed with 18.8 and 17.9 *g* an almost equal acceleration in the prone position (Fig. 2). This means that the abdominal content deadens the renal acceleration compared with the whole system. This effect was minimal in the side position: 20.0 and 20.5 *g*.

Maximal Differential Acceleration. Maximal differential acceleration between the skeleton and the frame (= car passenger and passenger cell) was 48.6 *g* in the prone position, 45.4 *g* contra-, and 38.5 *g* ipsilaterally. Between the skeleton and the kidneys however 26.8 *g* were found in the prone position, 28.4 and 21.0 *g*, respectively.

Maximal Differential Velocity. The maximal differential velocity between kidney and skeleton occurred most distinctly at 1.8 m/s in the prone position (Fig. 3). This means that the kidney travels during a frontal impact of approximately 20 *g* (≈ 30 mph car crash with safety belts on) with 1.8 m/s from its fixation point at the renal hilus.

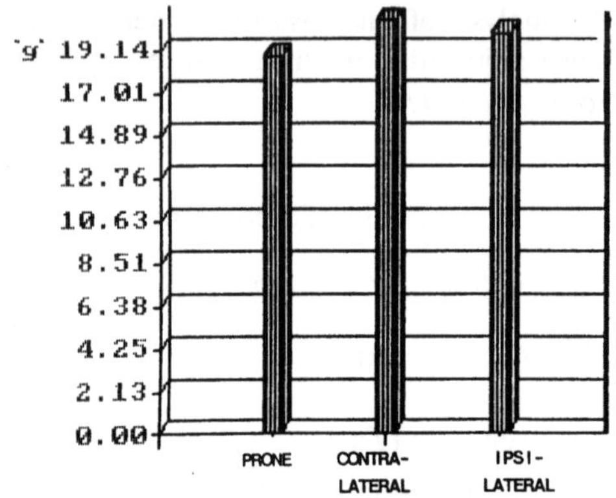

Fig. 2. Mean renal acceleration, measured in *prone* position or in the kidney *ipsi-* or *contralateral* to impact; (*g* force of gravity)

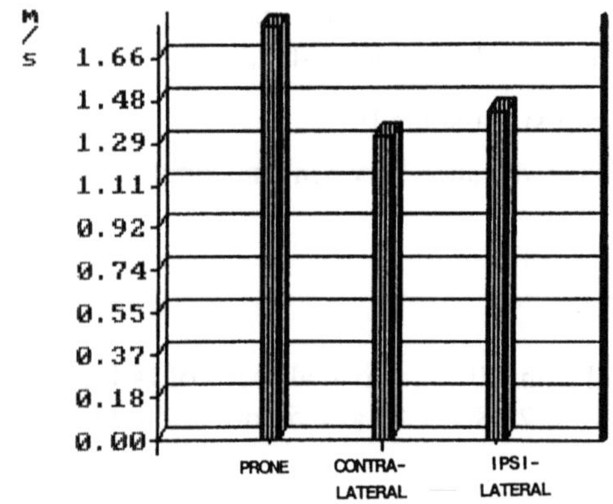

Fig. 3. Maximal differential velocity between kidney and skeletal reference point (= hilar fixation) in *prone* position, *ipsi-* or *contralateral* to impact

The maximal differential velocity reduced to 1.3 m/s in side collision and the contralateral kidney, and 1.4 m/s in the ipsilateral kidney.

Maximal Stretch Distance. During the crash the kidneys travelled in the prone position 30 mm from their point of fixation, that means, the renal vessels stretched this distance for a duration of about 50–60 ms (Fig. 4). Lateral impact moved the contralateral kidneys about 2.17 cm and the ipsilateral one, 2.40 cm.

Pressures. A peak pressure of 319.3 ± 26.1 mm Hg was found in the renal artery. The peak pressure in the ureter ranged up to 40 cm H_2O, starting from an initial pelvic pressure of 15 cm H_2O.

Renal Oscillation. The further analysis of the acceleration signals revealed that the kidneys oscillate in typical frequences during impact: 36.0 ± 2.7 Hz were found in the ipsilateral and 12.8 ± 0.4 Hz in the contralateral kidney. In the prone position the oscillating frequency was 17.1 Hz. The frame in comparison showed a typical frequency of 79.0 Hz.

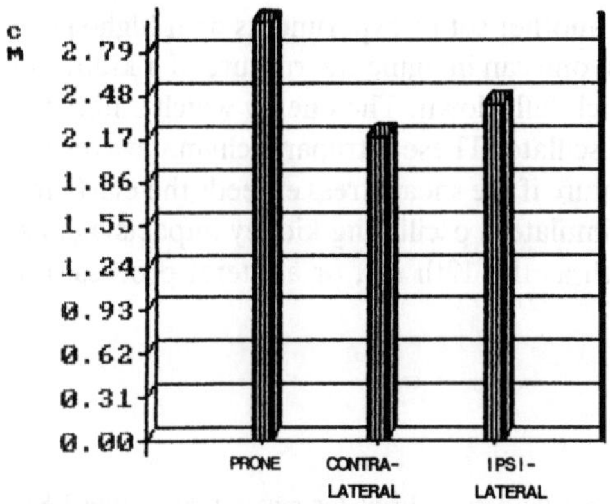

Fig. 4. Maximal stretch difference between kidney and skeletal reference point (= hilar fixation) in *prone* position, *ipsi-* or *contralateral* to impact

Discussion

For the first time real values of renal deceleration and velocity could be measured during critical impact. It could further be shown that approximal 85% of the maximal system deceleration is effective on the kidneys in the prone position. In the side position, however, the renal acceleration may reach up to 90% of the system deceleration in the kidney ipsilateral to the impact. It must not be overseen that in these experiments 40 cm of deformation distance was effective. In typical flank traumas, e.g., in bicycle riders or alpine skiers, when no deadening layer comes between the body surface and the ground, which is hard, extremely high accelerations may occur. Sheets of foamy material may be very effective as shock-absorbing kidney or hip protectors, e.g., in motorcycle garment (Aldman 1985).

Of special interest for the urologist are the injuries to the renal hilus. It could be shown in these experiments that the kidney travels with a speed of up to 1.8 m/s from its fixation point and stretches its hilar fixation to about 30 mm. Even in a relatively harmless impact of 22 *g* and a deformation distance of 40 cm, the maximal differential deceleration between kidney and skeleton ranged between 20 and 30 *g*. This means that under the conditions of these experiments, which were still in a subtraumatic range, a human kidney would tear with 2–5 kg at the renal hilus. According to our findings it can be assumed that this is the borderline for tissue elasticity, since hilar bleeding and histological changes in the tunica adventitia of the renal artery were seen, very similar to those found in aneurysmatic dissections.

It could be further demonstrated that the kidney can be stimulated through external forces to oscillate at different frequencies, which also depend on the position of the body relative to the force. The more directly the energy reaches the kidney, the higher is the frequency of these oscillations. In the prone position the whole abdomen and its contents acts as an additional, deadening deformation distance which reduces the acceleration to a great extent. Even more effective in respect to deadening is the fixation of the kidney contralateral to the impact in side position, due to its fixation to the thoracic wall. In direct flank traumas, however, enough energy may reach the contralateral kidney, causing a rupture of the parenchyma there, without any changes on the ipsilateral organ.

According to these observations and another set of experiments with high-speed movies of the rupture of isolated kidneys, one can imagine the rupture of a kidney as the bursting of a water-filled balloon which falls down: The energy which enters the blood-filled kidney causes the organ to oscillate. These intraparenchymal waves are reflected from the capsule and lead to rupture if the shear stress exceeds the elasticity. This situation may occur earlier if the stimulated, oscillating kidney impacts against a hard or sharp, e.g., bony obstacle such as the 12th rib, or a lateral process of a vertebral body.

References

Aldman A (1985) The protective effect of a specially designed suit for motorcyclists. 10th ESV-Conf, Oxford

Kallieris D, Mattern R (1984) Belastbarkeitsgrenze und Verletzungsmechanik des angegurteten Fahrzeuginsassen beim Seitenaufprall. In: Arbeitsgemeinschaft Industrieller Forschungsvereinigungen, FAT Schriftenreihe, 36

Nusholtz GS, Melvin JW, Mueller G, Mackenzie JR, Burney R (1980) Thoraco-abdominal response and injury. 24th Stapp Car Crash Conf

Improvement of In Situ Renal Protection Against Complete Ischemia Through the Replacement of Chloride by Aspartate in the HTK Solution of Bretschneider*

M. Kallerhoff[1], M. Blech[1], G. Kehrer[2], M. Langheinrich[2], U. Helmchen[3], H. J. Bretschneider[2], and R. H. Ringert[1]

Introduction

The cardioplegic solution, HTK (histidine-tryptophan-ketoglutarate) (Bretschneider et al. 1975, 1984; Bretschneider 1980), was primarily developed to improve myocardial protection, as compared with periods of ischemia, during artificial cardiac arrest in open heart surgery. It has since become a routine clinical procedure (Preusse et al. 1987). According to our results, this solution also significantly improves ischemic tolerance of *kidneys* (Kallerhoff et al. 1985a, b, 1986, 1987c). The superiority over simple ischemia or over the Euro Collins solution holds for "cold" as well as for "warm" ischemia (Kallerhoff et al. 1988a). Renal ischemic tolerance was increased from 15–20 min to 2 h at normothermia (Kallerhoff et al. 1986). There have now been several clinical applications of this method (Blech et al. 1988; Kallerhoff et al. 1988b).

The aim of the work presented here was to further improve renal ischemic protection by modifying this solution. The HTK solution (Table 1) is primarily optimized for sodium and calcium reduction and potassium and magnesium enrichement. This electrolyte composition reduces cellular energy consumption and allows a buffer concentration of almost 200 m*M* histidine/histidine-HCl at isoosmolarity. The cation composition, however, entails a chloride concentration of 50 m*M* (Table 1). In contrast, the intracellular chloride concentration is 5–15 m*M*. The result might be net influx of chloride into the cell during ischemia.

This led us to examine whether further improvement in kidney protection could be achieved by replacing the chloride in the HTK solution by aspartate. For myocardial protection, such an improvement was not found (Bretschneider et al. 1975).

Materials and Methods

The experiments were performed on 54 kidneys of mongrel dogs with a body weight between 28 and 32 kg. A detailed description of our experimental procedure (Kallerhoff et al. 1987c) and of the protective perfusion of the kidneys with HTK solution

* Supported by the DFG, SFB 330-Organprotektion
Dedicated, gratefully, to Prof. Dr. W. Knipper

[1] University of Göttingen, Dept. of Urology, Robert-Koch-Str. 40, 3400 Göttingen, FRG
[2] University of Göttingen, Dept. of Physiology, Humboldtallee 23, 3400 Göttingen, FRG
[3] University of Hamburg, Dept. of Pathology, Martini-Str. 52, 2000 Hamburg 20, FRG

Investigative Urology 3
Edited by H. Rübben et al.

Table 1. Composition of kidney protective solutions investigated (m*M*)

	HTK	HTK-"aspertate"
Sodium	15	15
Potassium	9	9
Calcium	0	0
Magnesium	4	4
Chloride	50	18
Aspartate	0	32
Tryptophan	2	2
K^+-α-ketoglutarate	1	1
Histidine/histidine-HCl	180/18	180/18
Mannitol	30	30
Osmolality (mOsmol/kg_{H_2O})	310	310
pH at 8°C	7.3	7.3
PO_2 (mm Hg) at 37°C	200	200

has been published (Kallerhoff et al. 1987a; Kehrer et al. 1985). The solutions investigated – the HTK solution and the HTK-aspartate solution (Dr. Franz Köhler Chemie, Alsbach, FRG) – are similar in composition except for their NaCl, KCl, and MgCl content. In the HTK-aspartate solution these substances have been replaced by Na^+-aspartate, K^+-aspartate, and Mg^{2+}-aspartate. This results in an unchanged cation composition, while the chloride content is reduced from 50 m*M* to 18 m*M*.

In each case, we compared the kidneys protected by one of the two solutions (11 HTK kidneys and 16 HTK-aspartate kidneys) with the individual contralateral kidneys (27 control kidneys). The arteriovenous oxygen consumption (V_{O_2}/min) was determined by multiplying the arteriovenous difference in oxygen content with the flow rate. The glomerular filtration rate (GFR) was calculated using the endogenous creatinine clearance. At the end of each experiment, the kidneys were excised, weighed, and dried until weight constancy was achieved. For comparisons, all functional parameters were related to the so-called edema-free normalized wet weight (ww) of 17%.

Tissue samples consisted of ⅔ renal cortex and ⅓ renal medulla. For determining content of adenine nucleotides and lactate, they were immediately homogenized in cold perchlorate acid and analyzed according to established procedure using Boehringer Mannheim test kits. Measurements were made by means of a filter photometer (1101 m, Eppendorf Instrument, Hamburg, FRG) and a double beam photometer (UV-210 A, Shimadzu, Japan).

For light and electron microscopy evaluation, the tissue was immersion-fixed in buffered 4% formaldehyde immediately following the 3-h postischemic reperfusion phase. The PAS reaction was used to prepare the tissue samples for light microscopical examination. Electron microscopy was performed on Araldite-embedded material that had been cut in 50–70 nm slices, using a Zeiss EM 10 microscope.

Results

The ischemic stress resulting from the duration of ischemia (120 min) and the mean temperature during ischemia (30°C) are approximately equal in the groups examined (Fig. 1).

The electromagnetically measured total renal blood flow was 200–300 ml/min · 100 g_{ww} for control kidneys. HTK- and HTK-aspartate-protected kidneys did not differ substantially in their blood flow, either from each other or from control kidneys (Fig. 2).

Under our experimental conditions, renal oxygen consumption in the control kidneys amounted to 6–6.5 ml/min · 100 g_{ww}. After HTK protection it amounted to 3.8 ml/min · 100 g following 15 min of reperfusion, rising to an average of 4.5 ml/min · 100 g within 2 h. Following the same protocol for HTK-aspartate-protected kidneys, renal oxygen consumption was 4.8 ml/min · 100 g_{ww} after a 15-min reperfusion, reaching 5.5 ml/min · 100 g_{ww} after 45 min and averaging 5.2 ml/min · 100 g_{ww} (Fig. 3).

The endogenous creatinine clearance was measured to determine the glomerular filtration rate (GFR). In control kidneys it was 40–50 ml/min · 100 g_{ww}. Following

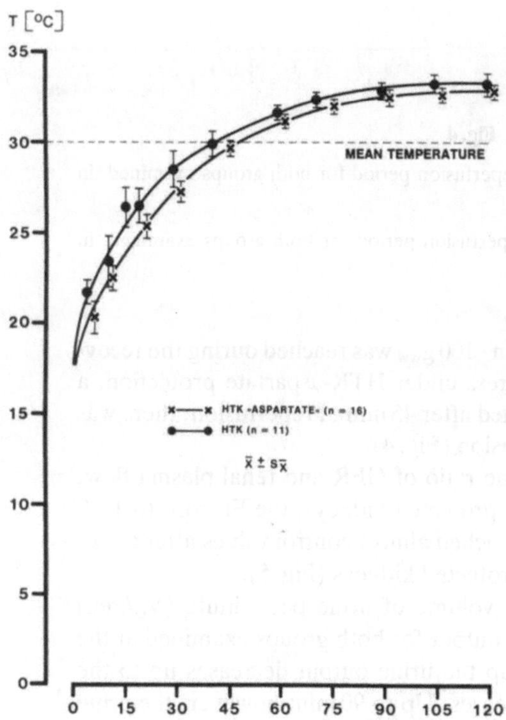

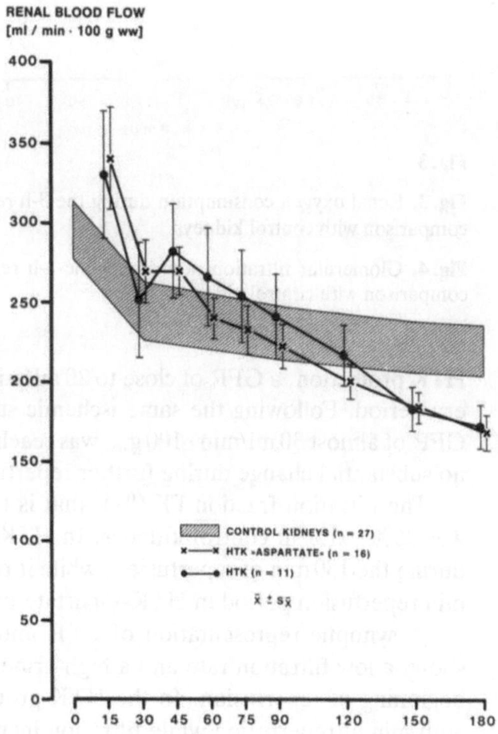

Fig. 1

Fig. 2

Fig. 1. Changes in temperature during ischemia for both groups examined

Fig. 2. Renal blood flow during the 3-h reperfusion period for both groups examined, in comparison with control kidneys

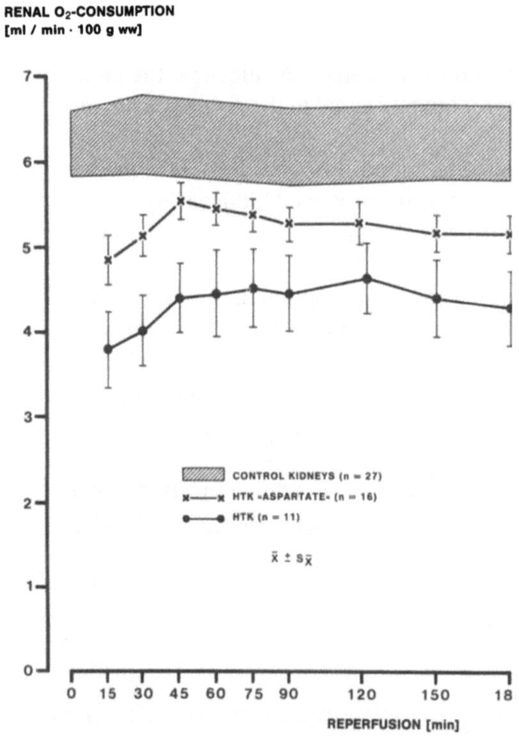

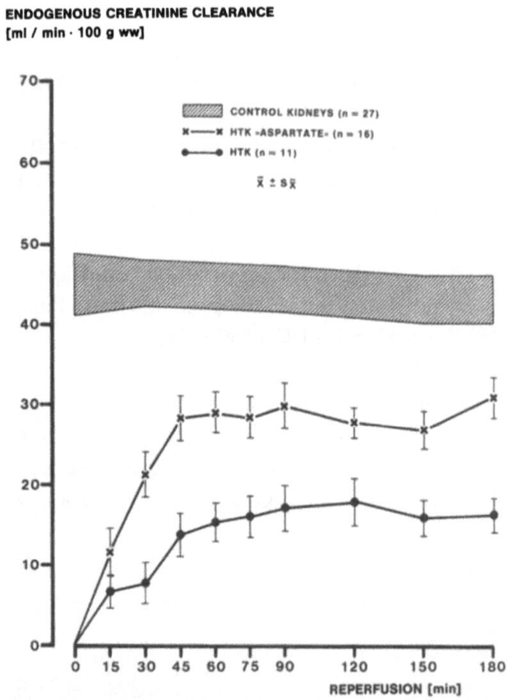

Fig. 3 **Fig. 4**

Fig. 3. Renal oxygen consumption during the 3-h reperfusion period for both groups examined, in comparison with control kidneys

Fig. 4. Glomerular filtration rate during the 3-h reperfusion period for both groups examined, in comparison with control kidneys

HTK protection, a GFR of close to 20 ml/min · 100 g_{ww} was reached during the recovery period. Following the same ischemic stress under HTK-aspartate protection, a GFR of almost 30 ml/min · 100 g_{ww} was reached after 45 min of reperfusion; there was no substantial change during further reperfusion (Fig. 4).

The filtration fraction FF (%), that is the ratio of GFR and renal plasma flow, was 25%–35% in control kidneys. In HTK-protected kidneys, the FF rose to 15% during the 180 min of reperfusion, while it reached almost control values after a 180-min reperfusion period in HTK-aspartate-protected kidneys (Fig. 5).

A synoptic representation of GFR and volume of urine per minute (V_U/min) shows a low filtration rate and a high urine output for both groups examined at the beginning of reperfusion. In the HTK group the urine output decreases up to the 30th min of reperfusion while filtration increases. Up to 90 min, however, the urine output increases again and then declines from the 90th to the 180th min of reperfusion. After HTK-aspartate protection urine output decreases from the beginning of reperfusion, while the GFR increases (Figs. 6, 7).

After 3 h of postischemic reperfusion, tissue samples for biochemical and morphological analysis were obtained from control kidneys as well as ischemically stressed

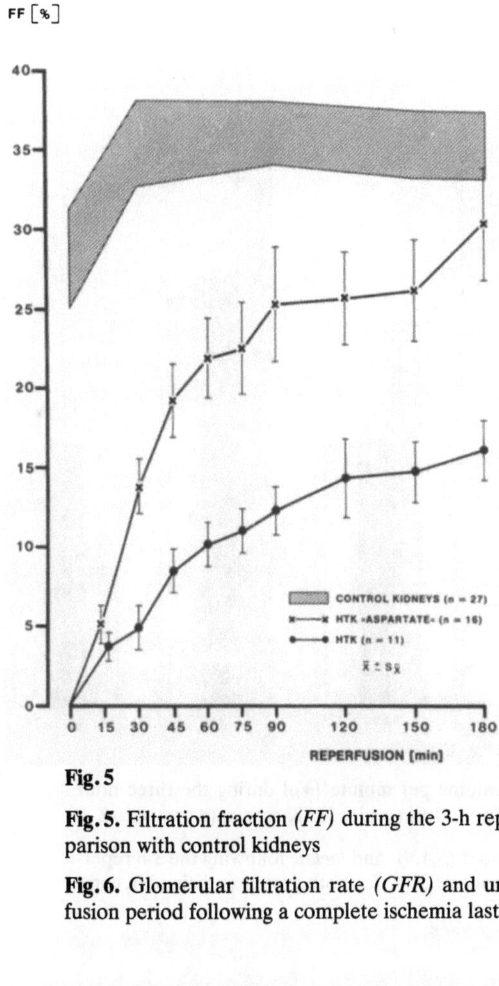

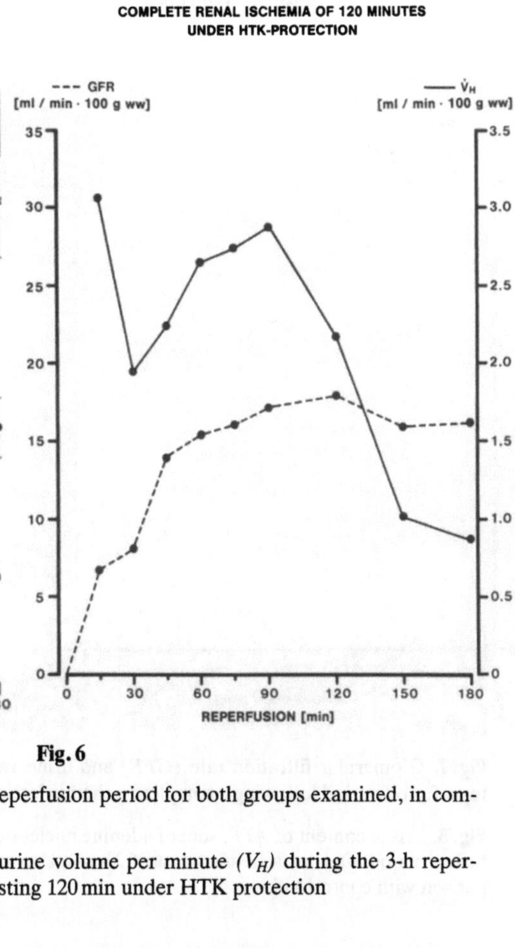

Fig. 5 **Fig. 6**

Fig. 5. Filtration fraction *(FF)* during the 3-h reperfusion period for both groups examined, in comparison with control kidneys

Fig. 6. Glomerular filtration rate *(GFR)* and urine volume per minute *(V_H)* during the 3-h reperfusion period following a complete ischemia lasting 120 min under HTK protection

kidneys (see Materials and Methods). In control kidneys, the adenosine triphosphate (ATP) content was 9 μmol/g_{dw}, the sum of adenine nucleotides (SAN) was 14.5 μmol/g_{dw}, and the lactate content was 6.5 μmol/g_{dw}. In both protected groups investigated, the ATP content was 6.5 μmol/g_{dw}, the SAN was 10 μmol/g_{dw}, and the lactate content amounted to 5–6 μmol/g_{dw} (Fig. 8).

For all 11 HTK and 16 HTK-aspartate experiments, morphological analysis was performed. The morphology shown is representative for the particular group with respect to the functional data. After a 120-min ischemia at 30°C under HTK protection and a 180-min reperfusion, the general appearance of the renal cortex shows regular glomeruli and an interstitial space that is not enlarged. Several proximal tubules contain flaky proteinaceous material (Fig. 9a). A detail of the same tissue shows a glomerulum with an unfolded capillary tuft. The proximal tubular epithelium shows a slightly edematous cytoplasm (Fig. 9b). In the electron microscopical detail one can recognize a horizontally cut proximal tubule, with two circumscribed brush border defects and with a localized cytoplasmic edema (Fig. 9c). Further enlargement reveals a proximal tubular cell with a small brush border defect, with a localized

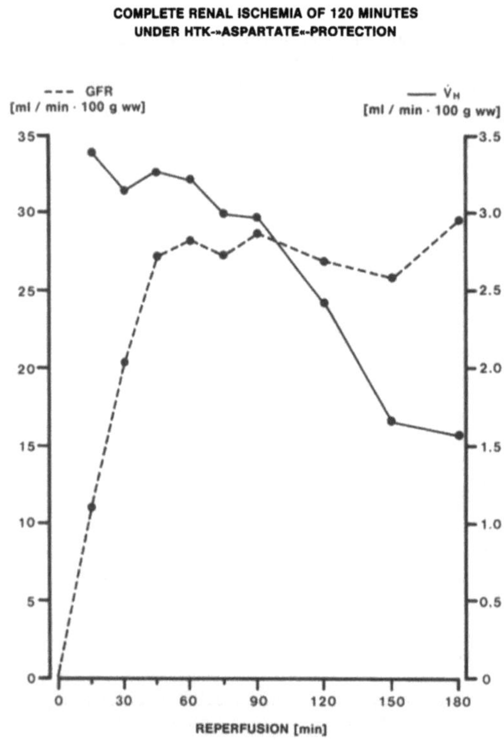

Fig. 7

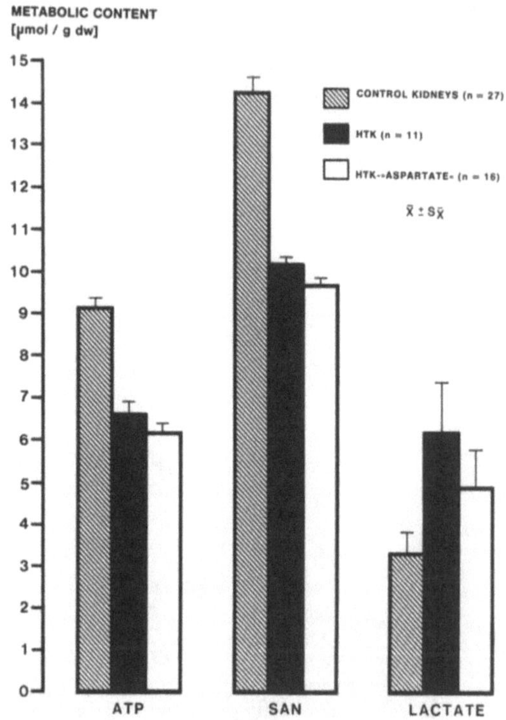

Fig. 8

Fig. 7. Glomerular filtration rate *(GFR)* and urine volume per minute *(V_H)* during the three hour reperfusion period following a complete ischemia lasting 120 min under HTK-aspartate protection

Fig. 8. Tissue content of *ATP,* sum of adenine nucleotides *(SAN),* and *lactate* following the 3-h reperfusion period after an ischemic stress of 2 h at an average of 30°C for both groups examined in comparison with control kidneys

cytoplasmic edema, with partially swollen mitochondria, and with a widened basal labyrinth (Fig. 9d).

Under the same procedure as described above, under HTK-aspartate protection the general appearance of the renal cortex shows regular glomeruli and a finely structured interstitial space, free tubule lumina, and well-preserved epithelium (Fig. 10a). On more detailed examinations, a normal glomerulum and well-preserved proximal tubules with regular cytoplasmic density can be seen (Fig. 10b). Electron microscopy shows a horizontally cut proximal tubule with a largely preserved brush border, normal cytoplasm, and a typicallly structured nucleus (Fig. 10c). Further enlargement reveals a proximal tubular epithelial cell with preserved brush border and with regular nuclear, mitochondrial, and basal labyrinth structures (Fig. 10d).

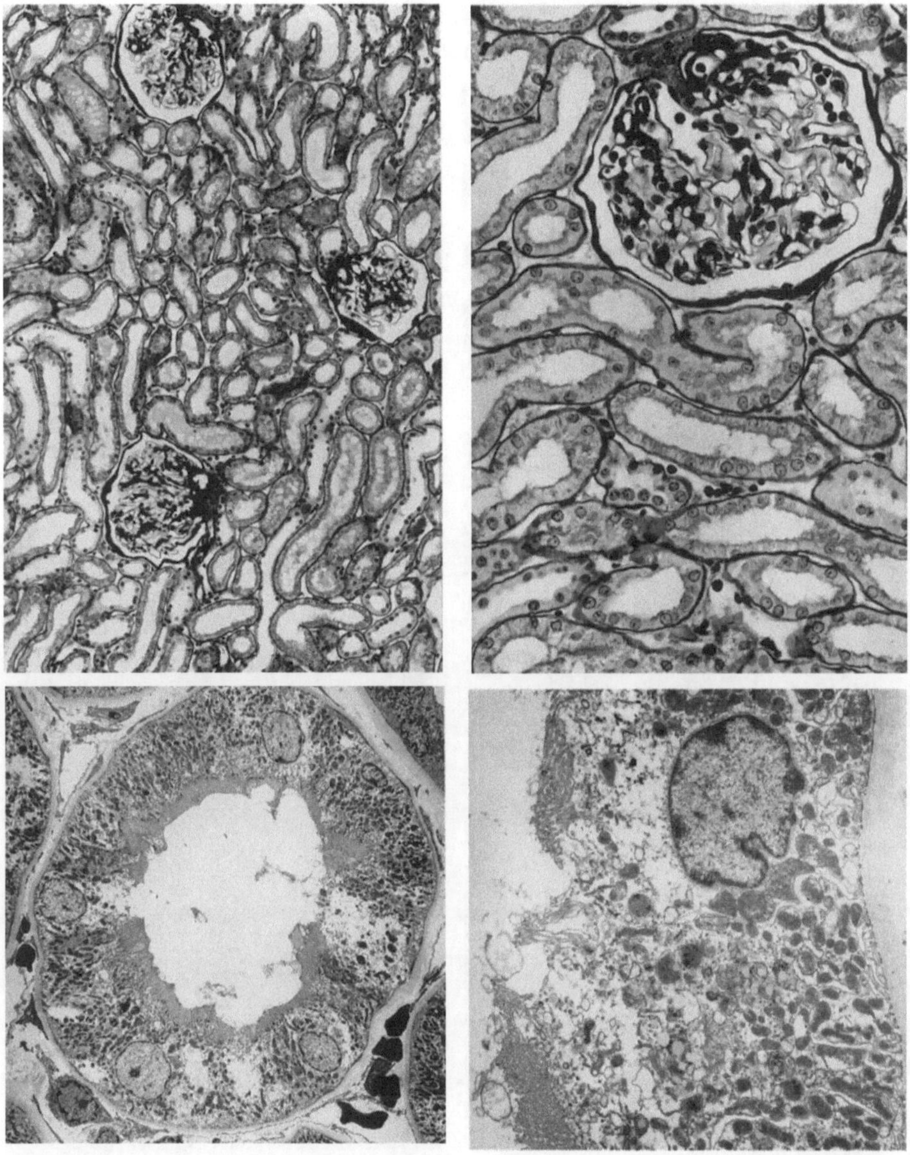

a b c d

Fig. 9a–d. Ischemia of 120 min at 30°C under HTK protection. **a** Overview: renal cortex with regular glomeruli and not enlarged interstitial space. Flaky, proteineous material in several proximal tubules. PAS, ×120. **b** Detail: glomerulum with unfolded capillary tuft. Proximal tubular epithelium with slightly edematous swelling of the cytoplasm. PAS, × 300. **c** EM: horizontal view of a proximal tubule with two circumscribed brush border defects and with localized cytoplasmic edema, ×1740. **d** EM: proximal tubular cell with a small brush border defect, with a localized cytoplasmic edema, with swollen mitochondria, and with a widened basal labyrinth. ×1992

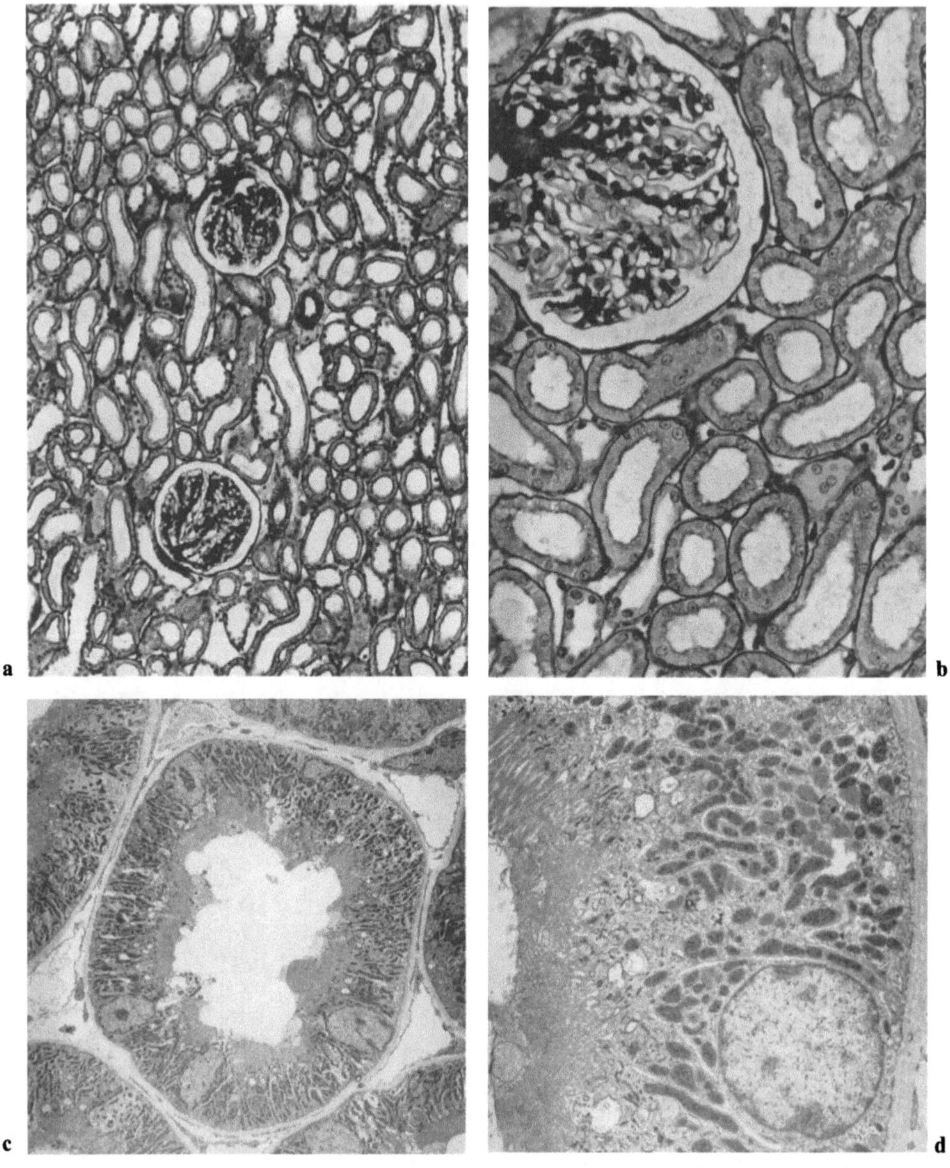

Fig. 10a–d. Ischemia of 120 min at 30°C under HTK-aspartate protection. **a** Overview: renal cortex with regular glomeruli and finely structured interstitial space, free tubule lumina, and well-preserved epithelium. PAS, × 120. **b** Detail: normal glomerulum. Well-preserved proximal tubules with regular cytoplasmic density. PAS, × 300. **c** EM: horizontally cut proximal tubule with largely preserved brush border and typically structured nucleus, × 1740. **d** EM: proximal tubular epithelial cell with preserved brush border and with regular nuclear, mitochondrial, and basal labyrinth structures, × 1992

Discussion

Kidney protection by systemic administration or addition to organ protection solutions of calcium antagonists or postischemic infusion of $MgCl_2ATP$ is methodically simple but of uncertain effect and has been a subject of controversy (Schrier et al. 1987; Siegel et al. 1980). Application of renal protective solutions through the renal artery, however, is hampered by the high potassium content of those solutions (Euro Collins Solution, Sacks solution): A potassium content of 115 m*M* or 126 m*M* contrasts with the normal plasma potassium concentration of about 4 m*M*. Nevertheless, there is a demand for organ preservation during renal surgery (Blech et al. 1988). We have, therefore, over several years adapted the cardioplegic solution HTK to in situ protection of kidneys (Kallerhoff et al. 1986, 1987c). We are aiming for a tested, clinically applicable procedure for organ preservation in renal surgery, similar to that in open heart surgery with myocardial potection (Preusse et al. 1987).

Several models exist for studying renal ischemia, its consequences, and its prevention. Our experimental protocol offers the advantage that by preischemic protective perfusion with the HTK solution, kidneys can be exposed to an unusually long period of ischemia at the high mean temperature of 30°C. The resulting high ischemic stress would always lead to complete tissue loss without HTK protection. The total interruption of blood flow results, on the one hand, in interrupted oxygen supply and, on the other hand, in preventing the removal of ischemic metabolites (e.g., lacate, H^+-ions). Renal ischemia is thereby distinguished from acute renal failure in circulatory shock, in which some renal tissue perfusion remains (Brezis 1984). Furthermore, our so-called acute reperfusion model has the crucial methodical advantage that it allows us to perform a postischemic functional examination over several hours, with high analytical precision (Kallerhoff et al. 1987c). In survival experiments, we were able to exclude a secondary, late deterioration of kidney function (Kallerhoff et al. 1986). With the model of acute reperfusion used here, we intended to apply recent insights into the physiology of chloride transport (Cassola et al. 1983; Greger 1985; Wingo 1986) to the low-sodium, calcium-free, magnesium-enriched, and histidine-buffered cardioplegic HTK solution. We investigated whether reducing the chloride content from 50 m*M* to 18 m*M* while substituting with the corresponding aspartate salts would further improve postischemic function and structural recovery, as critical indicators of a successful organ protection. We measured renal blood flow, renal oxygen consumption as an indicator of sodium resorption, glomerular filtration rate, and the filtration fraction. All parameters show substantial improvement with the HTK-aspartate solution in comparison with the HTK solution (Figs. 2–5). Glomerular filtration in HTK-aspartate-protected kidneys is significantly increased (28 ml, as compared with 18 ml); however, the urine output after HTK-aspartate protection declines steadily during reperfusion, indicating tubular functional recovery (Figs. 6, 7). There were no differences between the two groups concerning energy substrates or metabolism, as the similar content of ATP, SAN, and lactate shows (Fig. 8). By light microscopic as well as electron microscopic (EM) criteria, application of the HTK-aspartate solution further improved structural recovery (Figs. 9, 10).

We propose the following mechanism of action. (a) Applying the HTK-aspartate solution instead of the HTK solution does not lead to a further reduction in energy consumption during protective perfusion, i.e., while initiating "nephroplegia". During protective perfusion, the temperature of the solutions is below 10°C, the sodium concentration is low at 15 m*M*, and the solutions are calcium free. Therefore, few diffusion and transport processes take place, and renal oxygen consumption amounts to only 0.2 ml/min · 100 g_{ww} as compared with approx. 6 ml/min · 100 g_{ww} under normal blood perfusion conditions (Kallerhoff 1987a). (b) During ischemia, i.e., under in situ conditions at temperatures of 25°–37°C (Fig. 1), an intracellular edema may result from a passive inward flow of chloride from the extracellular to the intracellular space, accompanied for reasons of electrical neutrality by a sodium and passive water influx (Koyuncuôglu et al. 1982; Mason et al. 1981). The intracellular chloride concentration is 5–15 m*M*. Because the chloride concentration in the HTK solution is 50 m*M*, there is a substantial extracellular – intracellular gradient. Exchanging chloride by aspartate in the HTK-aspartate solution reduces the chloride concentration to 18 m*M* (Table 1) and thereby diminishes the gradient between the extracellular and intracellular space. This hypothesis is supported by the structural recovery following the application of the HTK-aspartate solution as compared with the HTK solution. HTK-aspartate protection, as opposed to HTK protection, does not entail a visible cytoplasmic edema (compare Fig. 10c, d with Fig. 9c, d). (c) According to Brezis et al. (1984), the degree of renal ischemic damage depends particularly on the discrepancy between oxygen demand and oxygen supply. Renal oxygen demand can be lowered most effectually by reducing sodium reabsorption (Deetjen and Kramer 1961; Mandel 1986); however, according to Greger (1985), the chloride transport in the ascending limb of Henle's loop is a critical energy-consuming process. Therefore, this component is highly susceptible to cell volume dysregulation by ATP deficiency and the resulting failure of the Na-K pump (Jones 1986; Katz 1986; Soltoff 1986). (d) Adding substrates for anaerobic metabolism to the HTK solution (Guder et al. 1986; Kallerhoff et al. 1987b) results in some metabolic and energetic improvements, but they could not be confirmed by functional analysis (unpublished data). Consequently, the best way of matching energy demand and supply during ischemia appears to be a reduction in energy demand, which is determined mostly by the activity of the ion pumps (Hochachka and Mommsen, 1983). (e) It is not clear at present whether reducing ammonium production by inhibiting glutaminase is of additional significance (Fitzpatrick et al. 1982; Vinay et al. 1986). (f) A specific amino-acid effect of aspartate on the glomerular filtration rate may be significant (Andrews and Bates 1986; Silbernagel et al. 1975; Verkh et al. 1986), but it is still unclear how aspartate might act when it is already washed out by blood during reperfusion.

The rationale for the HTK-aspartate solution can thus be summarized as follows: By exchanging chloride for aspartate, a reduction in chloride influx into the tubular cell may have been achieved. Second, the electrolyte composition allows high concentrations of an amino acid buffer (histidine/histidine-HCL), which, by precluding a decrease in intrarenal pH, prevents enzyme inhibition. This effect may be supported by aspartate (Riggs 1988). A metabolism is thereby maintained that corresponds to a large degree to the ischemic demand. The improved functional data as well as the better structural preservation as compared with the HTK solution support the arguments presented initially. By reducing the chloride in the HTK solution, the HTK-aspartate solution offers an effective improvement of renal in situ protection.

Acknowledgements. For translating this manuscript we wish to thank Mrs. F.v. zur Mühlen. For technical assistance we are indebted to Mrs. R. Dohrmann and Mr. E. Bürger. Further we are grateful to Mrs. U. Kneissler for preparing morphological samples and figures, and Mrs. E. Neumeyer for drawing the diagrams.

References

Andrews PM, Bates SP (1986) Dietary protein prior to renal ischemia dramatically affects post-ischemic kidney function. Kidney Int 30: 299–303

Blech M, Kallerhoff M, Kehrer G, von Romatowsky HJ, Mündemann-Schultz Ch, Helmchen U, Truss F, Bretschneider HJ (1988) Klinische Anwendung der kardioplegischen Lösung HTK nach Bretschneider zur in-situ Protektion der Niere. Urologe [Ausg A] 27: 44–48

Bretschneider HJ (1980) Myocardial protection. Thorac Cardiovasc Surg 28: 295–302

Bretschneider HJ, Hübner G, Knoll D, Lohr B, Nordbeck H, Spieckermann PG (1975) Myocardial resistance and tolerance to ischemia: physiological and biochemical basis. J Cardiovasc Surg 16: 241–260

Bretschneider HJ, Gebhard MM, Preusse CJ (1984) Cardioplegia – principles and problems. In: Sperelakis N (ed) Physiology and pathophysiology of the heart. Martinus Nijhoff, Boston, pp 605–616

Brezis M, Rosen S, Silva P, Epstein FH (1984) Renal ischemia: a new perspective. Kidney Int 26: 375–383

Cassola AC, Mollenhauer M, Frömter E (1983) The intracellular chloride activity of rat kidney proximal tubular cells. Pflügers Arch 399: 259–265

Deetjen P, Kramer K (1961) Die Abhängigkeit des O_2-Verbrauches der Niere von der Na^+-Rückresorption. Pflügers Arch 273: 636–650

Fitzpatrick JM, Monson JRT, Gunther PA, Watkinson LE, Wickham JEA (1982) Renal accumulation of ammonia: the cause of post-ischemic functional loss and the "blue line". Br J Urol 54: 608–612

Greger R (1985) Ion transport mechanisms in thick ascending limb of Henle's loop of mammalian nephron. Physiol Rev 65: 760–797

Guder WG, Wagner S, Wirthenson G (1986) Metabolic fuels along the nephron: pathways and intracellular mechanisms of interaction. Kidney Int 29: 41–45

Hochachka PW, Mommsen TP (1983) Protons and anaerobiosis. Science 219: 1391–1397

Jones DP (1986) Renal metabolism during normoxia, hypoxia, and ischemic injury. Ann Rev Physiol 48: 33–50

Kallerhoff M, Kehrer G, Siekmann W, Blech M, Gebhard MM, Helmchen U, Bretschneider HJ (1985a) Experimentelle Anwendung der Kardioplegischen Lösung HTK nach Bretschneider für eine in-situ Protektion von Nieren. In: Harzmann R et al. (eds) Experimentelle Urologie. Springer, Berlin Heidelberg New York, pp 180–188

Kallerhoff M, Hölscher M, Kehrer G, Kläß G, Bretschneider HJ (1985b) Effects of preservation conditions and temperature on tissue acidification in canine kidneys. Transplantation 39: 485–489

Kallerhoff M, Blech M, Kehrer G, Kleinert H, Siekmann W, Helmchen U, Bretschneider HJ (1986) Post-ischemic renal function after kidney protection with the HTK-solution of Bretschneider. Urol Res 14: 271–277

Kallerhoff M, Blech M, Kehrer G, Kleinert H, Langheinrich M, Siekmann W, Helmchen U, Bretschneider HJ (1987a) Short-term perfusion and "equilibration" of canine kidneys with protective solutions. Urol Res 15: 5–12

Kallerhoff M, Blech M, Kehrer G, Kleinert H, Langheinrich M, Siekmann W, Helmchen U, Bretschneider HJ (1987b) Effects of glucose in protected ischemic kidneys. Urol Res 15: 215–222

Kallerhoff M, Blech M, Kehrer G, Kleinert H, Langheinrich M, Siekmann W, Helmchen U, Bretschneider HJ (1987c) Nierenfunktionsparameter nach Ischämiebelastung unter der Euro-Collins-Lösung oder unter der kardioplegischen Lösung HTK nach Bretschneider. Urologe [Ausg A] 26: 96–103

Kallerhoff M, Blech M, Isemer FE, Kehrer G, Kleinert H, Helmchen U, Bretschneider HJ (1988a) Metabolic, energetic, and structural changes in protected and unprotected kidneys at temperatures of 1°C and 25°C. Urol Res 16:57–62

Kallerhoff M, Blech M, Kehrer G (1988b) Nierenprotektion in situ mit der HTK-Lösung nach Bretschneider. Verh Dt Ges Urologie 40 (in press)

Katz AI (1986) Distribution and function of classes of ATPases along the nephron. Kidney Int 29: 21–31

Kehrer G, Kallerhoff M, Probst R, Siekmann W, Blech M, Bretschneider HJ, Helmchen U (1985) Construction and experimental application of a catheter for selective arterial kidney perfusion in situ. Urol Res 13:85–89

Koyuncuôglu H, Wildmann J, Berkmann K, Matthaei H (1982) The effects of D-and/or L-aspartic acids on the total weight of body, the weights of certain organs, and their protein, triglyceride and glycogen contents. Arzneimittel-Forsch/Drug Res 32(II):738–741

Mandel LJ (1986) Primary active sodium transport, oxygen consumption and ATP: coupling and regulation. Kidney Int 29:3–9

Mason J, Beck F, Dörge A, Rick R, Thurau K (1981) Intracellular electrolyte composition following renal ischemia. Kidney Int 20:61–70

Preusse CJ, Schulte HD, Bircks W (1987) High volume cardioplegia. Ann Chir Gyn 76:39–45

Riggs AF (1988) The Bohr effect. Ann Rev Physiol 50:181–204

Schrier RW, Arnold PE, van Putten VJ (1987) Cellular calcium in ischemic acute renal failure: role of calcium entry blockers. Kidney Int 32:313–321

Siegel NJ, Glazier WB, Chaudry IH, Gaudio KM, Lytton B, Baue AE, Kashgarian M (1980) Enhanced recovery from acute failure by the postischemic infusion of adenine nucleotides and magnesium chloride in rats. Kidney Int 17:338–349

Silbernagel S, Foulkes EC, Deetjen P (1975) Renal transport of amino acids. Rev Physiol Biochem Pharmacol 74:105–167

Soltoff STP (1986) ATP and the regulation of renal cell function. Ann Rev Physiol 48:9–31

Verkh L, Freier DT, Celik C (1986) Changes in concentration of amino acids and other metabolites during hypothermic perfusion of the canine kidney. Cryobiology 23:366–370

Vinay P, Lemieux G, Gougoux A, Halperin M (1986) Regulation of glutamine metabolism in dog kidney in vivo. Kidney Int 29:68–79

Wingo CS (1986) Effect of acidosis on chloride transport in the cortical thick ascending limb of Henle perfused in vitro. J Clin Invest 78:1324–1330

Investigations on the Crystallization Tendency in Urine with AC-Impedance Measurements and Cyclic Voltammetry

R.-D. Huber[1], H. Hommel[2], and E. Matouschek[1]

Introduction

The electrophysical properties of the outer and inner phase limit layers of a system (molecule cluster, solvate envelopes, adsorbate layers, etc.) can primarily be held responsible for nucleation, crystal growth, and aggregation in solutions. Electric double layers are formed, which are only partly or indirectly accessible to measurement. In recent years a great number of investigations were carried out, dealing with stimulation (initiation) or retardation (inhibition) of crystallization by means of different components of urine during stone formation. However, all these methods clarify only partial aspects of crystallization and do not give a complete view of urine (Adelman and Goldman 1981; Adey and Lawrence 1984; Blank 1986; Hille 1984; Lipinski 1982; Pethig 1979; Robertson and Scurr 1986; Schanne et al. 1978; Schelter 1985; Scurr and Robertson 1986). Our investigations aim to find out whether it is possible to differentiate urine with a "high crystallization tendency" from urine with a "low crystallization tendency" by determining the complex impedance and using cyclic voltammetry.

Material and Methods

Transportation processes at limit layers (electrodes, membranes, cell tissues) dependent on environmental conditions like temperature, substances, pH value, etc. may be examined by measuring the complex impedance within a large frequency range (e.g., 0.01 Hz–100 kHz, AC-impedance spectroscopy, frequency response analysis). These measurements of impedance are mainly carried out potentiostatically. We disturb the system by a prechosen polarization (nominal potential), superimpose an alternative current and observe its response as frequency-dependent parts of the resulting potential and current changes. The frequency-dependent complex impedance contains a resistance with a real component (ohm resistance Z') and an imagined component (reactance Z''; $Z = Z' + jZ''$). The result of measurement can be represented in different ways; we chose the so-called BODE-plot: The impedance /Z/ and the phase angle Θ are represented dependent on frequency; high reactance appears as a negative phase angle Θ, i.e., the voltage follows the current by the phase angle Θ. The behavior of impedance can be interpreted by the means of a model based on electrode kinetics (a so-called equivalent circuit). As to the conditions in urine, the

[1] Department of Urology, Municipal Hospital of Karlsruhe, 7500 Karlsruhe, FRG
[2] Fraunhofer Institute, Pfinztal-Berghausen, FRG

Investigative Urology 3
Edited by H. Rübben et al.

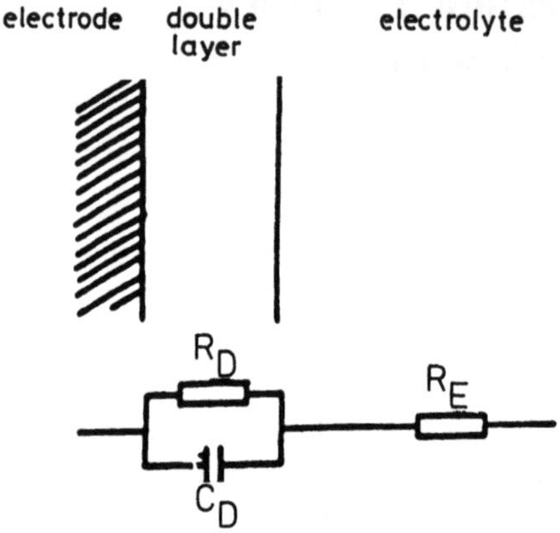

Fig. 1. Parallel RC-network as equivalent circuit of the electrical double layer between the electrode and electrolyte for urine. R_D, double layer resistance; C_D, double layer capacitance; R_E, electrolyte resistance

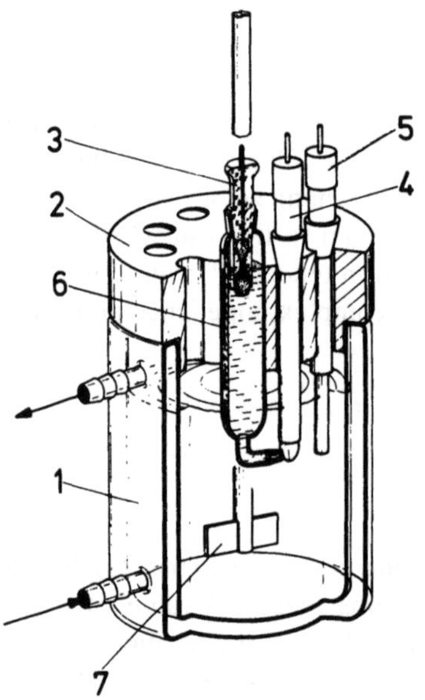

Fig. 2. Measuring equipment: *1*, glass vessel; *2*, Teflon cover; *3*, reference electrode (standard calomel electrode); *4*, counter electrode (gold electrode); *5*, working electrode (glassy carbon electrode); *6*, electrolyte bridge with 3.5 *M* KCl solution; *7*, stirring device

electric double layer between electrode and electrolyte can be represented by a parallel RC-network, preceeded by the electrolyte resistance R_E (Fig. 1).

We used an electrochemical AC-impedance measurement system with FFT (Fast Fourier Transform) technique in the frequency range of 0.01–11 Hz as well as a phase-sensitive Lockin detection in the frequency range of 5 Hz–100 kHz (EG & G Princeton Appl. Res. Corp., model 368-2) with computer analysis. The method used for measurements was the one involving three electrodes (Fig. 2).

An artificial polarization for simulation of different polarized limit layers may be freely selected via a positive or negative DC – the potential of the working electrode compared with the reference electrode. Inhibition is characterized by a high negative polarization tolerance of the system.

The same equipment was used to carry out a study of the cyclic voltammetry in a voltage range between −1.5 V and +1.5 V. Urine is submitted to polarization in a rapid cadence within this range and the resulting current is observed. The inhibition of a system appears as only a slight change of current within a wide voltage range.

We examined the urine of calcium oxalate stone "formers" as well as urine of stone-free people and artificial urine similar to those.

Results and Discussion

The urine of stone formers showed an definite susceptibility to DC-polarization in low frequency ranges of about 0.01–10 Hz. A polarization of −0.4 V results in an obvious decrease of reactance Z″ of their urine, while there is no change in reactance of the urine of stone-free people, even when it is highly supersaturated with calcium oxalate, up to a DC of −0.8 V. With the BODE-plot this is shown by the fact that in

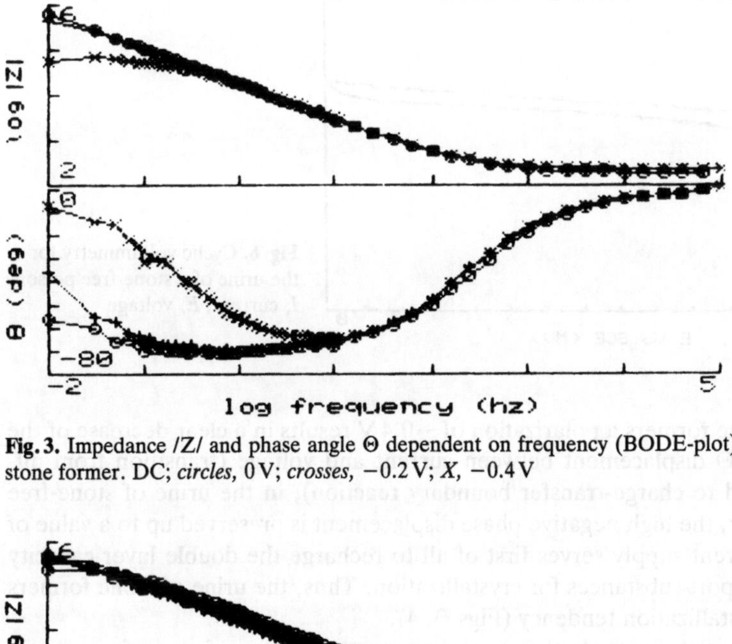

Fig. 3. Impedance /Z/ and phase angle Θ dependent on frequency (BODE-plot) for the urine of a stone former. DC; *circles*, 0 V; *crosses*, −0.2 V; *X*, −0.4 V

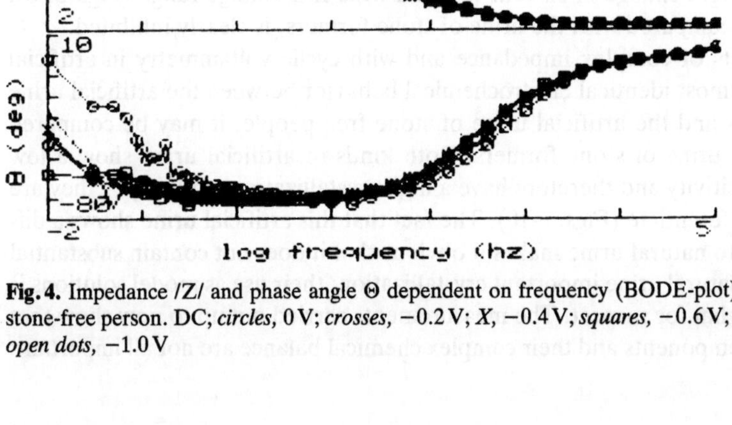

Fig. 4. Impedance /Z/ and phase angle Θ dependent on frequency (BODE-plot) for the urine of a stone-free person. DC; *circles*, 0 V; *crosses*, −0.2 V; *X*, −0.4 V; *squares*, −0.6 V; *solid dots*, −0.8 V; *open dots*, −1.0 V

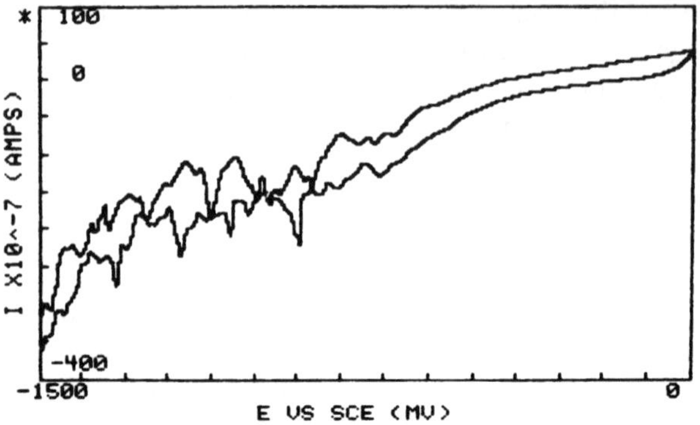

Fig. 5. Cyclic voltammetry for the urine of a stone former. *I*, current; *E*, voltage

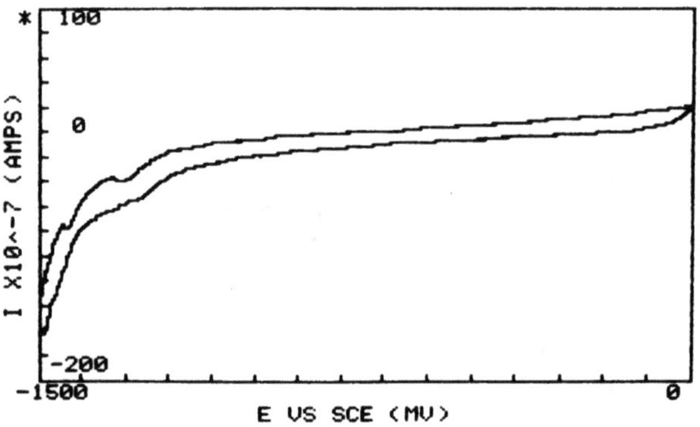

Fig. 6. Cyclic voltammetry for the urine of a stone-free person. *I*, current; *E*, voltage

the urine of stone formers a polarization of -0.4 V results in a clear decrease of the negative phase Θ displacement between current and voltage (transition from diffusion-controlled to charge-transfer boundary reaction); in the urine of stone-free people, however, the high negative phase displacement is preserved up to a value of -0.8 V; the current supply serves first of all to recharge the double layer capacity and not to transport substances for crystallization. Thus, the urine of stone formers has a higher crystallization tendency (Figs. 3, 4).

Cyclic voltammetry reveals that in the more stable urine of stone-free people there is only a slight change in current within a wide DC-voltage range (Figs. 5, 6), and the system, compared with the urine of stone formers, is clearly inhibited.

Measurements of complex impedance and with cyclic voltammetry in artificial urine show an almost identical electrochemical behavior between the artificial urine of stone formers and the artificial urine of stone-free people; it may be compared with the natural urine of stone formers. Both kinds of artificial urine show a low polarization sensitivity and therefore have a high crystallization tendency – they are impossible to differentiate (Figs. 7–10). The fact that this artificial urine shows a different behavior to natural urine makes it obvious that it does not contain substantial components of natural urine important crystallization; their use as model solutions is therefore somewhat for suspect. The measurements carried out up to now show that stone-forming components and their complex chemical balance are not all important;

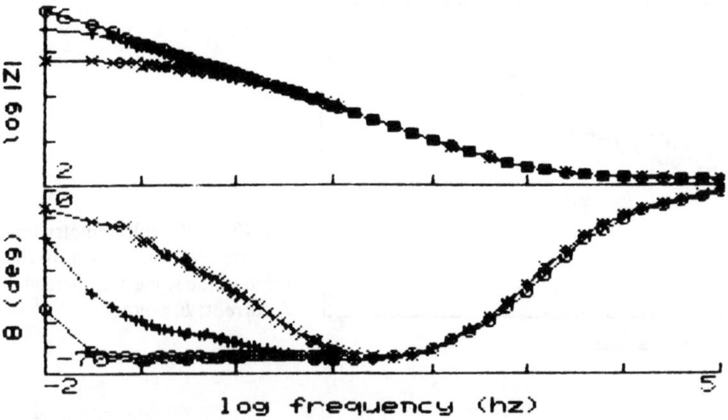

Fig. 7. Impedance /Z/ and phase angle Θ dependent on frequency (BODE-plot) for the artificial urine similar to the urine of the stone-former. DC; *circles*, 0 V; *crosses*, −0.2 V; *X*, −0.4 V

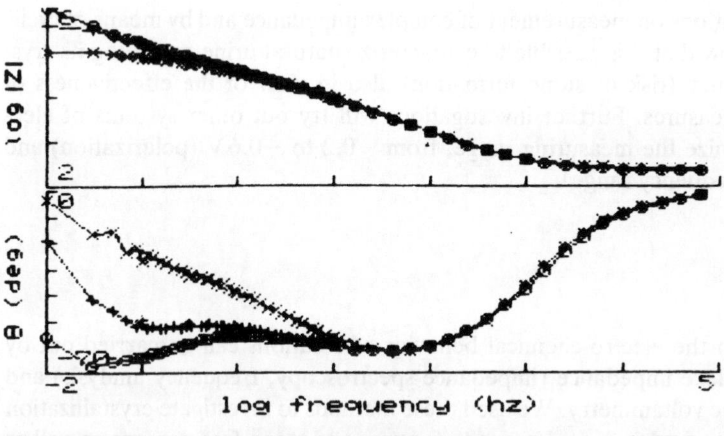

Fig. 8. Impedance /Z/ and phase angle Θ dependent on frequency (BODE-plot) for the artificial urine similar to the urine of the stone-free person. DC; *circles*, 0 V; *crosses*, −0.2 V; *X*, −0.4 V

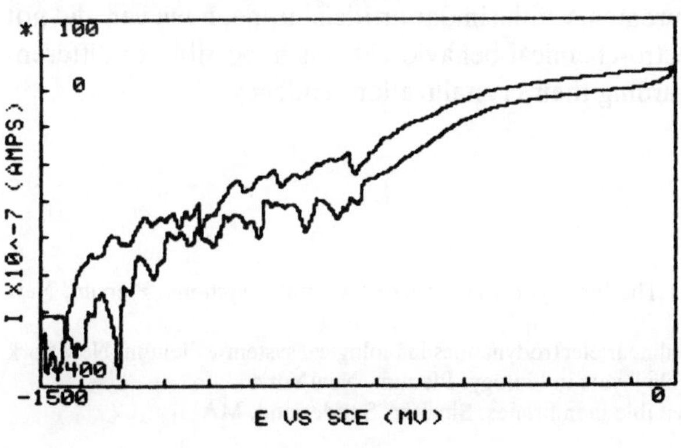

Fig. 9. Cyclic voltammetry for the artificial urine similar to the urine of the stone-former. *I*, current; *E*, voltage

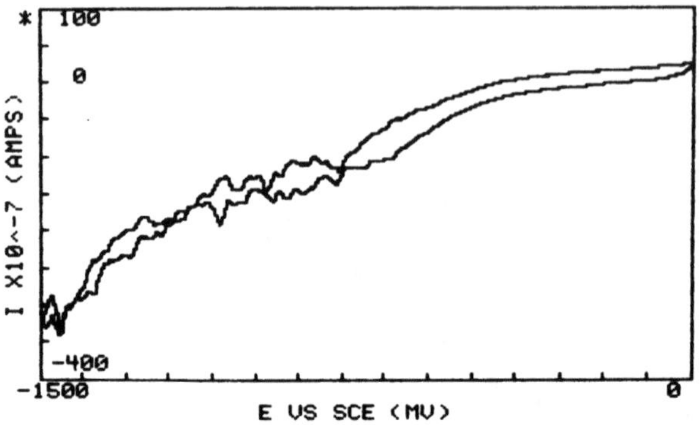

Fig. 10. Cyclic voltammetry for the artificial urine similar to the urine of the stone-free person. *I*, current; *E*, voltage

it may be presumed that components which are not recorded analytically (either inhibitors and/or promotors) can be found in stone-free people as well as in stone formers in different concentrations and that the interaction of all components results in an electrochemically different behavior of urine (i.e., at the inner and outer phase limit layers).

Our investigations on measurement of complex impedance and by means of cyclic voltammetry show that it is possible to characterize natural urine regarding its crystallization tendency (risk of stone formation) also in view of the effectiveness of metaphylactic measures. Further investigations will try out other systems of electrodes and optimize the measuring range, from −0.2 to −0.6 V (polarization) and 0.01 to 10 Hz (frequency range).

Summary

Investigations on the electro-chemical behavior of solutions can be carried out by measuring complexe impedance (impedance spectroscopy, frequency analysis) and by means of cyclic voltammetry. We used these methods to investigate crystallization tendency in urine of calcium oxalate stone formers and stone-free persons as well as in artificial urine similar to natural urine.

The urine of stone formers show a higher crystallization tendency compared to urine of stone-free persons, so that it is possible to differentiate urine in view of its risk of stone formation. Measurements with similar artificial urine, however, did not show any difference in its electro-chemical behavior; it was impossible to differentiate between these urines regarding their crystallization tendency.

References

Adelman WS, Goldman DE (1981) The biophysical approach to excitable systems. Plenum, New York

Adey WR, Lawrence AF (1984) Nonlinear electrodynamics in biological systems. Plenum, New York

Blank M (ed) (1986) Electrical double layers in biology. Plenum, New York

Hille B (1984) Ionic channels of excitable membranes. Sinauer, Sunderland, MA

Lipinski B (ed) (1982) Electronic conduction and mechano-electrical transduction in biological materials. Dekker, New York
Pethig R (1979) Dielectric and electronic properties of biological materials. Wiley, Chichester
Robertson WG, Scurr DS (1986) Modifiers of calcium oxalate crystallization found in urine. I. Studies with a continuous crystallizer using an artificial urine. J Urol 135 : 1322
Schanne OF, Ceretti E, Ruiz P (1978) Impedance measurements in biological cells. Wiley, New York
Schelter W (1985) Elektrische Eigenschaften biologischer Gewebe im Frequenzbereich 1 Hz–100 kHz. Dissertation, Universität Erlangen, FRG
Scurr DS, Robertson WG (1986) Modifiers of calcium oxalate crystallization found in urine. II. Studies on their mode of action in an artificial urine. J Urol 136 : 128

Autoradiographic Study of Oxalate in Rats

T. Sugimoto[1], H. Osswald[2], T. Kishimoto[1], K. Yamamoto[1], T. Kanazawa[1], H. Rübben[2], and T. Matsumura[1]

Introduction

We have already reported pharmacokinetic studies of oxalate in rats using radioisotopes; oxalate is more diffusible through biological membranes than inulin, and oxalate is excreted mainly by the kidney, although some is excreted by the liver (Sugimoto et al. 1988). Here, we checked these results in an autoradiographic study of oxalate in rats. Autoradiograms made after an injection of [^{14}C]oxalate were compared with those made after an injection of [^{14}C]inulin.

Materials and Methods

Six Sprague-Dawley rats weighing 200–250 g were used, three in the study of oxalate and the other three in that of inulin. The animals were anesthetized with ether and intravenously injected with either [^{14}C]oxalate or [^{14}C]inulin, at a dose of 5 μCi per 100 g of body weight. In both studies, one rat was killed 5, 30, and 90 min after the injection. The rats were immediately frozen in a mixture of dry ice and acetone and embedded in carboxyl methyl cellulose sodium. Then, the rats were sliced sagittally with a cryomicrotome. The whole body specimens were kept in contact with X-ray films for 2 weeks to make the autoradiograms.

Results

Autoradiograms at 5 and 30 min after the injection of [^{14}C]inulin showed that inulin accumulated mainly in the kidney and blood vessels (Fig. 1a and 1b). In contrast, in the autoradiograms at the same times after the injection of [^{14}C]oxalate, oxalate had accumulated not only in the kidney and blood vessels but also in the bone, liver, spleen, and muscles (Fig. 2a and 2b). The autoradiogram for 90 min after the injection of [^{14}C]oxalate showed that it had accumulated also in the bone, renal papilla, and the small intestine (Fig. 2c). At this time, no radioactivity from [^{14}C]inulin was observed except in the renal cortex (Fig. 1c).

Discussion

Oxalate is mostly endogenously generated (Madorsky and Finlayson 1977; Banwart et al. 1979) and excreted mainly from the kidney (Hautmann and Osswald 1983).

[1] Department of Urology, Osaka City University Medical School, Osaka, Japan
[2] Department of Urology and Pharmacology, RWTH-Aachen, 5100 Aachen, FRG

Investigative Urology 3
Edited by H. Rübben et al.

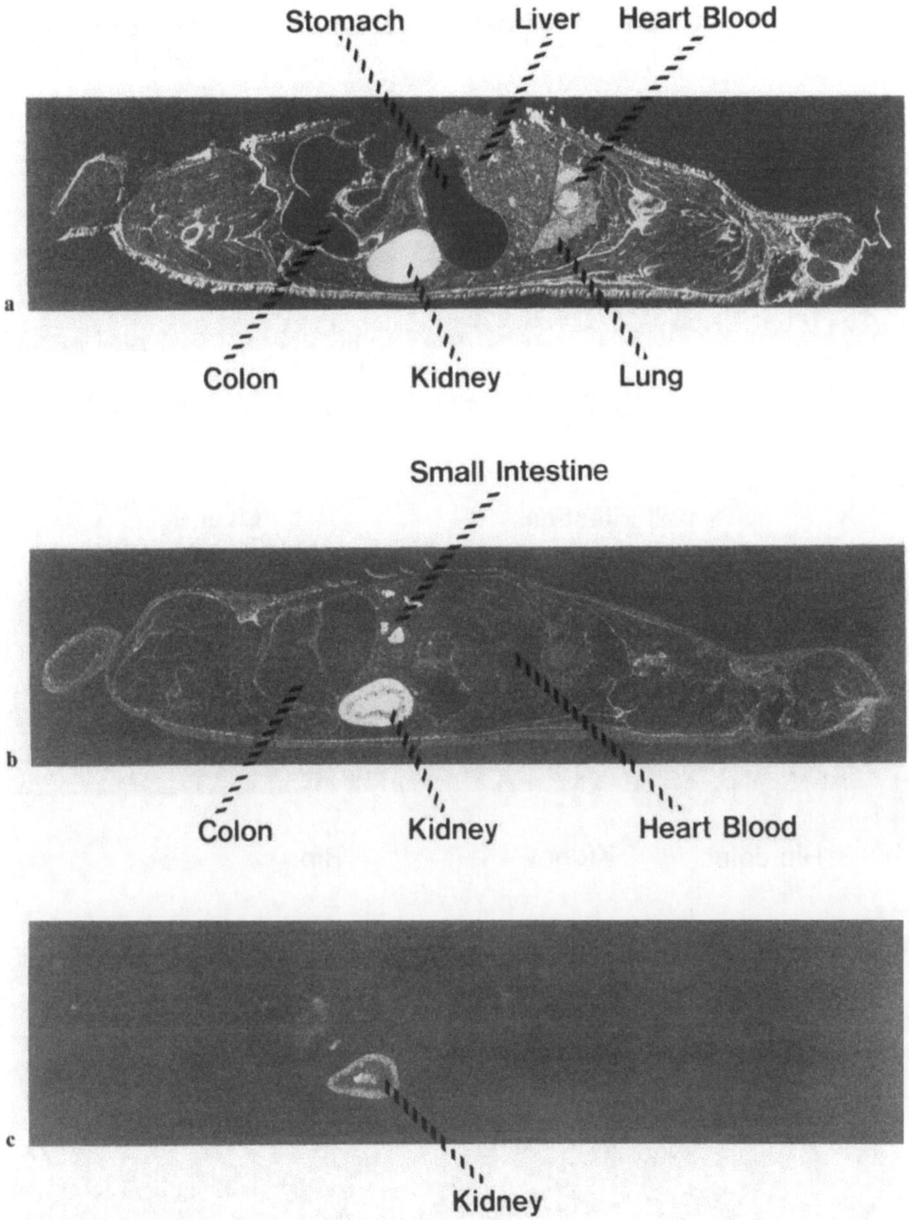

Fig. 1a–c. Autoradiograms showing the distribution of [^{14}C]inulin 5 min (**a**), 30 min (**b**), and 90 min (**c**) after injection

Animal experiments on the renal handling of oxalate have shown that the renal clearance of oxalate is about 1.3 times that of inulin (Knight et al. 1979). We had studied the pharmacokinetics of oxalate in rats, which suggested that oxalate was more diffusible through biological membranes because the total distribution volume of oxalate was 1.7 times larger than that of inulin, and that some part of the circulat-

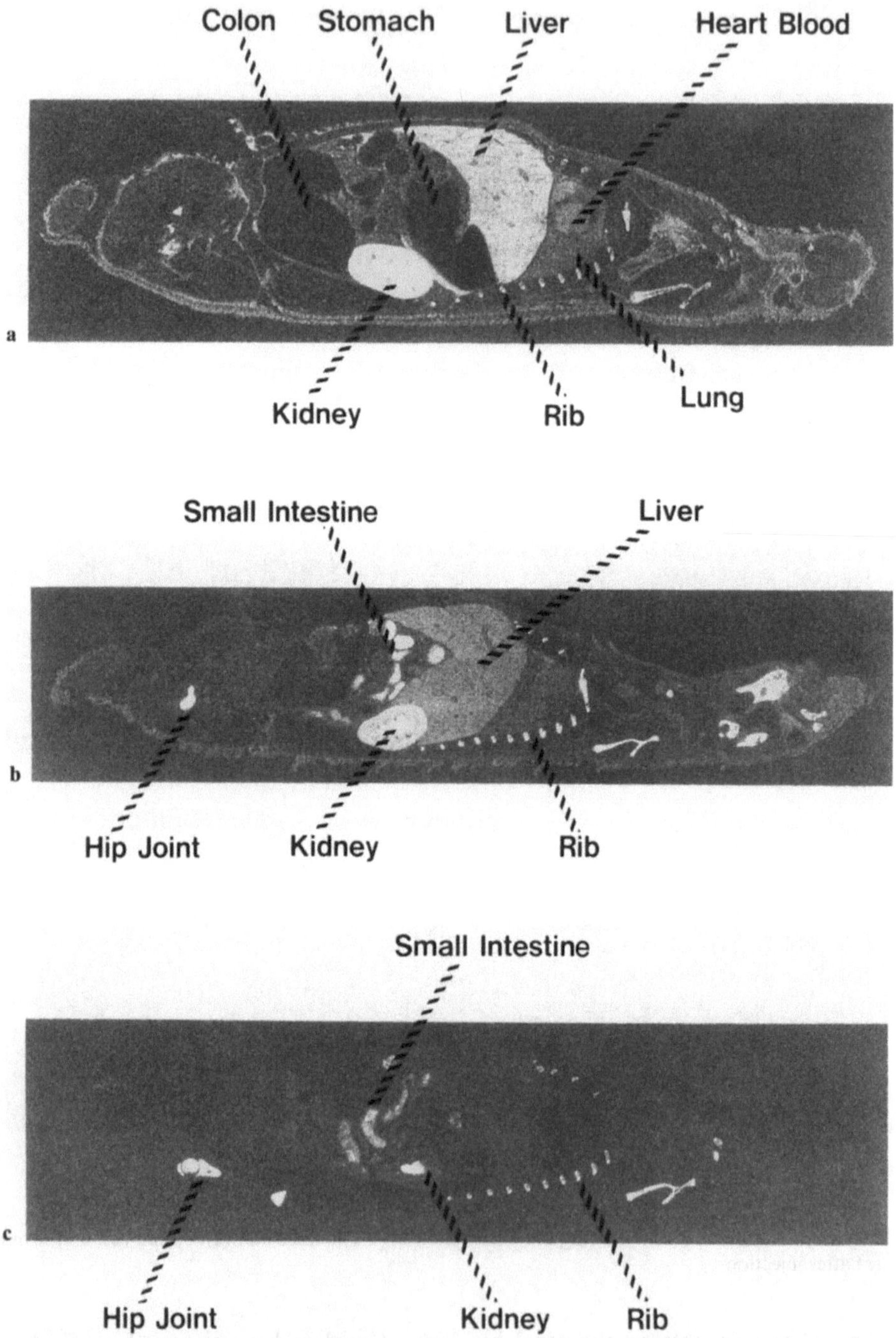

Fig. 2a–c. Autoradiograms showing the distribution of [^{14}C]oxalate 5 min (**a**), 30 min (**b**), and 90 min (**c**) after injection

ing oxalate was excreted by the liver because the recovery of [^{14}C]oxalate injected intravenously in the bile accounted for 2.3%–2.8%. In the present study, autoradiograms showed that [^{14}C]inulin activity accumulated mainly in the kidney and blood vessels. On the other hand, oxalate was distributed not only in the kidney and blood vessels but also in the bone, and the radioactivity in the liver, spleen, and muscles was much higher than that of [^{14}C]inulin. The radioactivity of [^{14}C]oxalate was also high in the small intestine. Thus, the results of the autoradiographic study supported the findings of our pharmacokinetic study.

References

Banwart C, Hagmaier V, Rutishauser G, Sieler H (1979) Absorption of oxalic acid in rats by means of a 14C method. Eur Urol 5:276–277

Hautmann R, Osswald H (1983) Concentration profile of calcium and oxalate in urine, tubular fluid and renal tissue – some theoretical considerations. J Urol 129:433–436

Knight TF, Senekjian HO, Weinman EJ (1979) Effect of para-aminohippurate on renal transport of oxalate. Kidney Int 15:38–42

Madorsky ML, Finlayson B (1977) Oxalate absorption from intestinal segments of rats. Invest Urol 14:274–277

Sugimoto T, Katoh Y, Matsumura T, Kishimoto T, Kanazawa T, Yamamoto K, Maekawa M (1988) Pharmacokinetic study on oxalate in rats. Acta Urol Jpn 34:1135–1139

Lactose-Induced Urolithiasis in the Rat

W. L. Strohmaier, K.-H. Bichler, and H. J. Nelde[1]

Introduction

Up to now the pathogenesis of idiopathic hypercalciuria has not been completely elucidated. The majority of patients are supposed to have primary intestinal hyperabsorption of calcium.

According to Bronner et al. (1986) there are two different intestinal calcium transport systems: first, a transcellular saturable process which is regulated by vitamin D and predominates in the proximal intestine; second, a nonsaturable, probably paracellular process similar in intensity throughout the whole intestine, which is vitamin D independent. Several authors (Insogna et al. 1985; Kaplan et al. 1977; Pak 1979) postulate increased 1,25-dihydroxycholecalciferol (1,25 DHCC) as the cause of absorptive hypercalciuria. On the other hand this is found only in a small part of these patients: 60% of our patients with absorptive hypercalciuria showed normal or even decreased 1,25 DHCC levels (Bichler et al. 1985; Schreiber et al. 1985).

In these cases one has to assume a primary epithelial hyperabsorption independent from vitamin D. There is either increased susceptibility of the saturable transport process to normal 1,25 DHCC or the nonsaturable, vitamin D-independent transport system absorbs more calcium.

To investigate absorptive hypercalciuria with primarily increased 1,25 DHCC there is the model of the spontaneously hypertensive rat (SHR) (Hsu et al. 1986; Lau et al. 1986). Looking for a similar model for absorptive hypercalciuria with low vitamin D levels, we found lactose-induced urolithiasis in the rat.

Materials and Methods

In the following pilot study 25 female Fü-Albino rats (Institut für Biologisch Medizinische Forschung AG, Füllingsdorf, CH-4402 Post Fränkendorf, Schweiz) were investigated. At the beginning of the study the animals' weight was 85 g. They were randomly divided into two groups: lactose diet ($n = 15$), or control diet ($n = 10$). The animals were kept on these diets for 9 months. Pair feeding was done, and the body weight was controlled weekly. At 3 and 9 months after the beginning, urine was collected. At the end of the study all animals were killed. Blood was taken from the aorta. Kidneys, ureters, and bladders were investigated for concrements and taken out for histological examination. In urine calcium, phosphate, magnesium, citrate, and Tamm-Horsfall protein were determined. The excretion of those parameters

[1] Department of Urology, University of Tübingen, 7400 Tübingen, FRG

Investigative Urology 3
Edited by H. Rübben et al.

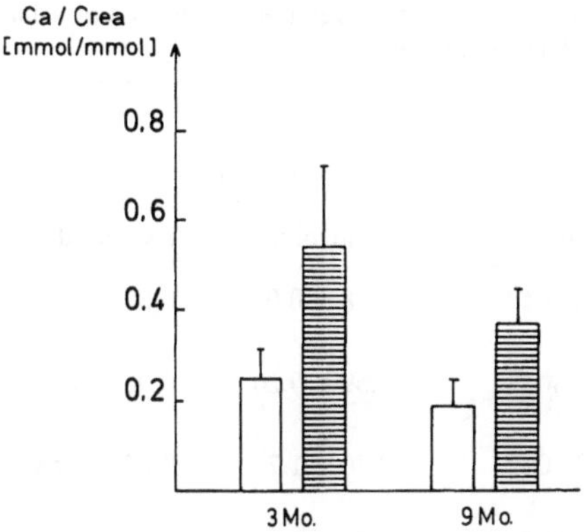

Fig. 1. Urinary calcium excretion with control diet (*open bar; n* = 10) and lactose diet (*hatched bar; n* = 15), $P \leq 0.02$ (Mann-Whitney test)

was related to urinary creatinine. In plasma calcium, phosphate, creatinine, 1,25 DHCC, and 25-hydroxycholecalciferol (25 HCC) were measured.

Kidneys were examined histologically (Voigt and Kossa staining) and by polarization microscopy.

Results

The body weight increased in both groups similarly: at the end of the study the animals weighed 300 g. On lactose diet urinary excretion of calcium increased significantly in both collecting periods (Fig. 1). Phosphate excretion was not significantly different (Table 1).

The lactose diet induced significantly increased magnesium excretion, especially in the second collecting period (Table 1).

The urinary excretion of citrate was increased, too; especially in the first collecting period there was a marked difference between the two samples (Table 1). The lactose diet induced an increased excretion of Tamm-Horsfall protein (Table 1).

Concerning plasma levels phosphate was elevated significantly with the lactose diet (Table 1). 1,25 DHCC was significantly decreased (Fig. 2), whereas 25 HCC, calcium, and creatinine were not changed (Table 1).

The animals on the lactose diet showed gravel in the urinary tract, and in the kidneys calcifications could be seen even macroscopically. The histological examination demonstrated marked calcifications in all animals on the lactose diet. They were located in the outer strip of the exterior zone of the medulla. As far as visible by light microscopy, the calcifications were located in the interstitium (Fig. 3). Polarization microscopy demonstrated calcium phosphate.

Discussion

First Gershoff and McGandy (1981) reported on apatite stones in rats on a lactose diet. These animals also demonstrated increased excretion of urinary calcium. Even 60 years ago it could be shown that lactose increases intestinal absorption of calcium

Table 1. Mean values, standard deviation, and levels of significance (Mann-Whitney test) of urine and plasma parameters with control diet ($n = 10$) and lactose diet ($n = 15$)

	Urine			
	After 3 months		After 9 months	
	Control diet	Lactose diet	Control diet	Lactose diet
Calcium (mmol/mmol)	0.24 ± 0.06	0.55 ± 0.20**	0.18 ± 0.06	0.38 ± 0.08**
Magnesium (mmol/mmol)	1.08 ± 0.18	1.44 ± 0.40*	0.59 ± 0.20	0.90 ± 0.20**
Phosphate (mmol/mmol)	8.76 ± 2.00	7.98 ± 2.10	8.30 ± 1.7	9.47 ± 1.18
Citrate (mmol/mmol)	0.07 ± 0.02	0.44 ± 0.88**	0.14 ± 0.02	0.18 ± 0.04*
Tamm-Horsfall (NE/mg)	0.04 ± 0.05	0.25 ± 0.12**	0.21 ± 0.14	0.44 ± 0.13**

	Plasma	
	Control diet	Lactose diet
Calcium (mg/dl)	10.24 ± 0.40	9.78 ± 0.43
Phosphate (mg/dl)	5.71 ± 0.32	6.54 ± 1.01*
Creatine (mg/dl)	0.98 ± 0.06	1.07 ± 0.25
1,25 DHCC (pg/ml)	51.0 ± 10.1	33.5 ± 7.2**
25 HCC (ng/ml)	27.5 ± 8.5	23.0 ± 7.1

* $P \leq 0.05$
** $P \leq 0.02$

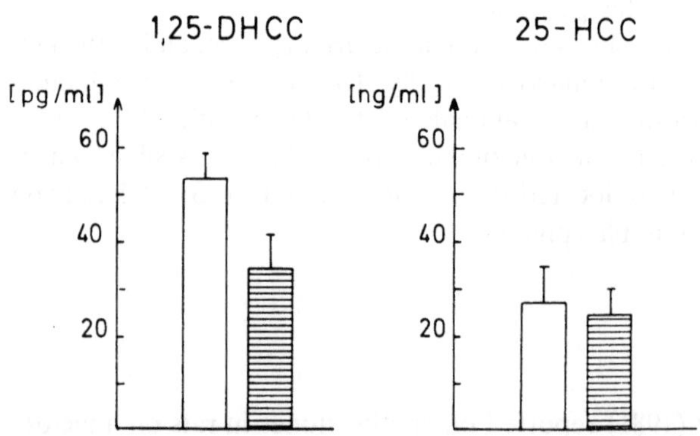

Fig. 2. 1,25-Dihydroxycholecalciferol *(1,25-DHCC)* and 25-hydroxycholecalciferol *(25-HCC)* with control diet (*open bar*; $n = 10$) and lactose diet (*hatched bar*; $n = 15$). Significant differences (Mann-Whitney test): 1,25 DHCC, $P \leq 0.02$; 25 HCC, not significant

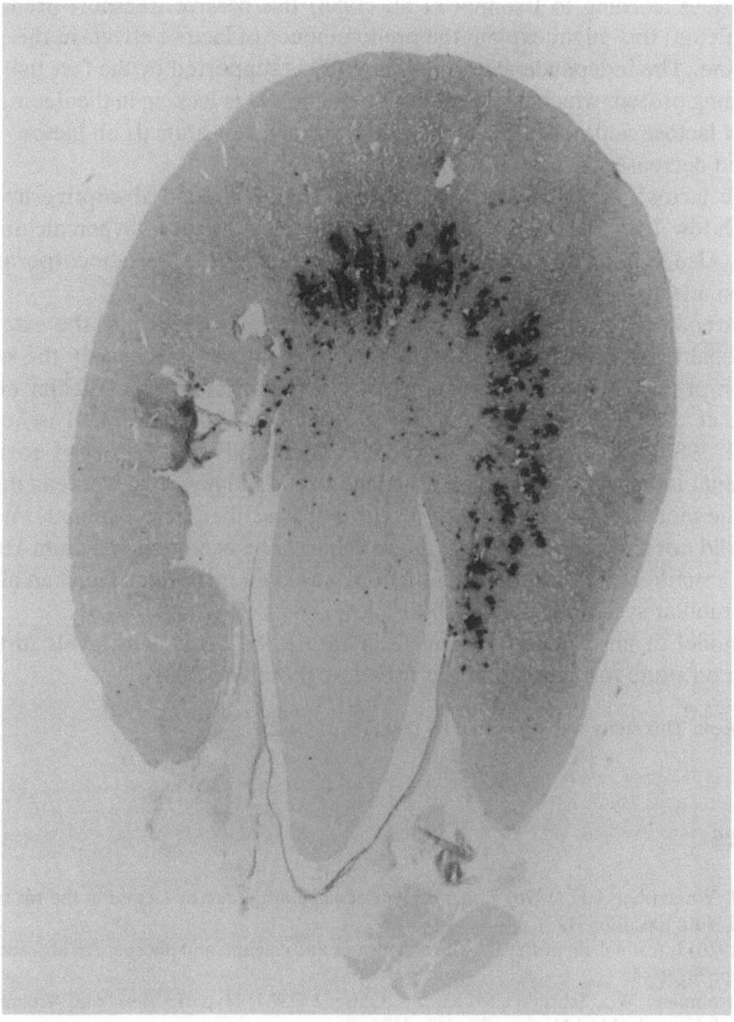

Fig. 3. Histological section of a rat kidney on lactose diet. Kossa staining, survey magnification × 320

(Bergheim 1926). The underlying mechanism, however, has not been elucidated sufficiently. Several hypotheses have been postulated: formation of an absorbable calcium lactose complex (Charley and Saltman 1963), reduction of intestinal pH (Bergheim 1926), and increased permeability of the intestinal membranes for calcium (Armbrecht and Wassermann 1976).

Investigations of Armbrecht and Wassermann (1976) and Lengemann et al. (1959) demonstrated that the formation of soluble complexes and intestinal pH reduction might not be the cause of increased calcium absorption. It could be shown that lactose acts predominantly in the ileum and independent of vitamin D. Furthermore, the application of dinitrophenol did not interfere with the lactose effects, thus indicating that lactose does not act on the active calcium transport system but on passive transport. According to Bronner et al. (1986) this passive transport predominates in the ileum; this might explain the predominance of lactose effects in this part of the intestine. The independence from vitamin D is supported by the fact that the calcium-binding protein which is dependent on vitamin D is lacking in the ileum, the major site of lactose action (Pansu et al. 1983). In fact, our animals on lactose diet demonstrated decreased 1,25 DHCC levels.

Thus, the lactose model seems to be comparable to human absorptive hypercalciuria with low 1,25 DHCC levels. A renal or osseous origin of hypercalciuria is improbable. Also, Sato et al. (1983) demonstrated an increased 45-Ca-incorporation into bones on a lactose diet.

The intrarenal calcifications were located only in the outer strip of the exterior medulla, probably in the interstitium. This type of calcification is exactly the same which can be produced by an atherogenic diet (rich in cholesterol) (Bichler et al. 1985; Nelde et al. 1985, 1987; Strohmaier et al. 1985) and acute renal ischemia (Hertle et al. 1985). Obviously the kidney reacts identically to a variety of noxious agents. In renal ischemia there is direct damage to the kidney cells, whereas this is unlikely in the model of lactose-induced urolithiasis described here. Animals on the lactose diet did not show increased creatinine values. The excretion of Tamm-Horsfall protein, a marker of distal tubular function, was even increased. Thus, an alteration of the tubular systems is improbable.

In this model of absorptive hypercalciuria with low 1,25 DHCC levels further investigation on stone formation and their therapy should be done.

Acknowledgement. This study was supported by DFG (Bi 159 4-2).

References

Armbrecht HJ, Wasserman RH (1976) Enhancement of calcium uptake by lactose in the rat small intestine. J Nutr 106:1265–1271

Bergheim O (1926) Intestinal chemistry. V. Carbohydrates and calcium and phosphorus absorption. J Biol Chem 70:35–45

Bichler KH, Strohmaier WL, Schreiber M, Korn S, Gaiser I (1984) Hyperkalziurie and Vitamin D Stoffwechsel. Fortschr Urol Nephrol 22:242–347

Bichler KH, Strohmaier WL, Schanz F, Nelde HJ, Gaiser I, Schulze E, Schreiber M (1985) Zur Wirkung von Kalziumanatagonisten (Nifedipin) auf die Nephrokalzinose und Kalziumausscheidung der Ratte. Urol Int 40:13–21

Bronner S, Pansu D, Stein WD (1986) An analysis of intestinal calcium transport across the rat intestine. Am J Physiol 250:G561–569

Charley P, Saltman P (1963) Chelation of calcium by lactose: its role in transport mechanisms. Science 139:1205–1206

Gershoff SN, McGandy RB (1981) The effect of vitamin A diet containing lactose in producing bladder calculi and tumors in rats. Am J Clin Nutr 34:483–489

Hertle L, Garthoff B, Chur C, Pötz B, Funke PJ, Senge T (1985) Limitierung des ischämischen Nierenschadens durch den Kalziumantgonisten Nisoldipin. In: Harzmann R, Jacobi GH, Weißbach L (eds) Experimentelle Urologie. Springer Berlin Heidelberg New York Tokyo

Hsu CH, Chen PS, Smith DE, Young CS (1986) Pathogenesis of hypercalciuria in spontaneously hypertensive rats. Miner Electrolyte Metab 12:130–141

Insogna KL, Broadus AE, Dreyer BE, Ellison AS, Gertner JM (1985) Elevated production rate of 1,25-dihydroxy vitamin D in patients with absorptive hypercalciuria. J Clin Endocrinol Metab 61:490–495

Kaplan R, Hausler M, Deftos L, Bone H, Pak CYC (1977) The role of 1,25-dihydroxy vitamin D in the medication of intestinal hyperabsorption of calcium in primary hyperparathyreoidism and absorptive hypercalciuria. J Clin Invest 59:756–760

Lau K, Langman CB, Gafter U, Dudeja PK, Brasitus TA (1986) Increased calcium absorption in prehypertensive spontaneously hypertensive rat. J Clin Invest 78:1083–1090

Lengemann FW, Wasserman RH, Comar CL (1959) Studies on the enhancement of radiocalcium and radiostrontium absorption by lactose in the rat. J Nutr 68:443–455

Nelde HJ, Bichler KH, Strohmaier WL, Schanz F (1985) Histopathologische Veränderungen in der Niere der Ratte unter atherogener Diät bzw. Nifedipinverabreichung. Fortschr Urol Nephrol 23:319–325

Nelde HJ, Bichler KH, Kriz W, Strohmaier WL (1987) Licht- und elektronenmikroskopische Untersuchungen über morphologische Veränderungen der Rattenniere bei Nephrokalzinose. Fortschr Urol Nephrol 25:393–398

Pak C (1979) Physiological basis for absorptive and renal hypercalciurias. Am J Physiol 237:F415–F421

Pansu D, Bellaton C, Roche C, Bronner F (1983) Duodenal and ileal calcium absorption in the rat and effect of vitamin D. Am J Physiol 244:G695–G700

Sato R, Noguchi T, Naito H (1983) Effect of lactose on calcium absorption from the rat small intestine with a non-flushed ligated loop. J Nutr Sci Vitaminol 29:365–373

Schreiber M, Bichler KH, Strohmaier WL, Gaiser I, Krug J, Nelde HJ (1985) Vitamin D metabolism in hypercalciuric patients. In: Schwille PO, Smith LH, Robertson WG, Vahlensieck W (eds) Urolithiasis and related clinical research. Plenum, New York, pp 315–318

Strohmaier WL, Bichler KH, Schanz F, Nelde HJ, Schreiber M (1985) Einfluß von Kalziumantagonisten auf die Ausscheidung von Kalzium und anderer für die Steingenese wichtiger Substanzen bei der Ratte. Fortschr Urol Nephrol 23:365–371

Investigation of Annual Rhythms for the Excretion of Calcium, Oxalic Acid, and Uric Acid in the 24-h Urine

A. HESSE[1] and F. BIERTH

In view of the varying climatic influences and the changing dietary habits of the population over the seasons of the year there is reason to believe that the risk of urolithiasis is subject to a seasonal rhythm. In this study, the 24-h urine of healthy women ($n = 30$) and healthy men ($n = 40$) was collected once each month for one year. The following parameters were determined: pH, specific weight, Na, K, NH_4, Ca, Mg, Cl, P, SO_4, creatinine, uric acid, oxalic acid, citric acid, titrable acid, glycosaminoglycan (GAG), relative supersaturation (EQUIL). Parallel to these, a dietary record was kept in each case in order to check the calcium and oxalate intake.

A statistically significant annual course was discovered for all the urolithiasis-related parameters. There were differences between the sexes. For example, the seasonal rhythm of Ca excretion (Fig. 1) and concentration peaks from August to November and is even more marked in men. In contrast to this, peaks for oxalic acid (Fig. 2) and uric acid (Fig. 3) were recorded from January to March. These results conform to those gained from evaluation of the diet records.

The citric acid and Mg excretions were highest in the summer and autumn months and were regarded as being seasonal protective factors. Women excreted more citric acid than men. When calculating the relative supersaturation all these results affect the Ca oxalate figure (Fig. 4). In autumn and winter the figures for relative supersaturation are at their highest.

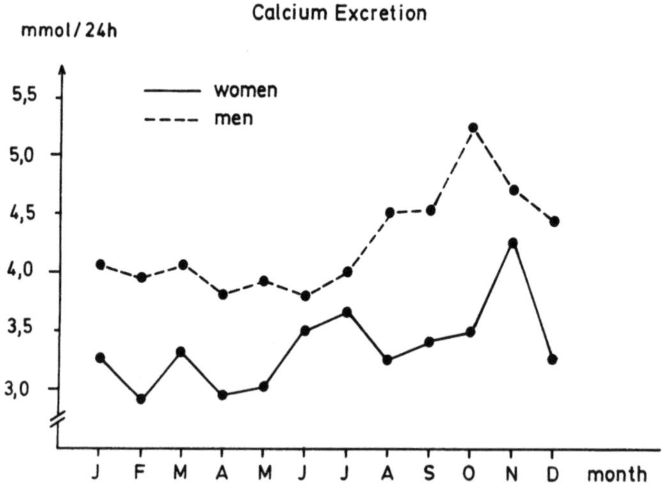

Fig. 1. Seasonal rhythm of calcium excretion in 24-h urine

[1]Experimentelle Urologie, Urologische Universitätsklinik, Sigmund-Freud-Str. 25, 3500 Bonn 1, FRG

Investigative Urology 3
Edited by H. Rübben et al.

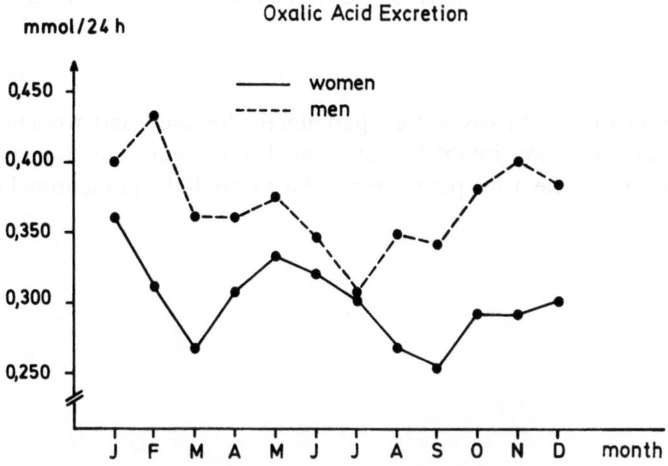

Fig. 2. Seasonal rhythm of oxalic acid excretion in 24-h urine

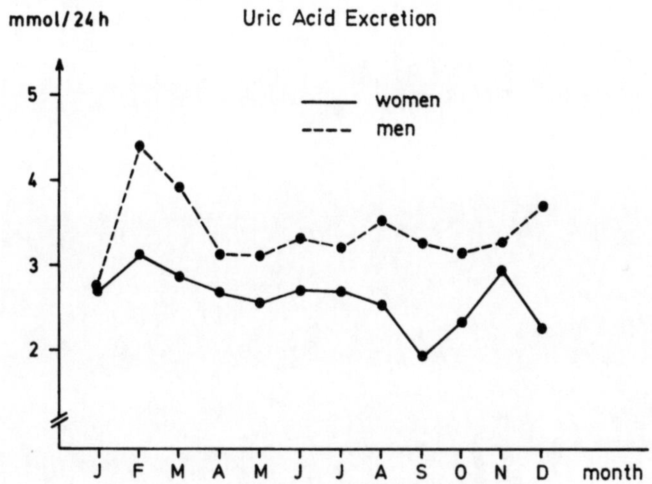

Fig. 3. Seasonal rhythm of uric acid excretion in 24-h urine

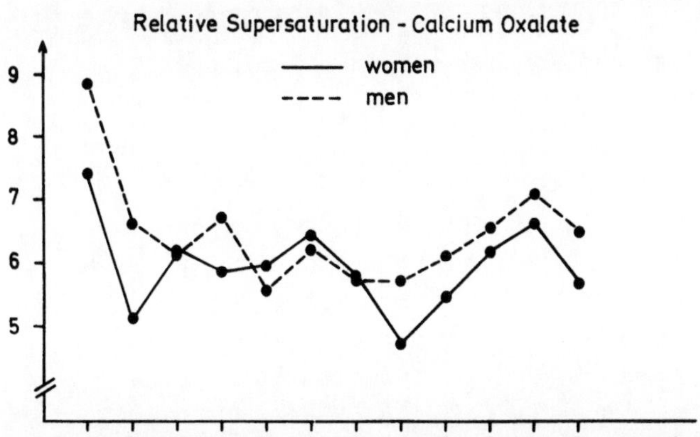

Fig. 4. Seasonal rhythm of supersaturation of calcium oxalate, calculated with EQUIL

Summary

The annual rhythm of urolithiasis-related parameters for men and women were studied in the course of a longitudinal study. Statistically significant courses were found for the majority of the urine parameters, which were linked to seasonal variations in diet.

Calcium Binding by Various Brans: In Vitro Experiment with ^{45}Ca

B. Gertz, A. Classen, and A. Hesse[1]

Introduction

Urolithiasis is a widespread disease. Most of the patients are recurrent stone formers, so there is a great need for a prophylactic treatment. Calcium is a main component of many urinary stones, and hypercalciuria is one important risk factor for urolithiasis. The urinary calcium excretion can be reduced by preventing the absorption of calcium in the intestine. Dietary fiber is said to bind calcium (McCane and Widdowsen 1942; Dintzis et al. 1985). Bran being a product rich in dietary fiber, we examined several types of bran for their calcium-binding capacity in vitro. It should be tested whether all brans are able to bind calcium and whether the binding is pH-dependent.

Materials and Methods

The principle of the assay is to mix bran with a solution of $CaCl_2$ and measure the not bound free calcium. By using the AAS low calcium-binding rates could not be recorded sufficiently; therefore, a new method using the radioactive isotope ^{45}Ca was developed.

Of each bran 1 g is mixed with a solution of $CaCl_2$ (50 mmol Ca/l) and a special amount of ^{45}Ca is added, followed by an incubation at 37°C. The radioactive calcium is bound in the same percentage as the nonradioactive calcium. The free ^{45}Ca can be measured by liquid scintillation counting. The amount of bound calcium is calculated from the amount of free radioactive calcium. Five brans [rice, rye, soy, wheat (fine), wheat (coarse)] were tested for their calcium-binding capacity at several pH, which are characteristic for the gastrointestinal tract (pH 2.2, pH 5–6, pH 7.3, pH 8.0). Adjustment of pH was accomplished by adding HCl and sodium citrate buffer or tris buffer.

Results and Discussion

Calcium binding was complete within about 6 h; only rye bran and wheat bran (fine) showed a small increase up to 10 h (Fig. 1). All brans bind calcium, but each to a different extent.

The results indicate that the calcium binding is pH-dependent (Fig. 2). At pH 2.2, typical for the stomach, all brans bind only weakly. A reason for this might be that at pH 2.2 all acids (e.g., uronic acids, phytic acid, and carboxyl groups) are undis-

[1] Urologische Universitätsklinik Bonn, Experimentelle Urologie, 5300 Bonn 1, FRG

Investigative Urology 3
Edited by H. Rübben et al.

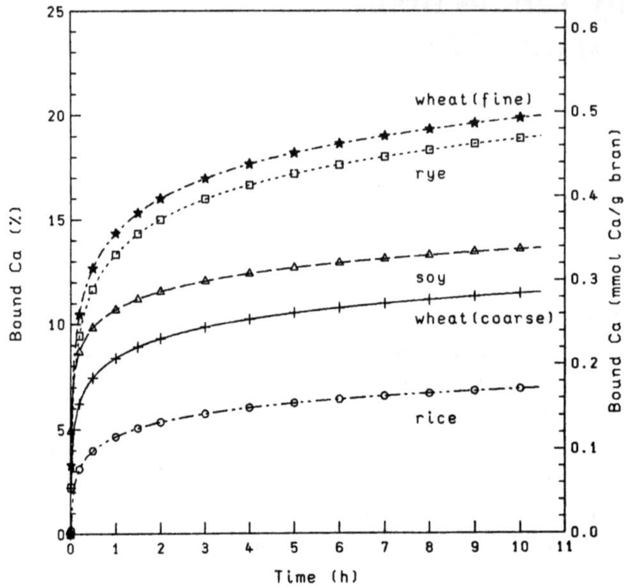

Fig. 1. Calcium binding by various brans (at pH 7.3, $n=9$)

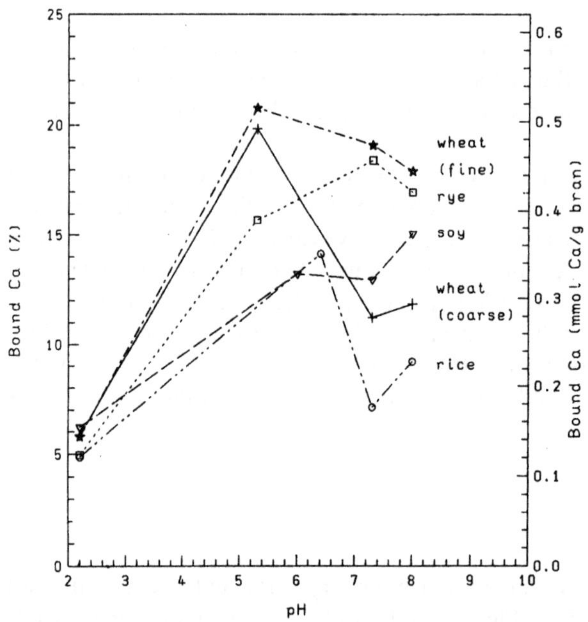

Fig. 2. Calcium binding by various brans (at different pH, $n=9$)

sociated, thus having no free binding sites for calcium. The 5% bound calcium might be a result of the inclusion of calcium in the network of dietary fiber. Rice bran shows the lowest calcium binding rate of all brans with a maximum at pH 6.4. In a slight alkaline environment soy bran has its highest calcium binding rate with 15 mg Ca/g bran, whereas rye bran binds under the same conditions about 18 mg Ca/g bran.

The calcium binding of wheat bran (coarse) is very pH-dependent with a maximum at pH 5.3 (20 mg Ca/g bran).

At all pH values wheat bran (fine) shows the highest calcium binding capacity (maximum 21 mg Ca/g bran). It binds about three times more calcium than rice bran.

These differences in the calcium-binding capacity of the five brans and the pH-dependence might be explained by the different chemical and structural compositions of the brans. Uronic acids (James et al. 1978), phytic acid (Davies 1979), or the whole bran (Reinhold et al. 1975) are thought to be responsible for the calcium binding by dietary fiber.

References

Davies NT (1979) Anti-nutrient factors affecting mineral utilization. Proc Nutr Soc 38:121–128

Dintzis FR, Watson PR, Sandstead HH (1985) Mineral contents of brans passed through the human GI tract. Am J Clin Nutr 41:901–908

James WPT, Branch WI, Southgate DAT (1978) Calcium binding by dietary fibre. Lancet 1:638–639

McCane RA, Widdowsen EM (1942) Mineral metabolism of healthy adults on white and brown bread dietaries. J Physiol 101:304–313

Reinhold JG, Ismail-Beigi F, Faradji B (1975) Fibre vs phytate as determinant of the availability of calcium, zinc and iron of breadstuffs. Nutr Rep Int 12(2):75–85

Application of High-Performance Liquid Chromatography for Determination of Cysteine and Cystine in Urine

H. Birwé and A. Hesse[1]

Introduction

Cystinuria is an hereditary metabolic disease characterized by recurrent urolithiasis resulting from excessive urinary excretion of the relatively insoluble amino acid, cystine (C-SS-C). Mostly cystinuria is detected subsequent to stone formation (Hesse and Schaefer 1987). The disorder requires a life-long therapy based on exact laboratory diagnosis.

Recent reports emphasize the potential use of high-performance liquid chromatography (HPLC) with precolumn derivatization in amino acid analysis. HPLC reduces analysis time and increases the sensitivity for quantitation of amino acids (Turner and Cooper 1982; Graser et al. 1985; Leah et al. 1986). Using *ortho*-phthaldialdehyde (OPA), the derivatization step is rather fast and simple to operate. One disadvantage of this method is the poor reactivity of cystine and its monomer, cysteine (C-SH). This problem is overcome by a special pretreatment of the samples. During a first step cystine is reduced to cysteine by dithiothreitol (DTT). The reduction is followed by the S-carboxymethylation of cysteine with iodoacetic acid. S-carboxymethylcysteine (CMC) yields a derivative with fluorescence intensity comparable to other amino acids.

This paper reports the analytical conditions and first results.

Materials and Methods

Apparatus. The chromatographic conditions are presented in Table 1. The sodium phosphate buffer was prepared weekly with *o*-phosphoric acid (85%) and sodium hydroxide (30%, both Suprapur, Merck Darmstadt, FRG). The buffer was filtered through a 0.45-µm pore size filter (Schleicher & Schüll, Dassel, FRG) and stored at 4°C. DTT (1.25 m*M*) and iodoacetic acid (10 m*M*) were diluted in the phosphate buffer.

Sample Preparation. Urine samples were collected into a beaker with sulfosalicylic acid (30%; 80 ml for a 2 l flask) to bring the pH immediately down to a level of 1–2. After centrifuging (4000 rpm, 10 min) and passing through a 0.2-µm pore size filter (Schleicher & Schüll), 10 µl (cystinuric urines require a further dilution) from this sample were diluted to 900 µl with the phosphate buffer, and 100 µl potassium borate (1 *M*, pH 10.4; Pierce, Oud Beijerland, Netherlands) was added.

[1] Experimentelle Urologie, Urologische Universitätsklinik, Sigmund-Freud-Str. 25, 5300 Bonn 1, FRG

Investigative Urology 3
Edited by H. Rübben et al.

Table 1. Chromatographic conditions

2 HPLC pumps (Pharmacia LKB 2150)
1 Gradient controller (Pharmacia LKB 2152)
1 High pressure mixer (Pharmacia LKB 2152-400)
1 Injection valve (Rheodyne 7125, 20 µl loop)
1 Fluorescence detector (Shimadzu RF 535)
1 Integrator (LDC/Milton Roy CI 10)

Stationary Phase:
Column: Spherisorb ODS II, 3 µ, 4.6 * 250 mm
Guardcolumn: Spherisorb ODS II, 5 µ, 4.6 * 10 mm (Grom, Herrenberg)

Mobile Phase:
12.5 m*M* Na-phosphate buffer pH 7.2
Eluent A: 0.35% Tetrahydrofurane (Merck) in PO_4
Eluent B: 50% Acetonitrile (J.T. Baker) in PO_4

Gradient:
0–9 min 0% B, 9–12 min to 100% B, 12–16 min
100% B, 16–19 min to 0% B, 19–30 min 0% B

Derivatization. Derivatization was done according to the diagram shown in Fig. 1. Analyzing the total cysteine, the prepared sample solution was treated with DTT (100 µl, 1.25 m*M*) to reduce cystine. After completion of this reaction, 100 µl iodoacetic acid (10 m*M*) to blocking the sulfhydryl group was added. Looking only for the cysteine content of the sample, the reduction step was omitted and instead of DTT another 100 µl of the phosphate buffer was added. The cystine content was then calculated by the difference of two chromatographic runs of one sample (see Fig. 1).

Quantitation. Peak identification was done by the retention times, and the analyte concentrations were calculated by peak areas.

Results and Discussion

Typical chromatograms of a standard (A) and an urine sample of a cystinuric patient analyzed for cysteine (B) and total cysteine (C) are shown in Fig. 2. Under the conditions described the calibration curve is linear from 0.5 to 500 pmol CMC on column (2.5 µ*M* to 2.5 m*M*; $r = 0.995$, $n = 12$).

The within-run precision for total cysteine ($n = 10$) is 9.3%, for cysteine ($n = 10$), 4.8%. Analytical recovery varied from 97.6% (SD = 2.1, $n = 20$; cysteine) to 101.6% (SD = 7.7, $n = 20$; total cysteine).

The values for total cysteine agreed well with results of the conventional amino acid analysis based on ion exchange ($n = 20$; $r = 0.998$).

The technique described allows a rapid and sensitive determination of cysteine in urine. The poor reactivity of cysteine and cystine with OPA is overcome by blocking the sulfhydryl group with iodoacetic acid.

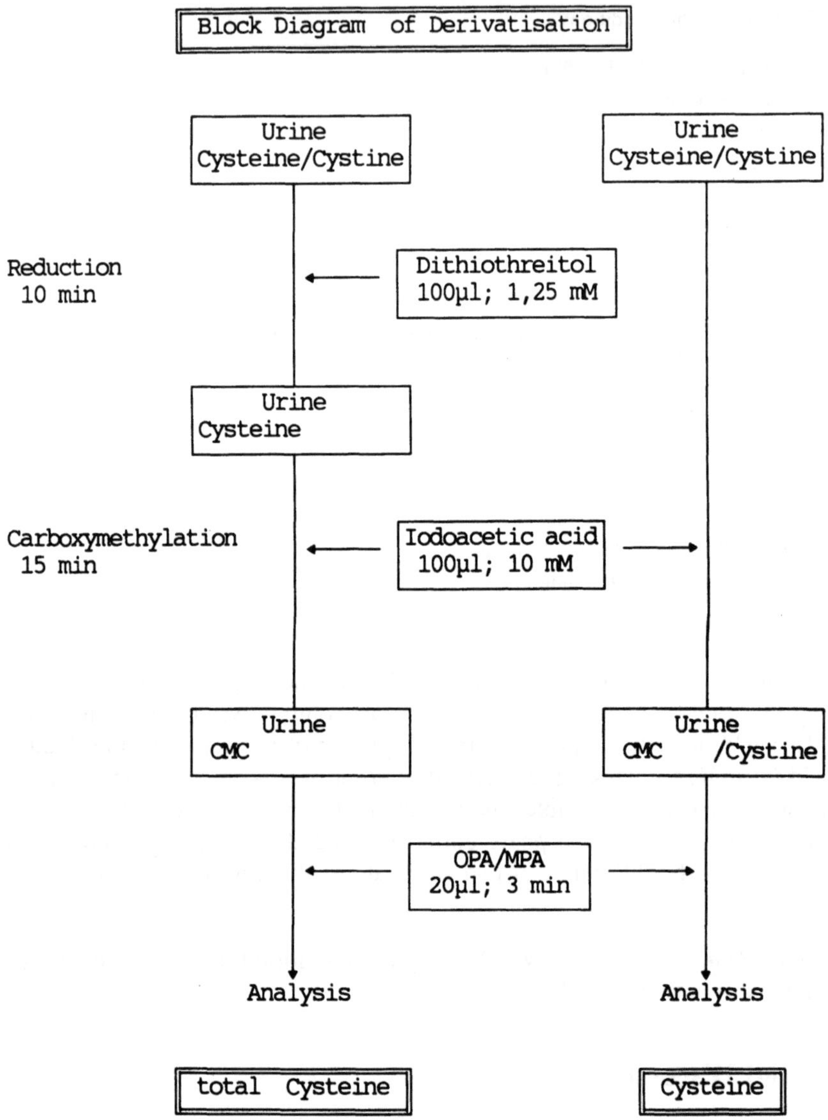

$$\text{Cystine } (\mu mol/l) = \frac{\text{total Cysteine } (\mu mol/l) - \text{Cysteine } (\mu mol/l)}{2}$$

Fig. 1. Block diagram of cysteine/cystine determination

Another difficulty arising is the rather fast oxidation of cysteine. Special precautions during collection and storage of urine – e.g., lowering of pH as soon as possible and storage at 4°C – must be undertaken to prevent oxidation. Using a conventional amino acid analyzer, no information about the cysteine content of a sample is available because all cysteine is oxidized to cystine (Asper and Schmucki 1982).

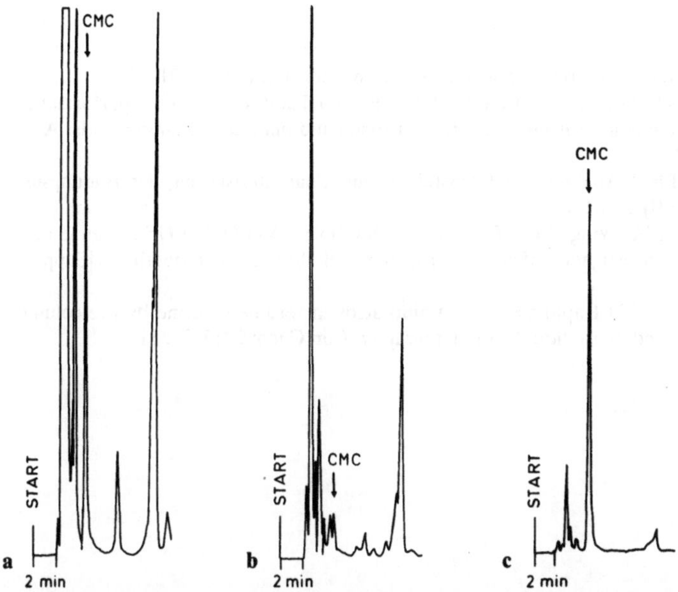

Fig. 2a–c. Chromatograms of a standard (**a**) and an urine sample analyzed for cysteine (**b**) and total cysteine (**c**; same urine as in **b**, further diluted 1 + 7). For conditions, see Table 1

Table 2. Cysteine and cystine concentrations in human urine ($\bar{x} \pm$ SD, µmol/l)

	Cysteine	Cystine
Normal persons ($n = 10$)	23.8 ± 8.5	90.7 ± 35.7
Cystinuric patient ($n = 1$, 10 samples)	33.5 ± 13.9	804.7 ± 237.7

Treating the samples in the above-mentioned way, a precise differentiation between cysteine and cystine is possible (see Fig. 1): one part of the sample is treated with DTT and iodoacetic acid while another part receives only iodoacetic acid.

Some results are presented in Table 2. The cysteine content of 23.8 µmol/l (normal people) agrees well with the few known values (25 µmol/l; Asper and Schmucki 1982).

The possibility of differentiation between cysteine and cystine is extremely important in diagnostic and therapy control of cystinuria because only cystine is relatively insoluble at normal urinary pH but not cysteine. Considering this, the method must allow the monitoring of a special therapy of cystinuria (high intake of ascorbic acid) changing the redox equilibrium of the cysteine – cystine system in the direction of the more soluble cysteine.

Acknowledgement. This work was supported by a grant of the Dr. Robert Pfleger Stiftung.

References

Asper R, Schmucki O (1982) Cystinurietherapie mit Ascorbinsäure. Urol Int 37:91–109

Graser T, Godel H, Albers S, Földi P, Fürst P (1985) An ultrarapid and sensitive high-performance liquid chromatographic method for determination of tissue and plasma free amino acids. Anal Biochem 151:142–152

Hesse A, Schaefer RM (1987) Analyse von Harnsteinen und Charakterisierung der Bildungsursachen. Urologe [Ausg B] 27:81–86

Leah JM, Palmer T, Griffin M, Wingad CJ, Briddon A, Oberholzer VG (1986) Urine amino acid analysis by HPLC in the investigation of inborn errors of metabolism. J Inher Metab Dis [Suppl 2] 9:250–253

Turnell DC, Cooper JDH (1982) Rapid assay for amino acids in serume or urine by pre-column derivatization and reversed-phase liquid chromatography. Clin Chem 28:527–531

Pathological-Anatomical Renal Alterations Following Application of Extracorporeally Produced Piezoelectric Shock Waves (Wolf-Piezolith): A Laboratory Animal Research Study

G. Seitz[1], D. Neisius[2], T. Gebhardt[2], and M. Ziegler[2]

Introduction

At the moment several techniques for extracorporeal shock wave lithotripsy (ESWL) are available (Chaussy 1980; Reichenberger and Naves 1986; Riedlinger et al. 1986). According to preliminary clinical studies, the treatment with the Piezolith 2200 (Wolf, Knittlingen) causes fewer side effects than other techniques (Ziegler et al. 1986). Animal studies dealing with the pathologic effects on renal tissue, caused by a higher number of piezoelectric shock waves (EPL), have not been published yet.

Materials and Methods

Thirteen adult beagle dogs (12–14 kg body weight) were treated with the Piezolith 2200 (Wolf, Knittlingen). Kidneys without stones received 2000, 3000, or 4000 shock waves in a single session (constant pressure: 900–1000 bar). The dogs were anesthetized for treatment with pentobarbital, and shock waves were focused on the pelvis of the kidney by ultrasound.

The dogs were killed 1–2 days, 7, or 14 weeks after treatment (Fig. 1). The kidneys were removed and lamellated into slices of 2-mm thickness, then they were examined macroscopically and histologically.

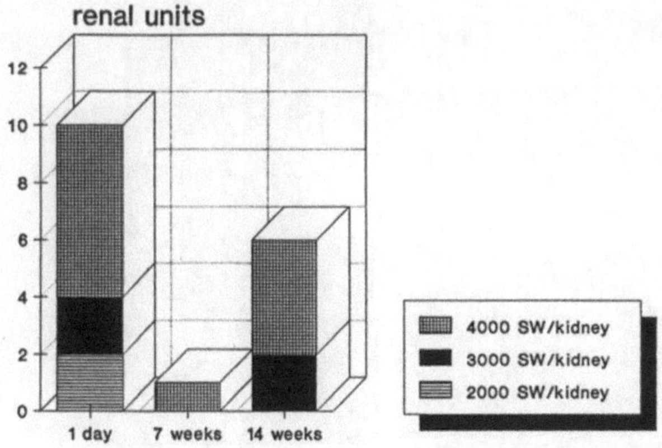

Fig. 1. Removal of organs after piezoelectric shock waves

[1] Institute of Pathology, Dept. of Gen. and Spec. Pathology, University of the Saarland, 6650 Homburg/Saar, FRG

[2] Clinic of Urology, University of the Saarland, 6650 Homburg/Saar, FRG

Investigative Urology 3
Edited by H. Rübben et al.

Results

Early Alterations. All kidneys examined (10) showed alterations of variable degree depending on the number of applied shock waves. There were neither perirenal nor subcapsular hematomas (Table 1). The size of intrarenal hematomas generally increased with the number of applied shock waves; after application of 4000 shock

Table 1. Early renal alteration after piezoelectric shock waves ($n = 10$)

	Shock waves		
	2000	3000	4000
Hematopyelon	0/2	1/2	3/6
Hematoma			
Intrarenal	2/2	2/2	5/6
Subcapsular	0	0	0
Perirenal	0	0	0
Papillary necrosis	1/2	1/2	4/6
Vascular lesion			
Veins (thrombosis)	0	1/2	2/6
Arteries (segmental necrosis)	2/2	1/2	4/6

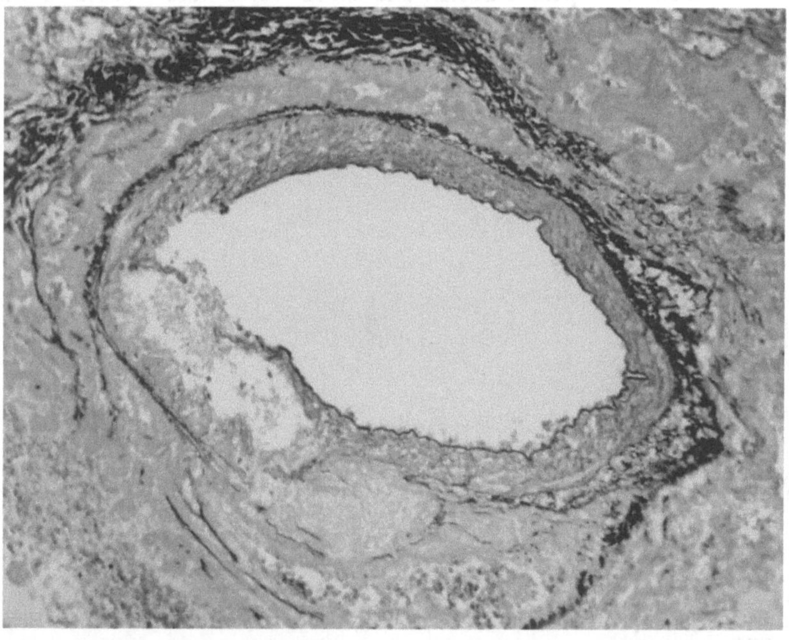

Fig. 2. Artery with media necrosis and destruction of lamina elastica interna and endothelium, 1 day after treatment with 2000 shock waves. Elastica van Gieson, ×140

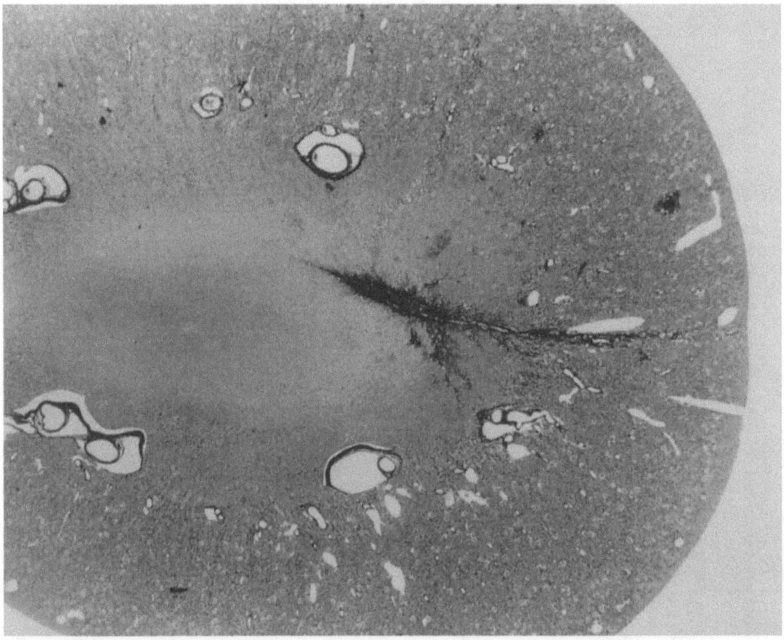

Fig. 3. Cordlike scar at the corticomedullary junction, 14 weeks after treatment with 4000 shock waves. Large field section, elastica van Gieson, × 3

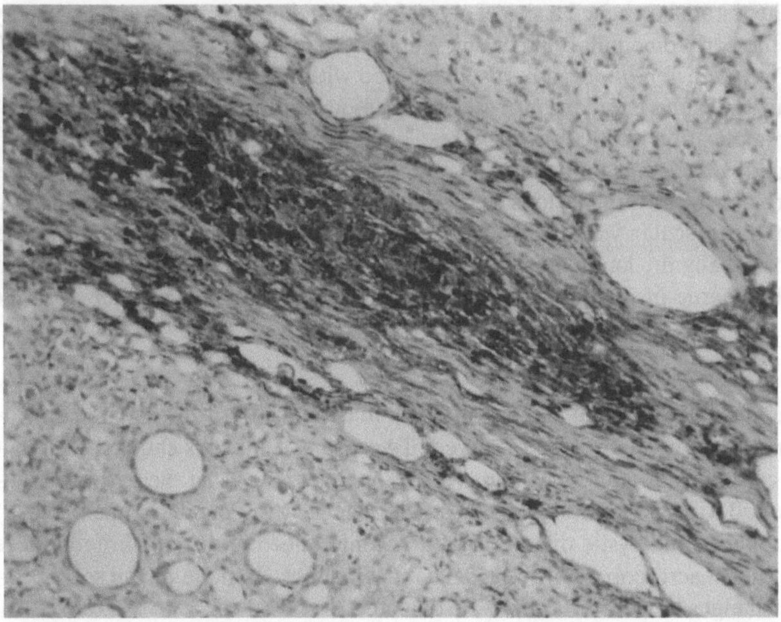

Fig. 4. Cordlike scar of renal parenchyma with clusters of siderophages, 14 weeks after treatment with 4000 shock waves. Turnbull blue, × 140

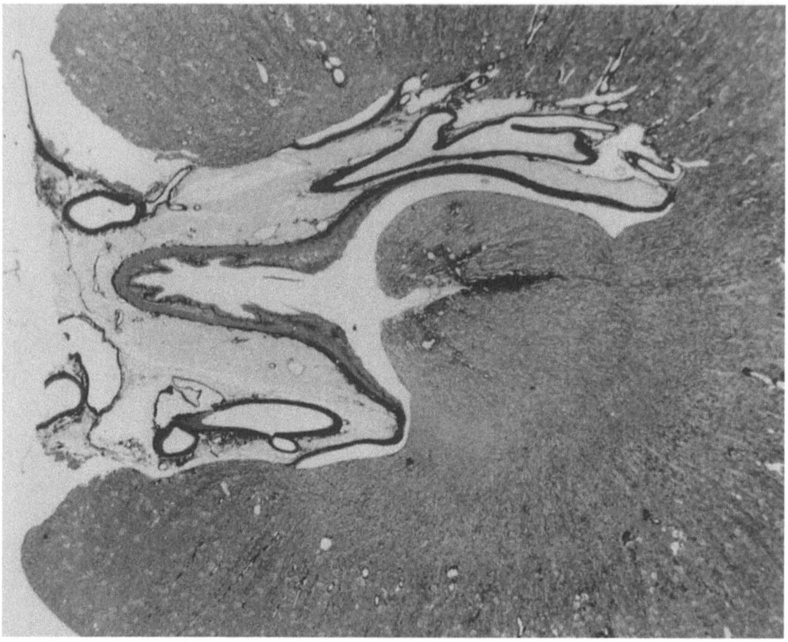

Fig. 5. Wedge-shaped defect of papillary apex, 14 weeks after treatment with 4000 shock waves. Large field section, elastica van Gieson, × 5

waves the hematomas reached a size of about 2.5 cm in diameter and were preferably sited near the corticomedullary junction. We found papillary necroses in 6 out of 10 kidneys: The extension of necroses also increased with the number of applied shock waves. Four times the papillary necroses were associated with hematopyelon, especially after application of 4000 shock waves.

Damage of vessels was found in small and midsized veins and arteries: three veins showed thrombosis. Arterial lesions were seen in seven kidneys: We found segmental necrosis of the vascular wall with hemorrhages and precipitates of protein in the media; occasionally the lamina elastica interna and the endothelium were destroyed (Fig. 2). The degree of the arterial lesion was independent of the number of shock waves.

Late Alterations. The residual extent was small in comparison with early renal damage. Two patterns of lesion were observed: Two out of 7 kidneys showed an about 1 cm long, cordlike scar (Fig. 3) with many siderophages (Fig. 4) at the corticomedullary junction. Twice we found a wedge-shaped defect of the papillary apex (Fig. 5) with siderophages and cystic dilatation of adjacent collecting ducts. Three kidneys showed neither macroscopic nor histologic abnormalities. In none of the seven kidneys could changes in veins or arteries be detected.

Discussion

There have only been a few laboratory animal research studies on renal damage after extracorporeal shock wave lithotripsy (Delius et al. 1986; Muschter et al. 1986; Newman et al. 1987). Systematic studies of canine renal damage after extracorporeal piezoelectric shock wave lithotripsy have not been published yet. Our macroscopic and histologic investigations demonstrate early and late renal alterations after EPL with 2000–4000 shock waves.

After application of a higher number of shock waves, we also observed more extensive intrarenal hematomas and more frequent bleeding into the pelvis, as has been reported by other authors (Delius et al. 1986; Muschter et al. 1987; Newman et al. 1987). In contrast to other investigators (Muschter et al. 1986, 1987; Newman et al. 1987), however, we could not find any perirenal or subcapsular hematomas. The intrarenal alterations are preferably localized near the corticomedullary junction. This may be due to the physics of the shock waves (dispersion of shock waves at the border of tissues with different density). Vascular damage is the most interesting early effect: In contrast to other authors, we only found single thrombosis of veins (Delius et al. 1986; Newman et al. 1987). Surprisingly, we detected segmental necroses of small and mid-sized arteries in 7 out of 10 kidneys.

To our knowledge, such alterations have not been described yet. Further investigations are necessary to find out whether these alterations are associated with the onset of arterial hypertension after ESWL. According to Williams et al. (1988) up to 8% of patients develop arterial hypertension after ESWL; its pathogenesis still remains unknown. Despite systematic investigation, we could not find late vascular lesions, which might have been derived from the early alterations mentioned above, e.g., segmental necrosis, hemorrhages, etc. After 3 months, only some kidneys showed small scars at the corticomedullary junction or at the papillary apex without decrease of renal function (Muschter et al. 1986, 1987). These late alterations, as far as detectable, are subtle in comparison with early damages.

Discussing the significance of the findings described above, it has been taken into account that minor alterations can be expected in humans. In our animal study, the distance from skin to renal pelvis is shorter than that in man. Furthermore, the animal kidney did not suffer from nephrolithiasis, thus there was no possibility of the absorption of energy by renal stones.

Acknowledgment. We thank Mrs. O. Klein for technical assistance.

References

Chaussy C (1980) Berührungsfreie Nierensteinzertrümmerung durch extracorporal erzeugte, focussierte Stoßwellen. Thesis submitted for the certificate of habilitation. Medical Faculty of the Ludwig-Maximilians-University, Munich

Delius M, Enders G, Xuan Z, Rath M, Liebig C, Brendel W (1986) Effect of shock waves on the kidney. First int symp on anesthesia and ESWL, Munich

Muschter R, Schmeller N, Kutscher K, Reimers I, Hofstetter A, Löhrs U (1986) Morphologische Nierenveränderungen durch die Anwendung der extracorporalen Schockwellenlithotripsie und ihr klinisches Korrelat. Verh Dtsch Ges Urol 38:303–304

Muschter R, Schmeller N, Reimers I, Kutscher K, Knipper A, Hofstetter A, Löhrs U (1987) ESWL-induced renal damage – an experimental study. Invest Urol 2:193–196

Newman R, Hackett R, Senior D, Brock K, Feldman J, Sosnowski J, Finlayson B (1987) Pathologic effects of ESWL on canine renal tissue. Urology 29:194–200

Reichenberger H, Naves G (1986) Electromagnetic acoustic source for the extracorporeal generation of shock waves in lithotripsy. Siemens Forsch Entwicklber 15:187–194

Riedlinger R, Ueberle F, Wurster H, Krauß W, Vallon P, Konrad G, Kopper B, Stoll HP, Goebbels R, Gebhardt T, Ziegler M (1986) Die Zertrümmerung von Nierensteinen durch piezoelektrisch erzeugte Hochenergie-Schallimpulse – Physikalische Grundlagen und experimentelle Untersuchungen. Urologe [Ausg A] 25:188–192

Williams C, Kaude J, Newman R, Peterson J, Thomas W (1988) Extracorporeal shock-wave lithotripsy: long term complications. AJR 150:311–315

Ziegler M, Kopper B, Riedlinger R, Wurster H, Ueberle F, Neisius D, Krauß W, Vallon P, Gebhardt T (1986) Die Zertrümmerung von Nierensteinen mit einem piezo-elektrischen Gerätesystem – erste klinische Erfahrungen. Urologe [Ausg A] 25:193–197

The Effect of Shock Wave Exposure on Kidney Function in Dogs

K. Yamamoto[1], T. Kishimoto[1], H. Iimori[1], M. Senjyu[1], T. Sugimoto[1], H. Ochi[2], and M. Maekawa[1]

Introduction

The comparable safety of extracorporeal shock wave lithotripsy (ESWL) has been shown by the results from the more than 50000 patients who have been treated with the Dornier kidney lithotripter around the world (Dornier Medizintechnik 1988; Drach et al. 1986). We started ESWL at our hospital in July 1985, and treated over 1000 patients with upper urinary tract stones using the Dornier kidney lithotripter HM3. The success rate included both patients who became stone-free and those whose stones were disintegrated into less than 4 mm. The success rate of 521 renal stone patients treated in the first 2 years was 87.1%, including 62.9% stone-free cases judged by KUB. Similarly, the success rate of 200 ureteral stone patients was 90.0%, including 76% stone-free cases. Common complications were pain and fever, which occurred in 16.3% and 13.5% of the patients, respectively. Most of these cases were not serious, and they recovered in a few days without special treatment (Yamamoto et al. 1983). However, macroscopic hematuria occurred in almost all cases, and a petechiae-like lesion was observed at the skin where the shock waves entered in about half of the patients. In addition, an elevation of the level of cell-escaped enzymes in the blood occurred, indicating hemolysis and myolysis (Kishimoto et al. 1986). Taking account of these facts, it may be possible that the kidney exposed to shock waves by focusing may be damaged to some extent. Therefore, we studied the effect of high energy shock wave exposure on the kidney in dogs.

Materials and Methods

Nineteen mongrel dogs weighing an average of 12.7 kg were used for this study. In 6 of them, systemic hemodynamics and regional blood flow were measured by the microsphere method during shock wave exposure. In 9 dogs, serial renoscintigraphies using $^{99}Tc^{m}$-DTPA were done, and the remaining 4 dogs were used for histological examination of the kidney.

All dogs were anesthetized with an intravenous administration of pentobarbital sodium at dose of 30 mg/kg, and a tracheal tube was inserted for ventilation with HFO jet ventilator (Mella Co.) using air, to minimize the respiratory movement of the kidney. The dog was placed in the supine position on the modified patient stretcher of the Dornier kidney lithotripter HM3. Twenty milliliters of 60% urographin was injected intravenously to visualize the kidney on the X-ray monitor. The

Departments of [1] Urology and [2] Radiology, Osaka City University Medical School, 1-5-7, Asahimachi, Abeno-ku, Osaka 545, Japan

Investigative Urology 3
Edited by H. Rübben et al.

lower pole of the left kidney was exposed to a total of 1000 shock waves generated at 20 kV.

Hemodynamic Study. A hemodynamic study was performed using carbonized microspheres having a diameter of 15 µm and labeled with 141-celium, 95-niobium, and 51-chromium (New England Nuclear Co.). They were injected into the left ventricle via the catheter introduced through the carotid artery before shock wave exposure and at 500 and 1000 shock waves. The injected microspheres were distributed peripherally according to blood flow rate and were trapped at the capillaries. The number of injected microspheres at each injection was about 440000.

Renoscintigraphy. Renoscintigraphy was performed by bolus injection of 10 mCi of ^{99m}Tc-DTPA before shock wave exposure and at 30 min, 1, 2, and 4 weeks after the exposure of 1000 shock waves.

Histological Examination. Histological examination was performed just after and 1 week after the exposure of 1000 shock waves. After fixation with 10% formalin and staining with hematoxylin and eosin and periodic acid-Schiff, microscopic examination was carried out.

Results and Discussion

Hemodynamic Study. The change in cardiac output measured by the microsphere method is shown in Fig. 1. Immediately after 500 shock waves, cardiac output increased, followed by a decrease after 1000 shock waves. These changes were not statistically significant, indicating that systemic hemodynamics were not altered so much during shock wave exposure. Percentage distribution of cardiac output to the kidney is shown in Table 1. Blood flow to each lesion measured was standardized as blood flow to 100 g of the tissue. Percentage distribution of cardiac output to the affected side slightly changed but not significantly; that to the contralateral side showed a slight decrease during treatment with no significance. The change in blood flow to the other organs is shown in Table 2. Blood flow to the colon overlying the affected part of the kidney decreased after 1000 shock wave exposure. In fact, small hematomas and bleeding were found in this lesion of the colon, suggesting that the

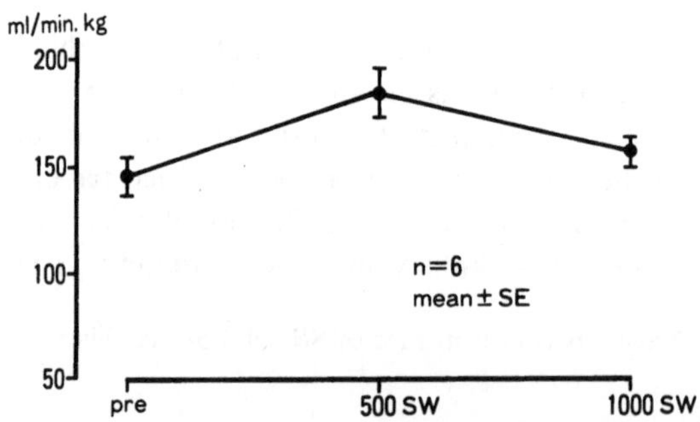

Fig. 1. Change of cardiac output

Table 1. Change of renal blood flow distribution (% CO/100 g) ($n = 6$)

		Pre	After 500 SW	After 1000 SW
Involved	Whole	27.2 ± 3.0	28.9 ± 2.8	24.3 ± 1.3
Involved	Upper half	27.3 ± 3.5	28.7 ± 2.6	24.7 ± 1.5
Involved	Lower half[a]	27.0 ± 2.6	29.0 ± 3.2	23.9 ± 1.3
Contralateral	Whole	32.7 ± 3.3	30.4 ± 2.6	26.4 ± 2.0
Contralateral	Upper half	33.1 ± 3.7	29.7 ± 2.6	26.5 ± 2.1
Contralateral	Lower half	32.4 ± 2.9	31.1 ± 2.8	26.4 ± 1.9

Values are means ± SE; SW, shock waves
[a] Discharged portion

Table 2. Change of blood flow distribution (% CO/100 g) ($n = 6$)

	Pre	After 500 SW	After 1000 SW
Right rectal muscle	0.41 ± 0.14	0.44 ± 0.11	0.49 ± 0.11
Left rectal muscle	0.31 ± 0.06	0.53 ± 0.12	0.47 ± 0.15
Right psoas muscle	0.25 ± 0.06	0.34 ± 0.09	0.22 ± 0.03
Left psoas muscle	0.28 ± 0.05	0.34 ± 0.05	0.26 ± 0.06
Spleen	14.2 ± 13.5	15.2 ± 2.56	11.3 ± 1.67
Right lobe of liver	4.1 ± 1.11	4.8 ± 1.28	4.5 ± 1.14
Left lobe of liver	3.9 ± 0.98	3.9 ± 0.95	3.8 ± 0.81
Colon (descending)	7.9 ± 1.55	5.4 ± 0.97	4.5 ± 0.84*

Values are means ± SE; SW, shock waves
* ($P<0.05$) significant difference from the pre value (paired *t*-test)

air-bearing hollow organ near the focus was damaged. However, blood flow to the other organs and tissues was stable during the treatment.

Renoscintigraphy. Renoscintigram using ^{99m}Tc-DTPA at 30 min after shock wave exposure is shown in Fig. 2. The arrow indicates the exposed site. In the early phase of scintigram, the accumulation of the tracer was delayed in the exposed site. Then an enlargement of the affected kidney was observed with a delay in excretion of radioactivity. These changes were also noted at 1 week after shock wave exposure to a lesser degree, and at 3 weeks after the exposure there was no significant difference in renoscintigrams between the two kidneys.

The time required to reach half of the maximum radioactivity, the so-called half-life time or $t_{1/2}$, in the excretory phase of the renogram is shown in Fig. 3. A delay in the half-time was observed in the affected kidney, especially in the lesion. These changes were still observed at 2 weeks after the exposure but recovered to the control level after 4 weeks.

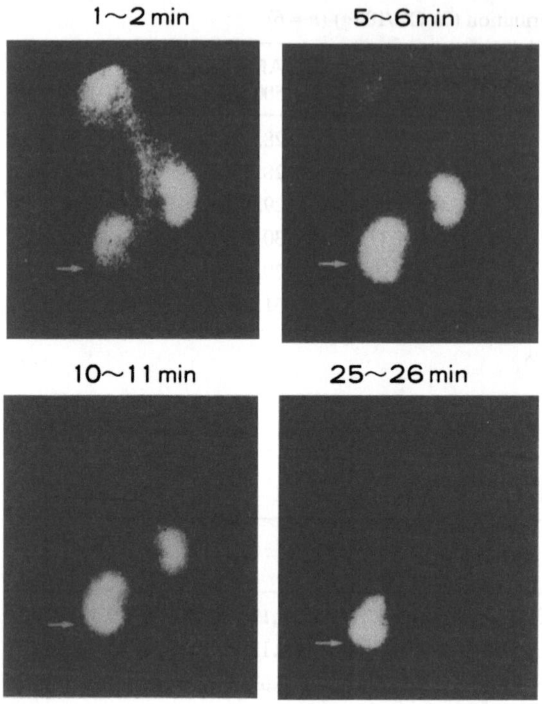

Fig. 2. Scintigram (^{99m}Tc-DTPA) just after shock wave exposure. *Arrow*, site exposed

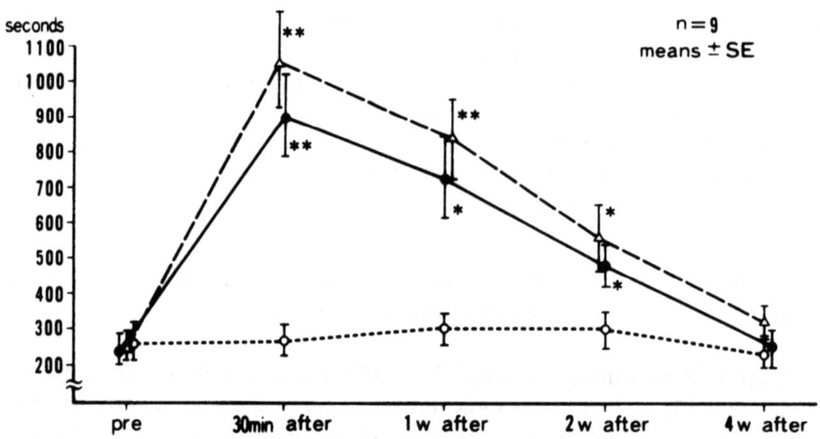

Fig. 3. Time from peak to half peak ($t_{1/2}$)

Histological Examination. The macroscopic view of the affected kidney just after shock wave exposure showed small subcapsular hematomas and hemorrhage in the parenchyma. The light microscopic view of the kidney stained with hematoxylin and eosin just after shock wave exposure showed bleeding in the peritubular space and in the intratubular space as well, and these findings were especially notable in the corticomedullary border and deep medulla. As for the glomerulus, almost no structural

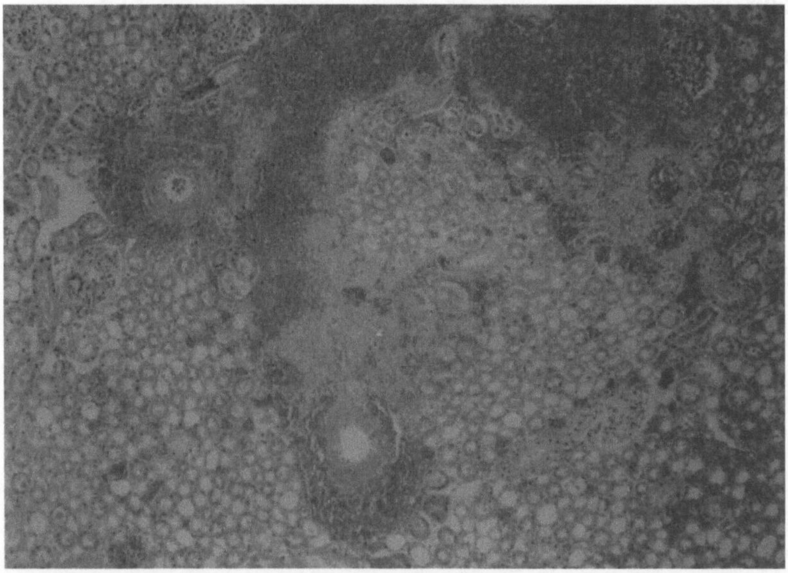

Fig. 4. Immediately after exposure to 1000 shock waves. H and E, ×100

change was shown, but for the tubules, vacuolation of the tubular epithelial cells was noted (Fig. 4). The basement membrane of the tubules and glomerulus judged by periodic acid-Schiff stain were intact, and vacuolation of the tubules was no longer seen after 1 week.

Accordingly, it is suggested that high energy shock waves focused on the kidney mainly caused an impairment in tubular function, partly by tubular cell compression owing to bleeding and partly by the direct damage to the tubular cells themselves, and that these morphological and functional changes of the affected kidney are reversible and recover within 4 weeks.

Summary

The effect of high energy shock wave exposure generated by the Dornier kidney lithotriper HM3 on the dog kidney was evaluated by the microsphere method, ^{99m}Tc-DTPA renoscintigraphy, and histology, and the following results were obtained.

1. Renal blood flow to the affected kidney increased slightly after 500 shocks followed by a slight decrease after 1000 shocks without statistical significance.
2. Renoscintigraphy using ^{99m}Tc-DTPA showed an enlargement of the affected kidney with delay in not only the accumulation but also excretion of the tracer.
3. Histological examination showed that there was bleeding in the peritubular space and vacuolation of the tubular cells without few structural change in the glomerulus.
4. Changes in both renoscintigraphy and histology were improved within 4 weeks. Therefore, the kidney was reversibly and temporarily damaged probably by contusion due to shock wave exposure.

References

Dornier Medizintechnik GmbH (1988) User letter 3:3
Drach GW, et al (1986) Report of the United States cooperative study of extracorporeal shock wave lithotripsy. J Urol 135:1127–1133
Kishimoto T, et al (1986) Side effects of extracorporeal shock-wave exposure in patients treated by extracorporeal shock-wave lithotripsy for upper urinary tract stones. Eur Urol 12:308–313
Yamamoto K, et al (1988) Extracorporeal shock-wave lithotripsy for stones in the urinary tract. Saishin-igaku 43:1716–1721

Urinary Proteins as Parameters of Renal Functional Changes After Extracorporeal Shock Wave Lithotripsy

D. M. WILBERT, W. L. STROHMAIER, S. H. FLÜCHTER, and K.-H. BICHLER[1]

Introduction

Currently extracorporeal shock wave lithotripsy (ESWL) is the method of choice for treatment of most renal and ureteral calculi. Very little is known about its immediate and long-term side effects. Occasional iodine hippuran clearance studies even revealed an increase of renal function when the values before and after ESWL were compared (Chaussy 1982).

From various animal experiments it is known that renal damage can occur when large doses (1000–6000 shock waves) of these high-energy pressure waves are directed towards the kidney. Major injury, as for instance intrarenal hemorrhage, vascular lacerations, and later extensive scarring, has been reported from these animal experiments (Muschter et al. 1987; Riedlinger et al. 1986). On the other hand, routine treatment does not seem to jeopardize renal function too much. In several studies, in only approximately 1% of the patients did perirenal or intrarenal hematomas lead to clinical symptoms (Knapp et al. 1988; Waldthausen et al. 1987). It is hard to believe that in the treatment of humans no alterations should occur, whereas in animal experiments extensive trauma, admittedly with large quantities of shock waves, is encountered.

It has been difficult to assess renal damage quantitatively after extracorporeal shock wave lithotripsy. Imaging techniques can show morphological changes early after ESWL, such as diminished perfusion, perirenal fluid collection, or edema of the kidney in 30%–50% (Knapp et al. 1988). Radionuclide scans do not show alterations regularly.

Therefore, this study was undertaken to evaluate urinary protein excretion after ESWL of renal stones to find possible means of assessing potential renal damage.

Material and Methods

In 17 patients urine samples were obtained before and up to 4 days after ESWL. To monitor glomerular function, immunoglobulin M (IgM), alpha-2-macroglobulin, and immunoglobulin G (IgG), and to monitor tubular function, beta-2-microglobulin, albumin, and Tamm-Horsfall protein (THP), excretions were determined in aliquots of 24-h urine samples and one 6-h sample immediately after ESWL by a routine laboratory enzyme immunological method for beta-2-microglobulin, and radial immunodiffusion for all other proteins. The mean and standard errors were plotted over time and expressed per gram creatinine.

[1] Dept. of Urology, Eberhard-Carls-University, Hoppe-Seyler-Str. 3, 7400 Tübingen, FRG

Investigative Urology 3
Edited by H. Rübben et al.

According to the method published by Bichler et al. (1973) Tamm-Horsfall protein is determined by first dialyzing an aliquot of 5 ml of urine overnight through a collodium membrane. Then 0.3% SDS solution (sodium-dodecylsulfate, Serva, Heidelberg) is added to the outer portion. In the meanwhile agarose gel disks are produced containing THP-specific antibodies (Behringwerke, Marburg). Then 6 µl of concentrated urine are filled into preformed wells, and immunoelectrophoresis is maintained for 2.5 h. The plates are colored with Coomassie brillant blue and the peaks measured and compared with appropriate standards.

Beta-2-microglobulin is determined with a commercially available enzyme-linked immunoassay (Behringwerke, Marburg). The beta-2-microglobulin of the aliquot and the beta-2-microglobulin-peroxidase conjugate compete for binding to an antibody attached to the wall of a plastic vial. Addition of hydrogen peroxide and chromogen leads to an enzymatic reaction resulting in loss of color intensity which can be measured with a photometer.

All other urinary proteins are determined by radial immunodiffusion on LC-partigen disks (Behringwerke, Marburg). If the screening of urinary protein content reveals less than 150 mg/100 ml, then the urine is concentrated through Minicon filters (Amicon Division, Danvers, USA). Afterwards, the urine is rediluted and 5 µl of different dilutions are administered on LC-disks which contain appropriate antibodies. Immunodiffusion is allowed to run for 3–5 days according to the molecular weight of the proteins. After termination the circles around the wells are measured and compared with standards.

All 17 patients had calyceal or renal pelvic stones on one side only. They did not receive catheters of any type prior to treatment nor were nephrotoxic agents, such as aminoglycosides or contrast media, administered during the study period.

Shock wave impulses varied from 700 to 2200 shock waves per session. The treatment was performed on a HM4 Dornier bathless lithotripter with a modified low pressure generator.

Results

An approximately tenfold increase of albumin excretion is found immediately after ESWL, which reaches normal values after 3 days. Beta-2-microglobulin also is raised

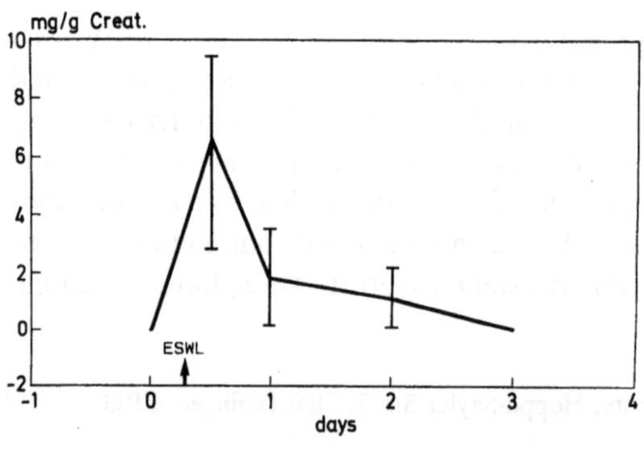

Fig. 1. Determination of immunoglobulin M before and after shock wave treatment *(ESWL)* in 24-h urine samples, expressed per gram creatinine. Mean and standard errors of the mean, $n = 17$

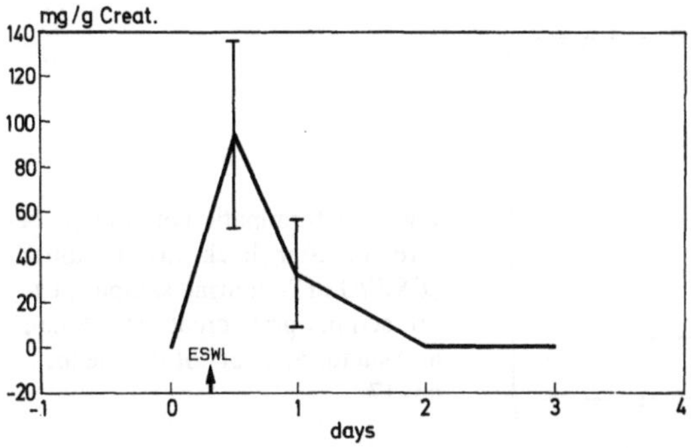

Fig. 2. Determination of immunoglobulin G before and after shock wave treatment *(ESWL)* in 24-h urine samples, expressed per gram creatinine. Mean and standard errors of the mean, $n = 17$

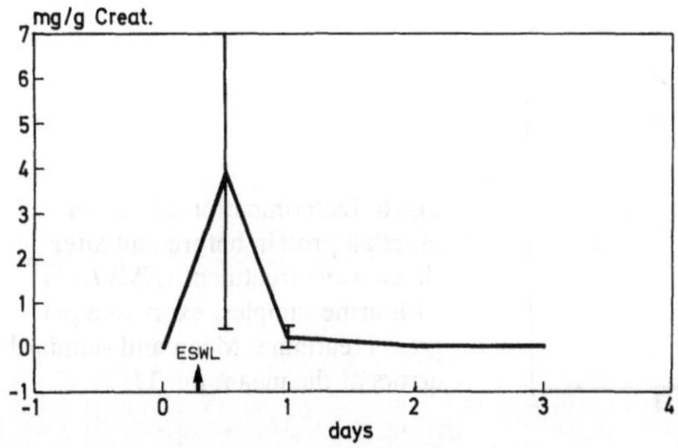

Fig. 3. Determination of alpha-2-macroglobulin before and after shock wave treatment *(ESWL)* in 24-h urine samples, expressed per gram creatinine. Mean and standard errors of the mean, $n = 17$

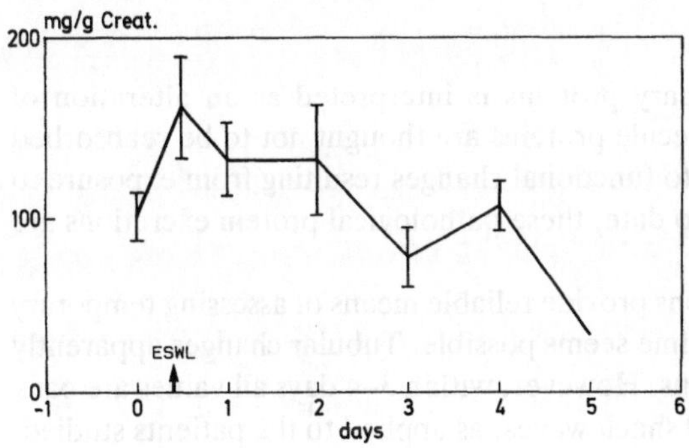

Fig. 4. Determination of beta-2-microglobulin before and after shock wave treatment *(ESWL)* in 24-h urine samples, expressed per gram creatinine. Mean and standard errors of the mean, $n = 17$

and gradually drops to normal values after 4 days. Interestingly beta-2-microglobulins were slightly elevated prior to ESWL, which is in keeping with results from the literature (Bichler et al. 1981). Tamm-Horsfall protein shows a pronounced decrease immediately after shock wave exposure, coming back to almost normal values after 4 days.

The larger molecule proteins IgM and alpha-2-macroglobulin, which under normal circumstances are found in the urine only in traces, show a tenfold increase and IgG, a twofold increase immediately after ESWL with normal levels after 3 days (see Figs. 1–6).

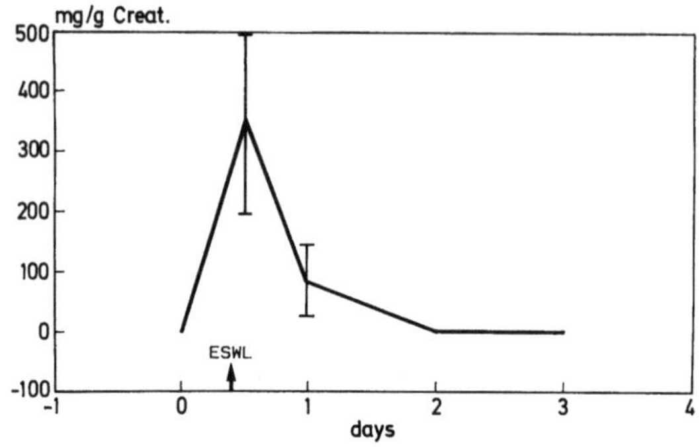

Fig. 5. Determination of albumin before and after shock wave treatment *(ESWL)* in 24-h urine samples, expressed per gram creatinine. Mean and standard errors of the mean, $n = 17$

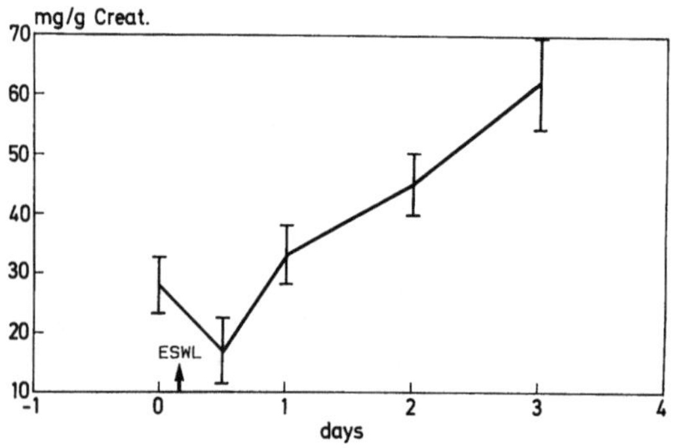

Fig. 6. Determination of Tamm-Horsfall protein before and after shock wave treatment *(ESWL)* in 24-h urine samples, expressed per gram creatinine. Mean and standard errors of the mean, $n = 17$

Discussion

An increase of large molecule urinary proteins is interpreted as an alteration of glomerular permeability. Small molecule proteins are thought not to be reabsorbed adequately by the tubular cells due to functional changes resulting from exposure to shock waves. As far as it is known to date, these pathological protein excretions are limited in time.

The urinary protein determinations provide reliable means of assessing temporary renal damage. Quantification over time seems possible. Tubular changes apparently last longer than glomerular alterations. However, within 3–4 days all values are back to normal. In the range of 700–2200 shock waves, as applied to the patients studied, we could not find a close correlation between the number of shock waves and the extent of the damage. This is conceivable when there are many variables to be taken into account. Accordingly, Ruiz Marcellan and Ibarz Servoi (1986) did not find a correlation between increased enzyme levels after ESWL and the number of shock waves applied. However, it is important to mention that in our study there was not a single patient who showed all proteins within normal limits after ESWL.

Kishimoto and coworkers (1986) studied the effects of shock waves by measuring urinary *N*-acetyl-β-D-glucosaminase before and after ESWL. They found a significant increase of this tubular enzyme for more than 4 days.

In 12 patients Gilbert and others (1988) found a significant proteinuria after ESWL, greater than 1.5 g/24 h no matter whether the kidneys were obstructed or not. Their mean number of shocks delivered was 1600 impulses at an average of 20 kV. They also stated that it seems unlikely for the proteinuria to result from bleeding as for instance from damaged urothelium. This is in keeping with the findings presented here, as for example the decrease of THP, a specific renal protein, supports the hypothesis of tubular alteration. Furthermore, increased urinary excretion of beta-2-microglobulin, as also shown in transplant patients, is considered a consequence of tubular damage as long as the serum creatinine is within normal limits.

Therefore the loss of urinary proteins seems to reflect a transient parenchymal trauma comparable to a renal contusion. The long-term effects of these findings require further evaluation.

For the clinical routine it seems safe to repeat the treatment after 3–4 days, after functional changes have returned to normal values.

References

Bichler KH, Haupt H, Uhlermann G, Schwick HG (1973) Human uromucoid – quantitative immunoassay. Urol Res 1:50–59

Bichler KH, Korn S, Lämmert J (1981) Beta-2-Mikroglobulinausscheidung bei Patienten mit Urolithiasis. In: Vahlensieck W, Gasser G (eds) Pathogenese und Klinik der Harnsteine, vol 8. Steinkopff, Darmstadt

Chaussy C (ed) (1982) Extracorporeal shock wave lithotripsy. Karger, Basel

Gilbert BR, Riehle RA, Vaughan ED (1988) Extracorporeal shock wave lithotripsy and its effect on renal function. J Urol 139:482–485

Kishimoto T, Yamamoto K, Sugimoto T, Yoshihara H, Maekawa M (1986) Side effects of extracorporeal shock wave exposure in patients treated by extracorporeal shock wave lithotripsy for upper urinary tract stone. Eur Urol 12:308–313

Knapp PM, Kulb TB, Lingeman JE, Newman DM, Mertz JHO, Mosbaugh PG, Steele RE (1988) Extracorporeal shock wave lithotripsy induced perirenal hematoma. J Urol 139:700–703

Muschter R, Schmeller NT, Reimers I, Kutscher KR, Knipper A, Hofstetter AG, Löhrs U (1987) ESWL – induced renal damage – an experimental study. In: Jacobi GH, Rübben H, Harzmann R (eds) Investigative urology, vol 2. Springer, Berlin Heidelberg New York

Riedlinger R, Ueberle F, Wurster H, Krauß W, Vallon P, Konrad G, Kopper B, Stoll HP, Goebbels R, Gebhardt T, Ziegler M (1986) Die Zertrümmerung von Nierensteinen durch piezoelektrisch erzeugte Hochenergie-Schallpulse. Urologe [Ausg A] 25:188–192

Ruiz Marcellan FJ, Ibarz Servoi L (1986) Evaluation of renal damage in extracorporeal shock wave lithotripsy by shock waves. Eur Urol 12:73–75

Waldthausen W, Schuldes H, Behrmann-Küster A, Nagel R (1987) Renale Hämatome nach ESWL – Verlaufsbeobachtungen. Akt Urol 18:193–197

Changes in Blood and Urine Chemical Parameters After Extracorporeal Shock Wave Exposure of Canine Kidneys

P. JAEGER and C. CONSTANTINIDES[1]

Introduction

Clinical observations such as the inevitable macrohematuria and the occasional renal hematomas have led investigators to the assumption that shock waves have more damaging effects on renal tissue than originally suspected. This assumption was confirmed in various experimental studies (Jaeger et al. 1988). Of great interest are the possible biochemical changes which might occur along with the morphological ones; if they do, are they to be considered as indications of permanent renal function deterioration or not.

Materials and Method

Eight mongrel dogs were exposed, under anesthesia, to 1500 shock waves of 18 kV, in the HM 3 human lithotropsy unit of Dornier. The shock waves were applied to the left upper renal pole and the right lower renal pole of each animal. Nephrectomy (plus two control animals) followed 1 and 24–36 h, 7–11 days, and 3–6 months after exposure. Laboratory parameters were controlled before and after exposure and before nephrectomy. The estimated serum and urine parameters are listed in Table 1.

Table 1. Parameters estimated

Serum parameters
Electrolytes: Na, K, Ca
Kidney: blood urea nitrogen, creatinine, LDH (?)
Liver: transaminases (SGOT, SGPT), alkaline phosphatase (AP)
Pancreas: alpha-amylase
Urine parameters
Quantitative: sodium (Na), potassium (K), creatinine (Cr)
Qualitative: glucose, leukocytes, nitrite, pH, urobilinogen, bilirubin, red blood cells, Hb

Results

Serum electrolytes (Na, Ca, K) were slightly decreased but, except for Ca, remained within normal limits. Those differences are not statistically significant. Serum electrolytes remained practically stable in late measurements as well (Table 2). Blood

[1] Urology Department, University Hospital, 8091 Zurich, Switzerland

Investigative Urology 3
Edited by H. Rübben et al.

Table 2. Serum electrolyte measurements

	Na	K	Ca
Normal	148 ± 5	4.8 ± 1.0	2.6 ± 0.2
Pre ESWL	147	3.8	2.60
Post ESWL			
1 h	142	3.5	2.26
24–36 h	146	3.9	2.32
7–11 days	146	3.7	2.43
3–6 months	148	3.8	2.60

Table 3. Serum blood urea nitrogen (BUN) and creatinine measurements

	BUN	Creatinine
Norm (mg%)	4.9 ± 1.5	90 ± 25
Pre ESWL	4.6	91
Post ESWL		
1 h	4.0	94
24–36 h	4.0	97
7–11 days	5.0	98
3–6 months	5.7	94

Table 4. Serum SGOT, SGPT, and alkaline phosphatase measurements

	SGOT	SGPT	Alkaline phosphatase
Norm (IU/l)	53 ± 40	43 ± 28	70 ± 5
Pre ESWL	16	38	84
Post ESWL			
1 h	223	205	71
24–36 h	167	158	179
7–11 days	27	66	166
3–6 months	9	46	67

urea nitrogen and creatinine in serum fluctuated minimally as well, without statistically significant differences. Stable values in late measurements indicate, through creatinine estimations mainly, a stable renal function after 6 months (Table 3).

From the estimated liver function parameters (SGOT, SGPT, and alkaline phosphatase), both transaminases expressed a marked increase after exposure, which was well above normal values. However, within a week, they returned to normal and remained normal even after 6 months. Alkaline phosphatase expressed a milder and

Table 5. Serum alpha-amylase and lactate dehydrogenase (LDH) measurements

	Amylase (U/dl)	LDH (IU/l)
Norm	930 ± 600	120 ± 80
Pre ESWL	822	48
Post ESWL		
1 h	680	331
24–36 h	1097	108
7–11 days	1192	130
3–6 months	1041	33

Table 6. Urine parameters (quantitative) measurements

	Na (mEq/l)	K (mEq/l)	Creatinine (mg%)
Norm	90 ± 72	70 ± 50	200 ± 100
Pre ESWL	131	70	211
Post ESWL			
1 h	79	29	33

delayed increase with values returning to normal more than 11 days after exposure. We should note here that those increased values were observed randomly and were not dependent on the side of shock wave exposure as one might expect but were registered even if only the left kidney was exposed to shock waves. However, no morphological changes in the liver could be found, so we think that the increase of liver parameter values is a result of renal cell damage, especially in the proximal tubules, since it is well-known that the measured enzymes exist in kidney cells as well. A typical example of this is the increase of those enzymes after kidney infarction (Table 4).

Serum amylase shows no significant early or delayed fluctuations. Lactate dehydrogenase, which is present in almost all cells and converts lactate to pyruvate, shows an early mild increase, which cannot be attributed to any specific organ but is an indication of cell damage (Table 5).

The main finding from the urine quantitative analysis is a remarkable decrease of urinary creatinine in immediate postexposure urine specimens. The electrolytes fluctuate nonspecifically within the normal limits. After 24 h, urinary creatinine returns to normal in all animals. The explanation of this finding, which is well related to similar urea changes, is difficult, since no 24-h urine specimens were collected. It may represent a transient decrease in creatinine glomerular filtration rate (Table 6). Qualitative urine estimations reveal a significant glucose excretion in all dogs immediately after exposure, a sign of renal parenchymal cell damage, especially in the juxtaglomerular region where glucose reabsorption takes place (Table 7).

Table 7. Urine parameters (qualitative) measurements

	Pre ESWL	Post ESWL
Lc	neg	neg
Nitrite	neg	neg
pH	7.38	7.44
Protein	unchanged	
Glucose	neg	+++(+)
Ketone bodies	neg	neg
Urobilinogen	no	no
Bilirubin	neg	neg
Blood	−(+)	++++
Hb	−(+)	+++

Discussion

The results of this study indicate that the exposure of canine kidneys to therapeutic amounts of shock waves leads to inevitable changes of certain serum and urine laboratory parameters. Those changes clearly indicate renal cell damage, which occurs mostly in the region of the proximal tubule. A functional deterioration of neighboring organs, such as liver and pancreas, was not detected. All values returned, however, quickly to normal.

If the decrease in urinary creatinine is in fact a result of decreased glomerular filtration, then, in spite of the remarkable morphological changes, only a marginal, transient renal cell damage from shock waves can be documented.

Summary

We exposed the left upper and right lower renal pole of 8 mongrel dogs to 1500 shock waves of 18 kV in our extracorporeal human lithotripsy unit and we estimated various serum and urin parameters one hour, 24–36 hours, 7–11 days and 3–6 months after the exposure (2 control animals included). In serum we observed a transient decrease of calcium (Ca), an immediate increase of lactate-dehydrogenase (LDH), transaminases (SGOT and SGPT) and a delayed increase of alcaline phosphatase (AP). Creatinin (Cr), blood urea nitrogen (BUN), sodium (Na), potassium (K) and amylase remained within normal limits. In urine a decrease of creatinin and an increase of glucose excresion were noted. We believe that those changes represent a relatively mild and transient damage of renal cells and do not reflect the occasionally heavy morphological changes observed after shock wave exposure.

Reference

Jaeger P, et al (1988) Morphological changes in canine kidneys following extra-corporeal shock wave treatment. Urol Res 16: 161–166

Application of High Energy Shock Waves to Single Cells

D. M. Wilbert[1], O. Schofer[2], and H. Riedmiller[1]

Introduction

Extracorporeal shock wave lithotripsy has been in clinical use since 1980 with several hundred thousand patients treated to date. Striking complications, like perirenal hematomas, are rare with a range of approximately 0.5%–1.5%. High dose applications in pigs and dogs have shown devastating effects on renal parenchyma with intrarenal hemorrhage and later fibrosis (Muschter et al. 1987). However, very little is known about shock wave effects on single cells like cellular blood components. Chaussy and coworkers (Chaussy 1982; Eisenberger et al. 1977) could show an increase of free hemoglobin after exposing canine erythrocytes to shock waves. Russo and associates (1986) found a profound influence of shock wave exposure on rodent experimental tumors, virtually extinguishing the tumor cells.

In the early 1970s when diagnostic ultrasound was introduced into clinical practice, there was much concern about possible side effects on cells on a biochemical level or by fracturing chromosomes. It is known that the energy level of diagnostic ultrasound waves is much less than that of shock waves.

Methods and Results

To examine further a possible influence of shock waves on cells, a set of experiments was carried out looking at different cell functions. As the shock wave source a serial type electromagnetic applicator was used as installed in the Siemens Lithostar lithotripsy unit, delivering approximately 200 bars pressure in the focal zone at 17.2 kV. Blood was drawn from 8 humans and either full blood for the red cell exposure or ficoll-separated leukocytes and lymphocytes exposed to varying numbers of shock waves in a small sterile container specially developed for these experiments.

The exact focal positioning of the test tubes was assessed by fluoroscopy after submersing the tubes in a water bath.

In a first experiment full blood was exposed to an increasing number of shocks at a constant kV setting. This experiment was paralleled by another set in which the number of shocks was kept constant and the generator voltage was increased from 17 to 20 kV. All these assays were performed in triplicate and then the free hemoglobin measured in the serum, utilizing the cyan-methemoglobin method. It revealed an increasing amount of free hemoglobin with increasing numbers of shocks or higher generator voltage (Wilbert et al. 1987).

[1] Dept. of Urology and [2] Dept. of Pediatrics, Johannes Gutenberg University Mainz, Langenbeckstr. 1, 6500 Mainz, FRG

Investigative Urology 3
Edited by H. Rübben et al.

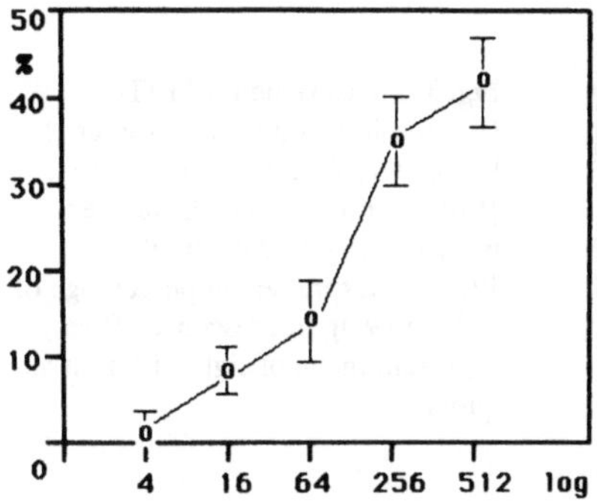

Fig. 1. 51-Chromium release from lymphocytes after shock wave exposure. Amount of tracer released expressed as percentage of total amount of radionuclide incorporated initially. Shock wave exposure from 4 to 512 impulses at 17.2 kV. $n = 8$, mean ± SEM

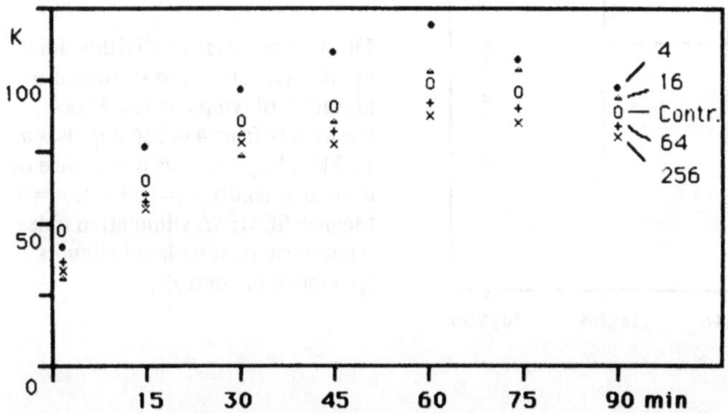

Fig. 2. Influence of high energy shock waves on catalase enzyme activity after stimulation with zymosan, which was initiated at time 0. Exposure of granulocytes (15 mill cells/ml) with 4 to 256 impulses at 17.2 kV. Optical measurement from 0 to 90 min. *K*, chemoluminescence (1/100 counts per 10 s; *Contr*, controls; $n = 8$

In the next experiment human lymphocytes were labelled with 51-chromium, then the cells exposed to 4–512 shocks and the amount of chromium assessed in the supernatent after centrifuging the cells down (Schmolke and Vorlaender 1982). With increasing energy delivery, more and more released chromium was detected (Fig. 1).

As a parameter of intracellular metabolism the leukocyte catalase activity was measured after stimulation with zymosan, a test which is generally used for assessment of nonspecific macrophage activity. After exposure to different numbers of shock waves, no significant changes of the catalase activity could be found as compared with untreated control cells (Fig. 2).

As another important aspect of cellular integrity, possible alterations of surface antigens were tested by labelling antigens of different lymphocyte subpopulations with monoclonal antibodies, countercoupled with fluorescin. Flow cytometric measurement of the presence of antigens did not show any loss of antigenicity as compared with nonexposed control cells (Fig. 3).

Finally, undisturbed reduplication of lymphocytes was examined by measuring [^{3}H]thymidine uptake after stimulation with several mitogens such as concanavalin A or phytohemagglutinine (PHA). After shock wave exposure, no significant de-

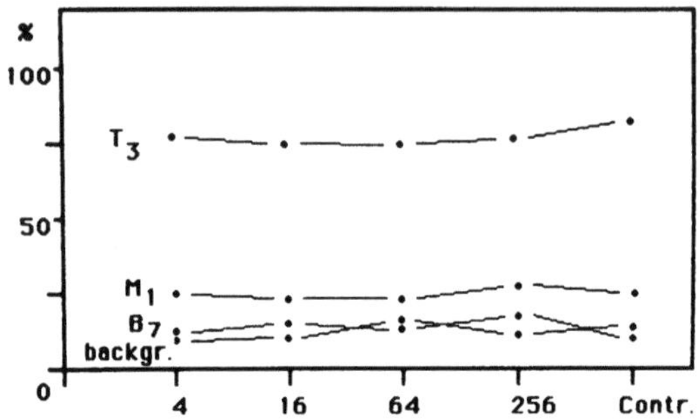

Fig. 3. Measurement of FITC (fluorescin-isothiocyanatisomer I)-labelled surface antigens before *(Contr)* and after shock wave exposure with 4 to 256 impulses at 17.2 kV. Expressed in percentage of cells showing fluorescence. *Dots* represent mean of eight different aliquots

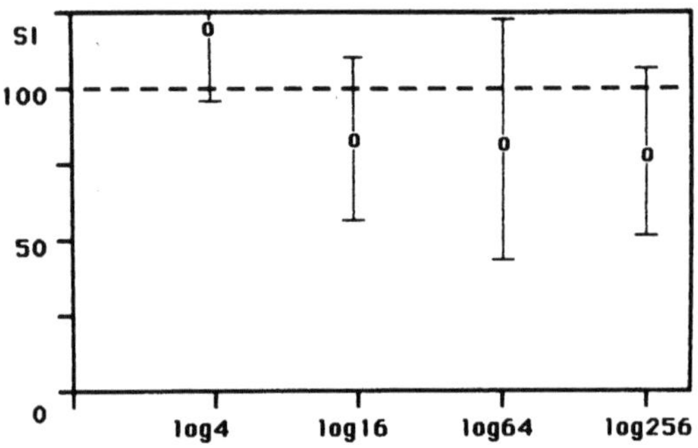

Fig. 4. Percentage of [^{3}H]thymidine uptake indicating undisturbed proliferation of lymphocytes. Shock waves vary from 4 to 256 impulses at 17.2 kV. Expressed as percentage of untreated controls (= 100%), $n = 8$. Mean ± SEM; *SI,* stimulation index (cpm mean of stimulated aliquots/cpm mean of controls)

crease of the stimulation index, expressed in percentage of the controls, was found (Fig. 4).

Complete sets of chromosomes were examined microscopically after exposing human leukocytes to 256 shocks. Here, among 1288 chromosomes, not a single fractured chromosome could be found.

However, after the initial finding of increasing free hemoglobin and even more after increasing release of radiolabelled chromium, these phenomena were further examined to find a morphological base.

Therefore, electron microscopy was carried out after high dose exposure from 256 to 4056 shock waves. This revealed some vacuolization of the exposed cells in the peripheral cytoplasm. However, this finding was also present in the unexposed cells. Cytoplasmic subcellular structures such as mitochondria remained undisturbed.

Discussion

From these experiments we have concluded that all cell functions such as enzyme activity, surface antigenicity, and reduplication remain unchanged after high dose shock wave exposure. However, the permeability of the cellular membrane is altered depending on the energy applied. This results in release of hemoglobin or ingested chromium as shown in the experiments above. In preliminary experiments the same is true for tumor cells investigated (results not shown). Therefore, to date it is felt that there is no logical basis for exposure of tumor cells to shock waves other than for the possible enhancement of permeability to cytotoxic agents. Second, with increasing shock wave exposure it is conceivable that specific cell functions related to stable membranes may become disturbed temporarily. This finding is well in keeping with other results, either looking at urinary protein excretion or urinary enzymes (Ruiz Marcellan and Ibarz Servio 1986) after shock wave exposure of the kidney. These hypotheses, as established by these experiments with leukocytes, await confirmation with other cell types as well.

References

Chaussy C (ed) (1982) Extracorporeal shock wave lithotripsy. Karger, Basel

Eisenberger F, Chaussy C, Wanner K (1977) Extracorporale Anwendung von hochenergetischen Stoßwellen – ein neuer Aspekt in der Behandlung des Harnsteinleidens. Akt Urol 8:3–15

Muschter R, Schmeller NT, Reimers I, Kutscher KR, Knipper A, Hofstetter AG, Löhrs U (1987) ESWL-induced renal damage – an experimental study. In: Jacobi GH, Rübben H, Harzmann R (eds) Investigative urology. Springer, Berlin Heidelberg New York, pp 193–196

Ruiz Marcellan FJ, Ibarz Servio L (1986) Evaluation of renal damage in extracorporeal lithotripsy by shock waves. Eur Urol 12:73–75

Russo P, Stephenson A, Mies C, Huryk R, Heston WDW, Melamed MR, Fair WR (1986) High energy shock waves suppress tumor growth in vitro and in vivo. J Urol 135:626–628

Schmolke B, Vorlaender K-O (1982) Standardtechniken zur Bestimmung zellulärer Immunreaktionen. In: Vorlaender K-O (ed) Immunologie, 2nd edn. Thieme, Stuttgart, pp 91–228

Wilbert DM, Jungbluth A, Rosenkranz T, Reichenberger H, Rumpelt H, Riedmiller H, Alken P, Hohenfellner R (1987) Experimental evaluation of a new electromagnetic shock wave source. In: Jacobi GH, Rübben H, Harzmann R (eds) Investigative urology. Springer, Berlin Heidelberg New York, pp 193–196

Evaluation of Optical Feedback for Preventing Tissue Damage in Dye Laser Lithotripsy

S. Thomas, R. Engelhardt, W. Meyer, and J. Pensel[1]

Introduction

Microsecond laser pulses are beneficial for laser lithotripsy because they can be coupled into and transmitted through very thin caliber fibers (200 μm core diameter). The interaction between the laser pulse at the fiber tip and the target object is both thermal and mechanical and relies more on the power density than on the wavelength. If the fiber tip is in direct contact with a urinary stone, a plasma is initiated by the high energy density of the laser pulse (> 100 J/cm^2). Oscillations of the plasma bubble result in mechanical shock waves that lead to stone disintegration. The quality of the distal fiber surface is uncritical in this process. For this reason highly flexible fiber application systems utilizing a 200 μm quartz fiber without accessory devices to facilitate plasma formation can be used with microsecond lasers for lasertripsy.

The biological side effects of microsecond pulses have not been investigated thoroughly to date. The short pulses yield high power densities, yet the average power is relatively small; thermal effects are therefore believed to be minimal,

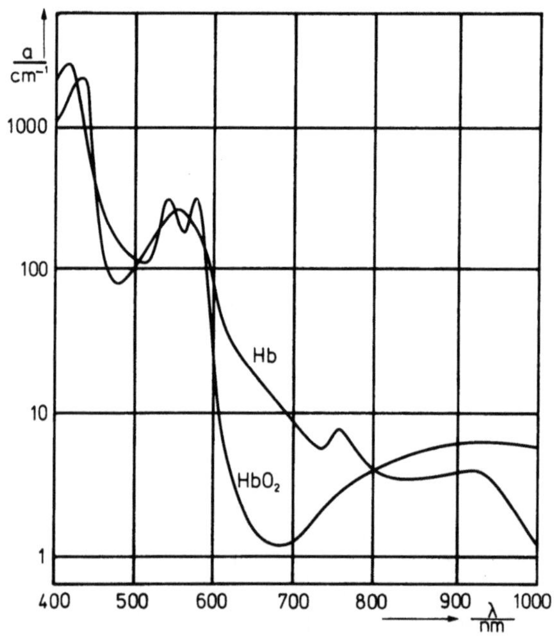

Fig. 1. Absorption spectra of oxygenated *(HbO_2)* and deoxygenated *(Hb)* hemoglobin solution in physiological concentration (150 mol · l^{-1})

[1] Medizinisches Laserzentrum Lübeck, Peter-Monnik-Weg 9, 2400 Lübeck, FRG

Investigative Urology 3
Edited by H. Rübben et al.

whereas mechanical effects in tissue caused by the plasma-induced shock wave are obvious. In a fundamental investigation Watson compared the influence of wavelength and pulse length on the fragmenting efficiency and the resulting fragment size. The optimal parameters were shown to be a wavelength of 504 nm with a pulse length of 1 μs (Watson et al. 1987a). A further benefit of this wavelength is the fact that hemoglobin has a relative absorption minimum around 500 nm (Fig. 1), minimizing tissue absorption that might lead to side effects.

An assessment of tissue reaction to direct application of microsecond pulses has only been made once. Watson applied 25–30 mJ laser pulses ureteroscopically to a pig ureter and could only see small petechial bleeding at the irradiated sites. Long-term effects were minimal; the lesions could not be clearly identified 4–6 weeks later (Watson et al. 1987b).

Our initial observations under comparable conditions of exposure show more extensive, even transmural hematoma (Thomas et al. 1988). The results of a series of in vitro and in vivo experiments on microsecond lasers for lithotripsy encouraged the development of an optical feedback regulation that will yield full laser energy only if fiber contact to a stone is given. The feedback regulation allows pulse energies that are actually required to disintegrate all kinds of urinary calculi to be used in clinical endoscopy without causing adverse effects to the surrounding tissue.

Results

In Vitro Fragmentation

The pulse energies for fragmentation of human urinary calculi were tested with a flashlamp pumped dye laser (Vuman Lasers Ltd/own modification) with a mean pulse duration of 2 μs. Apart from Cumarin 314 (504 nm), which Watson showed to have optimal efficiency for laser lithotripsy, Rhodamine 6G (590 nm) with its high energy yield and Rhodamine 700 (720 nm) which generates radiation similar to that of an alexandrite laser were used.

Another reason for investigations at 720 nm is that hemoglobin absorption is several-fold lower at this wavelength than at 590 nm and that tissue damage by direct absorption might thereby be diminished. Since absorption of stone material rapidly decreases with longer wavelengths, higher pulse energies are required for stone fragmentation at this wavelength.

Stone fragmentation in vitro was performed under identical conditions on human urinary calculi of various compositions (Struvit, uric acid, calcium oxalate monohydrate, calcium oxalate dihydrate, and Brushit). The stones were fixed under normal saline solution and exposed to laser pulses through a 200 μm quartz fiber in direct contact with the stone.

Fragmentation could only be seen after plasma formation and is easily identified by a bright flash of white light followed by an acoustic clap. The energy threshold for plasma formation did not correlate with stone disintegration in all stones. At the threshold energy a plasma was only obtained irregularly. Effective fragmentation required an energy rise of approximately 20% over the plasma threshold at 500 nm and 600 nm and of 60% at 720 nm. Only after this increase did we see a reliable, macro-

LIB / Disintegration Threshold in mJ

	Struvit	Uric Acid	Weddelit	Whewellit	Brushit
504 nm	35/40	35/50	35/40	35/50*	35/40
590 nm	40/40	40/50	40/40	40/50*	40/40
720 nm	50/50	50/80	50/50	50/80*	50/50

* only if stone is held tight in a Dormia basket with central fiber guidance

Fig. 2. In vitro fragmentation of urinary calculi of various compositions: plasma threshold and fragmentation threshold (mJ) are stated in dependence of the wavelength (λ). *LIB*, laser-induced breakdown

scopically visible fragmentation that we determined to be valid subjective criterion for the fragmentation threshold.

This threshold showed strong dependence on the wavelength of the laser and on the chemical composition and crystal structure of the stone.

All stones showed plasma formation with pulse energies of 30 mJ at 504 nm, 35 mJ at 590 nm, and 50 mJ at 720 nm, some even at lower energies. Struvit and dihydrate stones began to disintegrate at these pulse energies; uric acid and monohydrate stones did not fragment despite plasma formation. An increase of pulse energy to 40 mJ (504 nm), 45 mJ (590 nm), and 80 mJ (720 nm) enabled reliable fragmentation in stones of all compositions (Fig. 2). Brushit and monohydrate stones were particularly resistant to lasertripsy, even at higher pulse energies. Larger stones tended to be accelerated away from the fiber tip without breaking. By immobilizing the stone in a modified Dormia basket with a central fiber guide, minute fragments could be chipped off, and complete stone disintegration was achieved after a great number of pulses. Fragment size and mean fragmentation time did not differ with all three wavelengths once the necessary fragmentation energy was used.

In Vivo Animal Experiments

Effective lasertripsy with microsecond pulses required fairly high pulse energies of 40–80 mJ, higher than the energies investigated for biological side effects so far. We therefore determined macroscopic and histologic effects caused by microsecond pulses using the parameters actually necessary in clinical application.

In vivo experiments were done on a surgically exposed rabbit bladder, which is similar to the human ureter in histologic structure and strength. The lesions could be marked for later histological evaluation.

In six rabbits the bladder was opened by ventral incision and distended between six marginal sutures. The urine was flushed from the bladder and replaced with normal saline solution. Lesions with one, five, and fifty pulses were administered grid-like to a large area of the left and right bladder wall in two rabbits with each of the investigated wavelengths. Endoscopic irradiation with the same parameters were done in four further animals. The irradiation geometry was varied in different animals, so that in one case the fiber end was 1 mm away from the tissue, in a second

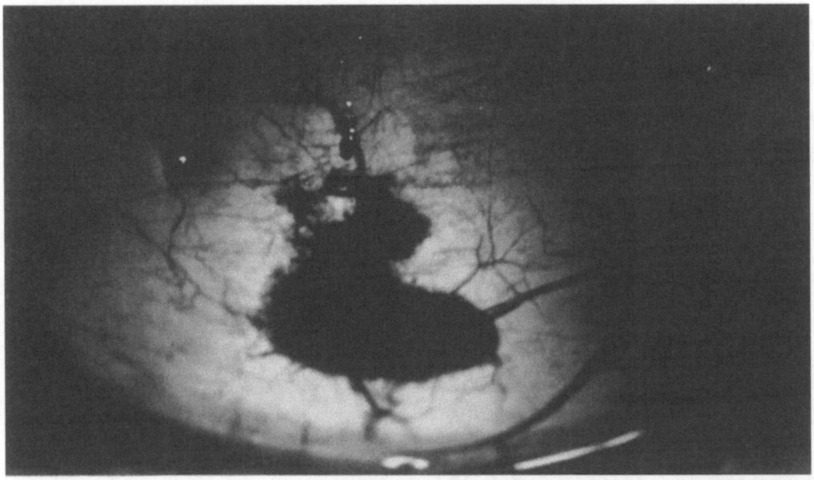

Fig. 3. Transmural hematoma caused by laser-induced breakdown in a rabbit bladder (40 mJ, 590 nm)

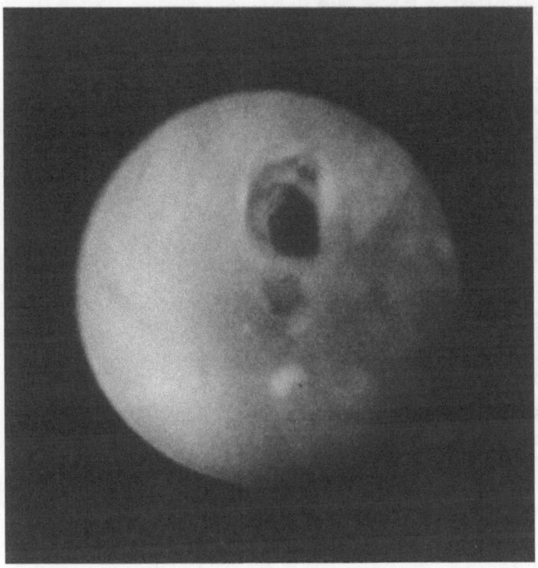

Fig. 4. One partial and one complete perforation of the bladder wall (rabbit), each caused by a single 40 mJ laser pulse without active optical feedback regulation

the fiber tip barely touched the tissue, and in the third the fiber was advanced to the tissue under slight pressure. The pulse energies were set to the threshold energy for effective fragmentation at the specific wavelength (504 nm, 40 mJ; 590 nm, 45 mJ; 720 nm, 80 mJ). One animal of each series was killed immediately, the others after 2–4 weeks.

Macroscopic effect and histological evaluation of acute specimens revealed a uniform reaction of tissue to microsecond laser pulses independent of the wavelength yet with differences in the mode of application.

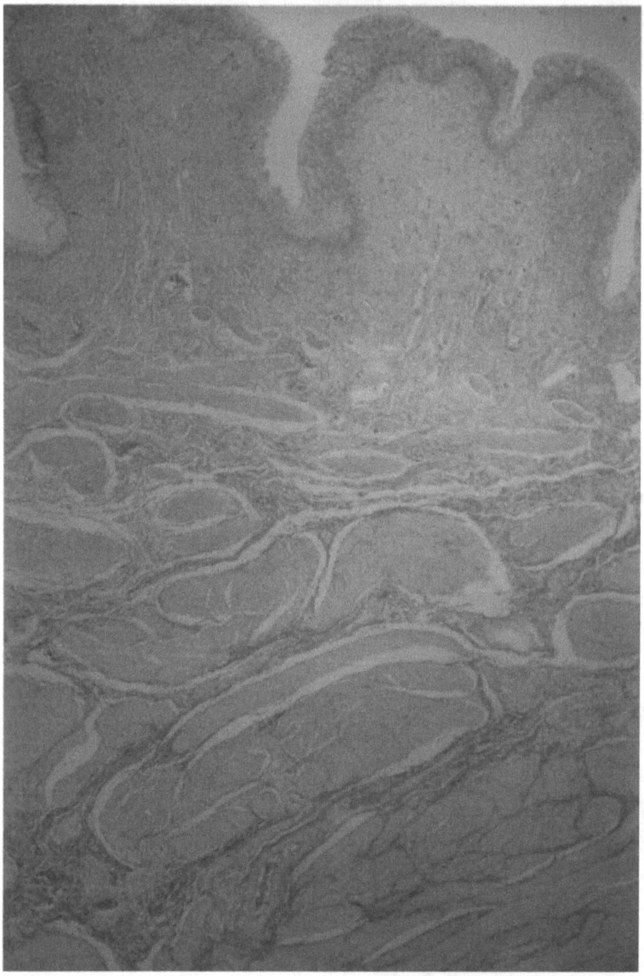

Fig. 5. Histological examination 4 weeks after application of single pulse lesions (40 mJ, 590 nm): thickening and fibrosis of the suburothelial stroma with fibrotic disarrangement of the muscle layers. Van Gieson, × 16.8

With noncontact irradiation at a distance of more than 1 mm, the power density of the laser pulse diminished by its divergence to the extent that breakdown did not occur and therefore no adverse effects were seen.

Direct tissue contact of the 200-µm fiber without pressure did not always lead to breakdown. Pulse energies below the plasma threshold (i.e. < 35 mJ) showed only minor mechanical effects. Even at fragmentation energy levels, plasma formation was only observed at every third to fifth pulse; in these cases macroscopic bleeding always occurred. Histology showed epithelial loss and extensive suburothelial bleeding.

Direct contact of the fiber with tissue under the slightest pressure caused the fine fiber tip to penetrate or perforate the muscular layers of the organ. Irradiation al-

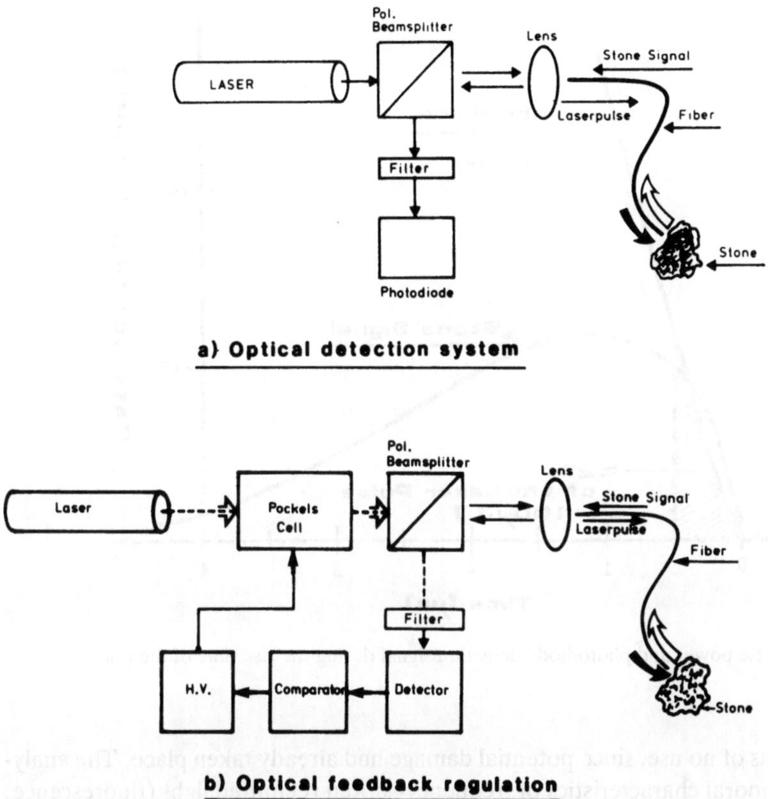

Fig. 6a, b. Experimental setup for passive optical stone detection (**a**) and for an active optical feedback regulation of the laser pulse (**b**)

ways led to macroscopic bleeding even though plasma formation did not take place with every pulse. Once a plasma did form, and an extensive, transmural hematoma occurred, appearing as a large subserosal hematoma (Fig. 3). In several cases, a single breakdown resulted in a minute perforation clearly not caused mechanically by the fiber itself (Fig. 4).

Histological examination at 4 weeks in these cases always showed patches of fibrosis within the muscular layers (Fig. 5).

Optical Feedback Regulation

The alarming results of our animal experiments led us to devise a system that can detect fiber contact with a calculus before the plasma threshold is reached and that can switch off the laser pulse if no stone is detected.

A single 200-µm quartz fiber was used to transmit laser energy to the target and to guide light back to a detection system. The reemitted light was coupled out of the optical axis of the laser by a polarizing beam splitter. By using intracavity polarization only a minor percentage of laser energy was lost and approximately 50% of the reemitted light could be diverted to the detection system. Analysis of the plasma

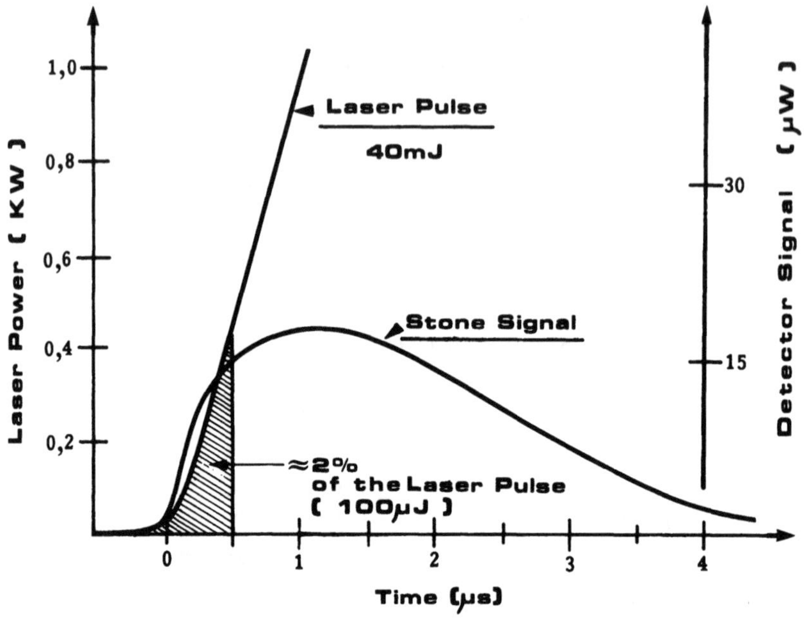

Fig. 7. Laser pulse power and photodiode detection signal during the rise time of the pulse

flash itself was of no use, since potential damage had already taken place. The analysis of the temporal characteristics of frequency-shifted reemitted light (fluorescence, scattering, black body radiation) was a more sensitive method and was possible at power densities well below the breakdown threshold. Using only the first part of a laser pulse at the fragmentation threshold we analyzed the reemitted light during the rise time of the laser pulse to determine the target in front of the fiber tip (Engelhardt et al. 1988a).

The temporal progress of the detection signal is registered (Fig. 6a) by a fast photodiode at a wavelength greater than 750 nm after passing filters (long pass interference filter 750 nm, negative interference filter).

Figure 7 shows power versus time of a 40 mJ laser pulse with a mean duration of 2 µs. Within the first 0.5 µs the pulse only reaches a power of about 400 watts. The resulting power density at the end of a 200 µm fiber is far below the breakdown threshold.

The temporal progress of detection signals of different targets using a 40 mJ laser pulse at 590 nm is shown in Fig. 8.

The upper half of the figure demonstrates the laser pulse, the lower half shows typical signals at different distances of the fiber tip from a Struvit stone and for a breakdown of tissue (dotted line). In this experimental arrangement a signal additional to the plasma flash is typically seen only if a stone and not tissue is in the vicinity of the fiber tip. The physical origin of the reemitted light during the first 0.5 µs of the pulse is not yet known.

The characteristic diagnostic return signal has been utilized for two different and complementary mechanisms to facilitate clinical lasertripsy and avoid potential tissue

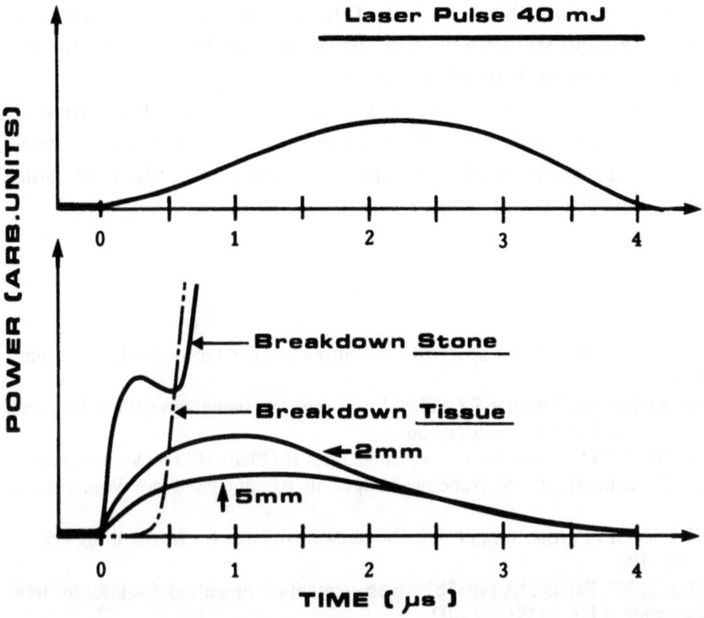

Fig. 8. Characteristic diagnostic return signals registered by the photodiode at different fiberstone distances *(solid line)* and of a breakdown of tissue *(dotted line)* compared with the temporal progress of a 40-mJ laser pulse.

damage (Engelhardt et al. 1988b). The first is passive, monitoring the distance of the fiber tip to the stone by generating an acoustic signal, in which the tone rises in proportion to the registered photodiode signal at t = 0.3 μs. This gives the surgeon additional information, since the resolution of thin caliber endoscopes often does not allow definite controlled positioning of the fiber.

The second mechanism is active and conceived to rule out tissue damage altogether. If the photodiode signal at t = 0.3 μs does not reach a certain threshold, the laser pulse is interrupted by an optical switch (Pockels cell) (Fig. 6b). The tissue will then only be exposed to about 20% of the maximum pulse energy (≈ 10 mJ), which is far below the breakdown threshold for both stone and tissue.

Both feedback mechanisms are unproblematical under clinical conditions. Their reliability and the biological effects of interrupted pulses are currently being tested in animal experiments before first clinical trials are undertaken.

Discussion

The use of microsecond laser pulses in lasertripsy offer the great advantage of very thin and highly flexible application systems. Potential tissue damage necessitates optical control of the lithotripsy progress by ureteroscopic instrumentation of the ureter. Even though small caliber instruments are sufficient to pass a 200-μm core fiber, the traumatic aspect of ureteroscopy is well-known. A controversial question still remains to be answered: Does the reduction of the ureteroscope diameter, from 11.5 F, which will allow a rigid sonotrode probe to be passed, to 7.2 F, justify the additional expenditure and technical problems of a lasertripsy system?

The optical feedback regulation by pulse interruption is a significant step forward in the development of a blind lasertriptor. Clinical evaluation will demonstrate its capability and determine the position of lasertripsy in comparison with such established and inexpensive methods as ultrasonic lithotripsy.

References

Engelhardt R, Meyer W, Hering P (1988a) Spectroscopy during laser-induced shock wave lithotripsy. SPIE Proc 906

Engelhardt R, Meyer W, Oehlert P, Thomas S (1988b) Laser-induced shock wave lithotripsy with microsecond pulses. Laser and Optronics 20(4):36–39

Thomas S, Pensel J, Oehlert P, Baretton G, Meyer W, Engelhardt R (1988) Mikrosekundenpulse in der Laserlithotripsy: Brauchbarkeit und Nebenwirkungen in Abhängigkeit der Wellenlänge. Laser 2:36–42

Watson G, Murray S, Dretler SP, Parrish JA (1987a) The pulsed dye laser for fragmenting urinary calculi. J Urol 138:195–198

Watson G, Murray S, Dretler SP, Parrish JA (1987b) An assessment of the pulsed dye laser for fragmentation in the pig ureter. J Urol 138:199–202

Technical Development, Biologic Effects, and Clinical Application of Laser-Induced Shock Wave Lithotripsy

R. Hofmann[1], R. Hartung[1], H. Schmidt-Kloiber[2], and E. Reichel[2]

Introduction

Extracorporeal shock wave lithotripsy (ESWL) provides a noninvasive treatment for most of the renal and ureteric calculi (70%–80%). ESWL has brought a tremendous change in the management of patients with urinary stones. Patient morbidity is lessened compared with other methods of stone removal and only 10%–20% of all patients need subsequent stone particle manipulation by secondary percutaneous or transurethral methods (Lingeman et al. 1987). Impacted or very hard amorphous calculi in the ureter, however, especially when they are not surrounded by fluid for ESWL shock wave coupling to the stone, can only be crushed in situ in about 50%, while the other half needs flushing up to the kidney and disintegration in the kidney pelvis. This procedure has to be done with ureteral catheters or an endoscope, so that direct access to the stone is necessary. Disintegration of ureteral calculi into tiny stone fragments and flushing out of the ureter can be realized with the help of laser-induced shock waves and cavitation, initiated by the so-called laser-induced breakdown (LIB).

Laser energy from a pulsed neodymium-YAG laser (Nd-YAG laser) with a pulse duration in the nanosecond range is changed into mechanical energy as shock waves by creation of a localized plasma.

A high intensity Nd-YAG laser was developed for intracorporeal laser-induced shock wave lithotripsy (LISL) of ureteral and kidney calculi.

Physical and Technical Aspects of Laser Induced Shock Wave Lithotripsy

Laser-induced shock waves with an extremely steep shock wave front and a high pressure amplitude are generated by localized optomechanic energy conversion from a Q-switched nanosecond pulsed Nd-YAG laser (Hofmann and Schütz 1984; Schmidt-Kloiber et al. 1985). At the interface between the surface of the calculus and the surrounding liquid, an electrical breakdown – LIB – is created by increasing the power density of the laser beam. At the focus part of the fluid vaporizes, and a tiny plasma-filled bubble is generated. By expansion and attenuation of this localized plasma, a shock wave front is emitted and propagated in the medium. Expansion and cooling of the plasma results in an oscillating plasma bubble, which causes cavitation in a liquid. The threshold intensities of these liquids for LIB lie apart from the threshold energy in the stone material or in the optical quartz fibers. This results in two advantages: operational independence from stone properties and hence from its composition and great security in guiding laser pulses through optical fibers.

[1] Dept. of Urology, Technische Universität München, Klinikum re. d. Isar, Munich, 8000 Munich, FRG
[2] Dept. of Experimental Physics, Karl-Franzens-Universität, Graz, Austria

Investigative Urology 3
Edited by H. Rübben et al.

With a Nd-YAG laser of 1064 nm, 8-ns pulse duration, and a single pulse energy of 20–80 mJ, shock waves can be created with peak pressures of 1000–10000 bar in less than 4 ns. This is some what higher pressure as compared with the maximum pressure at the second focus spot in ESWL lithotriptors (200–1300 bar) (Begun et al. 1987).

Shock waves reaching an area with different sound wave impedance – e.g., urinary calculi – are partly reflected. At the front of the calculus compressive, and at the rear tensile pressure is generated with consecutive disintegration of the stone.

The combination of the extremely short discharge time of the pulse with plasma formation and cavitational effects results in a small temperature rise around the LIB. The medium applied energy is at maximum several watts, so that in practice no thermic effects are involved. The interval between two short term pulses is so high (50 Hz repetition rate, 8 ns pulse duration) that thermic effects due to a series of pulses can be ruled out. The ratio of a nanosecond pulse (8×10^{-9} s) to 50 Hz repetition rate (50 pulses/s) – as applied in our laser system – would equal in a more comprehensive, enlarged scale a pulse of 1-s duration followed by a pause of 28.9 days. This comparison enlightens the laser principle using an extremely short pulse with a steep high intensity shock wave followed by a comparably long pause.

For intracorporeal application of the LIB, the laser energy has to be transmitted through small, preferably highly flexible fibers. Therefore, the mean energy density has to be chosen so small that no LIB can occur within the light guide, but high enough that an LIB is generated at the exit side of the fiber (30–70 mJ). Coupling of the Q-switched laser energy into a 600-, 400-, or 200-µm quartz fiber was performed by a specially designed tube into the plane end of the fiber. Focussing of the laser pulses at the fiber tip was achieved by a unique, optically shaped fiber end.

Optimal stone disintegration is performed within the LIB seen at the fiber tip as a light cone, resulting in an elongated, irregular pressure field. Fragmentation also can be heard as a series of slightly clicking sounds.

Influence of Irrigation Solutions and Laser Pulse Energy on Stone Fragmentation

Optimal parameters for intracorporeal LISL have been found to be 8-ns pulse duration, 50 Hz repetition rate, and 50 mJ single pulse energy (600 µm fiber). Constant irrigation and drainage of stone powder is mandatory to keep vision and efficacy of the laser treatment optimal.

Increasing the concentration of sodium chloride (1.4% compared with 0.9%) results in an increased efficacy of LISL, while two solutions-magnesium chloride and iron-dextran complex – improve laser-induced shock wave pressure about 10-fold. In particular, 1 mg/l Fe^{3+} proved to be optimal. The effect of metallic solutions on the LIB in liquids is not fully understood so far; however, a self-focussing effect of the laser beam in a metallic solution can be assumed. The already focussed laser beam with high peak pressures can thus be intensified even more, creating a smaller focus and smaller stone fragments. The stone particles created are all smaller than 1 mm or even stone powder, while the most frequent size of voided particles using an extracorporeal unit is 0.8–1.5 mm with usually one fragment being 1.4–2.0 mm. In ESWL even larger fragments are encountered with hard stones such as uric acid or calcium-oxalate monohydrate (Riehle et al. 1987).

Biologic Effects of Laser Irradiation

Biologic effects of laser irradiation were evaluated by irradiation of cell cultures, whole blood, and urothelium of bladder, ureter, and kidney parenchyma (Hofmann et al. 1988). Laser light from a Nd-YAG laser (8-ns pulse duration) was irradiated onto the tissue surface either as a single pulse or a pulse series of 20 Hz. Single pulse energy ranged from 50–120 mJ and was up to four times higher as compared with patient application. Focussing of the laser pulses onto the tissue was performed by a small apparatus, built of a biconvex lens in a cylindrical tube and a fixed-up plexiglas cone. The length of the plexiglas cone was designed in such a way that focussed laser pulses hit the tissue surface when the device was set upon the tissue.

Irradiation of Tissue Cultures. Irradiation of tissue cultures was performed (fibroblasts, allogeneic renal cancer cells). Pulse energy varied from 50 to 84 mJ with up to 600 focussed pulses. Only directly hit cells in the focus were destroyed and flushed off the glass during irradiation, while all cells surrounding the focus were vital and grew further in the culture.

Irradiation of Whole Blood. Irradiation of whole blood was performed focussing the laser beam into a flask filled with 20 ml whole blood. No significant hemolysis after laser exposure for up to 15 min was generated.

Irradiation of Live Tissue. Kidney, ureter, and urinary bladder in pigs were exposed transperitoneally. The ureter and the bladder were opened, the lumen held open with threads, and the urothelium irradiated.

Urothelium was exposed to focussed irradiation in three pigs to study the immediate effects of the laser beam. Laser energy varied from 50 to 84 mJ with 20 pulses for evaluation of the depth of the lesion. These animals were killed immediately following irradiation. The exposed areas were enclosed by nonresorbable threads for easier macroscopic and microscopic identification of the lesion. Macroscopically, the area of irradiation could be found sometimes as a tiny point in the urothelium. Four of 18 tissue sections showed a small "ruptured cone" with a maximum depth of 40 μm, while no thermic lesion could be found with serial cuts of 5 μm in the defined area. The electron micrograph revealed a conelike defect of about 40–50 μm depth and 100 μm width (Figs. 1, 2).

Late effects were studied in another four pigs with irradiation of 60 or 80 mJ single pulse energy for 10 and 30 s and 30 mJ for 10 and 30 s. The exposed area was examined 2, 4, 8, and 12 days later. Histologic evaluation was performed using elastica-van Gieson and elastica-Ladewig staining as well as electron microscopy.

No macroscopic lesions could be seen on the pig urothelium. Serial cuts (5 μm) showed no histologic change, especially no thermic damage, necrosis, or hemorrhage. Electron microscopy also did not reveal any tissue alteration.

Biologic effects on the urothelium are limited to a tiny mechanical rupture (100 μm width, 40 μm depth) of the tissue without creating thermic effects or a hole through the ureteral wall. This mechanic effect of the shock wave is still confined to the urothelial mucosa. Inadvertent laser irradiation of the urothelium during LISL in patients therefore does not cause any side effects or harm.

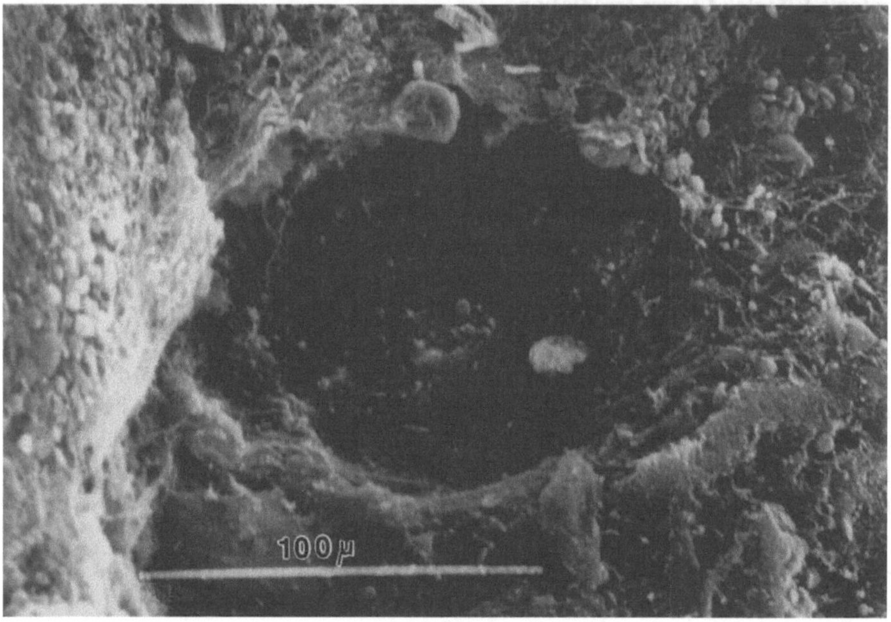

Fig. 1. Electron micrograph of the ureter immediately after laser application (60 mJ, 20 pulses), × 600. Note scale: the cone is about 100 µm wide and 40 µm deep

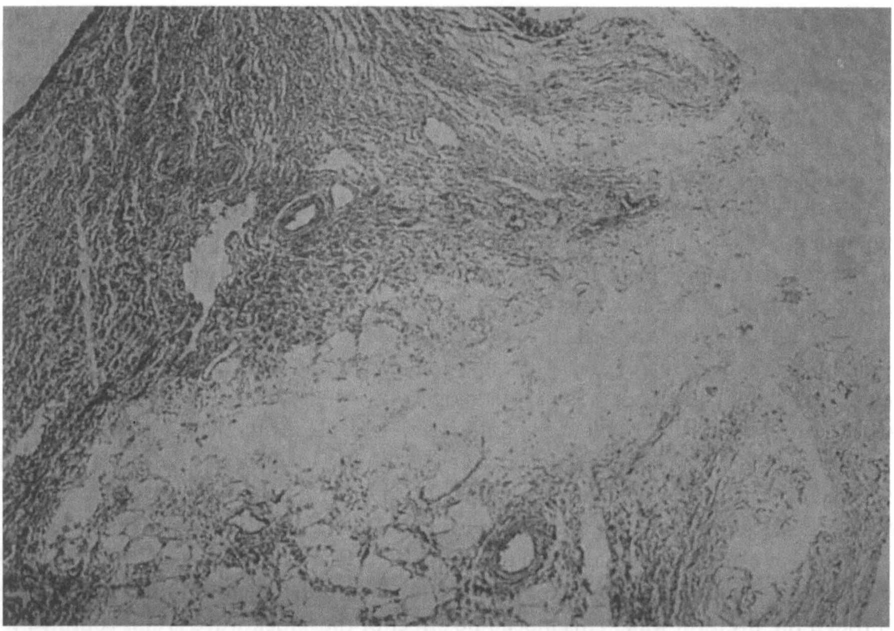

Fig. 2. Kidney parenchyma after focussed Nd-YAG laser irradiation (60 mJ, 20 pulses, 8 ns). Maximum depth of the mechanic rupture cone is 40 µm. No thermic effects are involved

Genetic Effects. Possible mutagenic effects of the Nd-YAG irradiation of 1064 nm wave length was evaluated by irradiation of Chinese hamster ovarian cells (CHO cells), human fibroblasts, and leukocytes. Sister chromatid exchange and chromosomal breaks were not significantly increased following laser application, thus ruling out mutagenic effects of this laser quality.

Clinical Application

Patients and Stone Localization. A total of 61 patients with 63 calculi have been treated. Only stones which did not pass spontaneously out of the ureter after at least 4 weeks' conservative treatment, obstructive ureteral stones, and ureteral and kidney stones not suitable for ESWL treatment or those which failed ESWL fragmentation were selected. Of 61 ureteric stones 40 were obstructing the ureter with consecutive upper urinary tract dilatation. Two stones were in the kidney pelvis, another two in a calix. The ureteric stones had been impacted for an average of 2.5 months (1–48 months). Stone size varied from 3 × 5 mm to 8 × 35 mm. Forty-three patients had general anesthesia; 14 ureteral and all 4 kidney stones were fragmented under local anesthesia.

Endoscopy. An 11.6 or 9 F ureteroscope was inserted into the bladder and advanced directly into the ureter in 14 patients. In another 47 patients a flexible 4 F ureteral catheter was passed into the ureteral orifice and to the stone. In front of the orifice, the endoscope was turned 180° and advanced into the ureter by constant retorsion of the instrument. The ureteral stent was used as a protection of the roof of the ureteral orifice and as a guide to the stone.

Intraoperative Stone Disintegration and Irrigation. During laser stone disintegration sufficient irrigation is essential as stone powder impairs the efficacy of LISL. Especially in obstructing ureteric calculi, good irrigation and drainage is mandatory, as the irrigation fluid is blurred earlier. The focussed shock waves of the laser do not propel the calculus in the ureter; however, vigorous inflow of the irrigation fluid can flush up the stone, particularly when the calculus has been partly fragmented. In seven patients with nearly obstructing stones with an dilated upper urinary tract, a 3 F Dormia basket was passed along the stone, the stone fixed in the basket and then fragmented by the laser beam. In three obstructing stones the calculus was first partly disintegrated by LISL, the residual concrement fixed within the Dormia basket and then disintegrated.

The 600- or 400 µm fiber was directly advanced in the ureteroscope. LISL was done under constant vision, using an irrigation solution (saline or iron-III-dextran solution, 1 mg/l). The calculus was brought into the focus of the laser with the help of a red helium-neon pilot laser and the stone fragmented with 30–70 mJ single pulse energy at the fiber tip, 20–50 Hz repetition rate and 8 ns pulse duration.

Results

From June 1987 to May 1988 61 patients with 63 ureteral stones underwent laser stone fragmentation. In 52 patients the stone was disintegrated completely into very

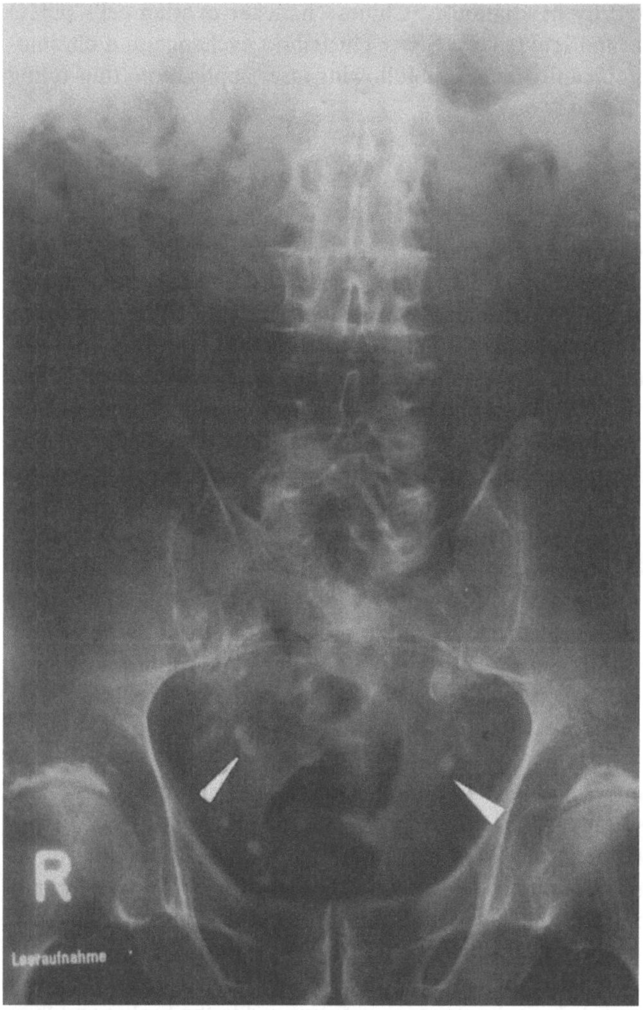

Fig. 3. Bilateral prevesical stones in a 66-year-old man

tiny particles, which were flushed out through the ureteroscope. In 6 patients with ureteral calculi the stone was reduced to a size small enough to be taken out by forceps together with the ureteroscope, as the small residual stones tend to move up in the ureter. These 58 stones were composed to amorphous calcium oxalate monohydrate ($n = 28$), crystalline ca-ox-dihydrate ($n = 19$), struvite ($n = 4$), and uric acid ($n = 7$). Five stones of amorphous calcium oxalate monohydrate were too hard to be completely disintegrated by the laser within reasonable time despite a single pulse energy of 60–70 mJ. Two calculi were further fragmented by ultrasound, also after a considerably long time (30 min), and the stone parts removed by a basket or forceps. Three stones were flushed up to the kidney and taken out percutaneously.

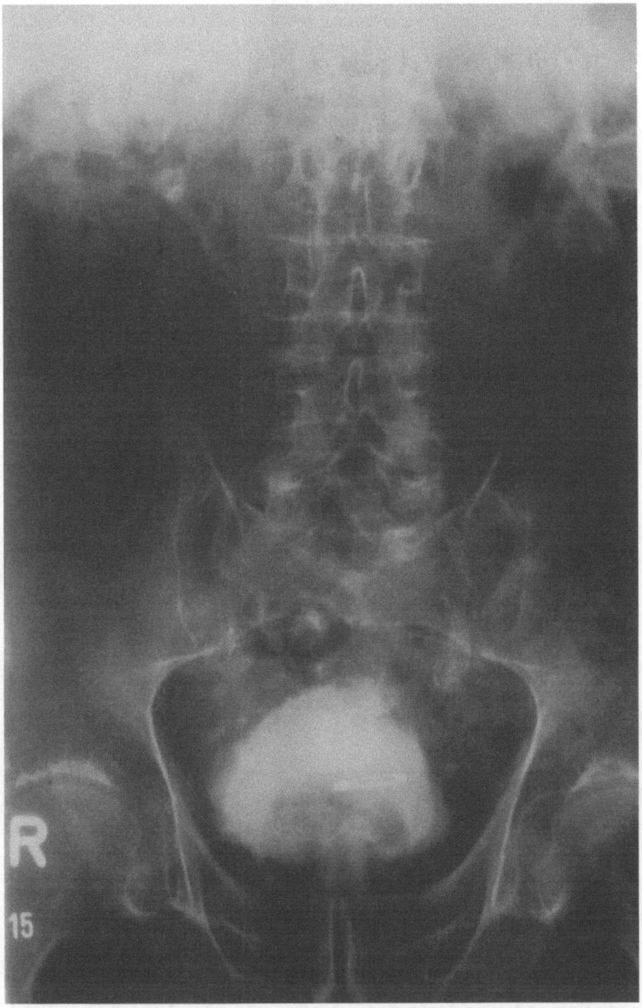

Fig. 4. IVP showing extremely delayed excretion of contrast medium (120 min) with hydronephrosis on the right side

In six patients a suction tube for the stone powder was used, but this procedure was given up, as sucking off the tiny stone particles (size less than 0.5 mm) was considered unnecessary. Stone disintegration under constant vision using only inflow of an irrigation solution was sufficient. Tiny stone particles or blurred liquid was flushed away by constant inflow and eventually drained out through the outflow of the ureteroscope.

LISL was performed within 20 s to 5 min irradiation time (1000–15000 pulses). The total operation time for the first ten patients was 36.7 min, which was reduced to 19.9 min for the following patients due to increasing operative experience with LISL. One fibre could be used for an average of 3.4 stone fragmentations. Fiber damage at

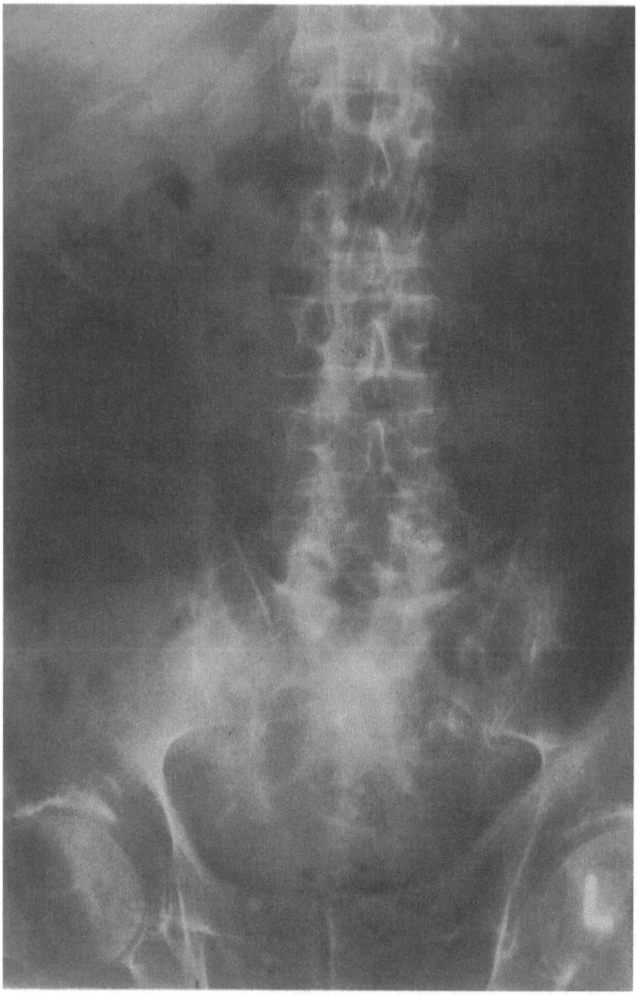

Fig. 5. KUB film after laser irradiation on both sides in one operation under local anesthesia. Total laser application time is 5 min

the tip depends on the energy used and the operative skill. Laser energy can increase all the way to 70 mJ/pulse. At high energy, the probability of an LIB in the fiber itself is increased, however laser energy of up to 50 mJ at the fiber tip does not damage the end; if fiber damage does happen, it is mainly caused by little cracks in the polished fiber tip resulting from stone particles. No harm was done to the ureteral wall by inadvertent laser irradiation in two cases or the manipulation with the ureteroscope or the laser fiber itself.

All patients were free of stones immediately following LISL, proven by plain X-ray film postoperatively and an IVP some weeks later. No ureteral stricture was found. All patients were left free of an ureteral stent postoperatively. No patient developed hydronephrosis, which could have made temporary stenting of the ureter

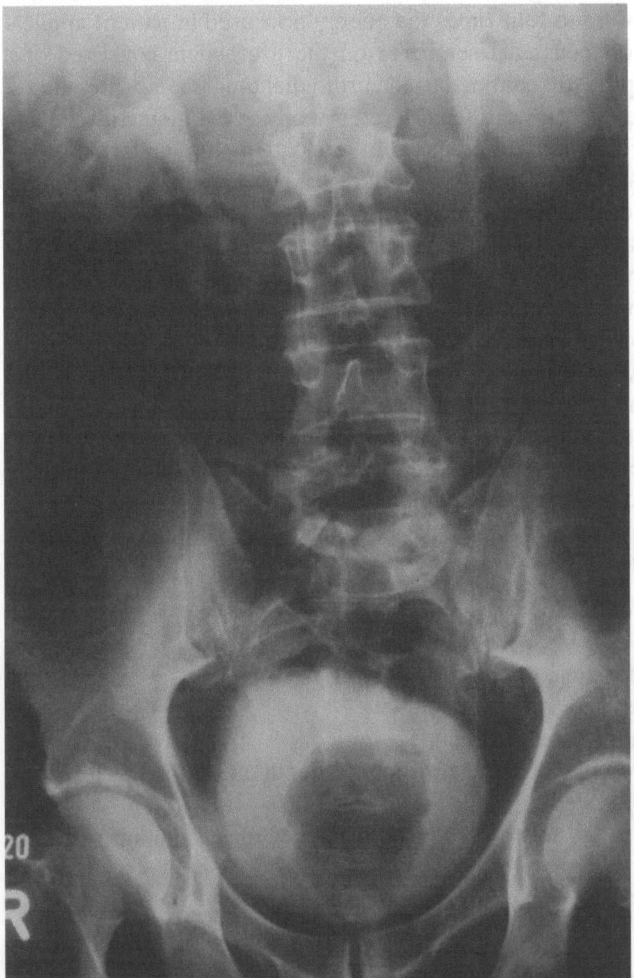

Fig. 6. IVP 2 months after laser stone disintegration. Note normal function of both kidneys compared with preoperative IVP

necessary. Four stones in the ureter were flushed up during LISL due to the inflow of the irrigation solution. Three calculi were fragmented still in the ureter, while one stone was extracted percutaneously (Figs. 3–6).

Discussion

Q-switched laser pulses from a Nd-YAG laser disintegrate calculi by transformation of laser energy into mechanical energy as shock waves. Laser energy with nanosecond pulses can be coupled into currently available 200-, 400-, or 600-μm quartz fibers with a maximum single pulse energy of up to 70 mJ (600 μm fiber).

Extensive animal studies using this laser type did not reveal any serious tissue damage with an energy of up to four times the energy now used in patient application. Immediate effects of focussed laser beam on the urothelium consisted of a craterlike hole (40 μm depth) still confined to the urothelial mucosa. No late effects, especially no thermic side effects, were seen. Ureteroscopy at the moment seems to be the most critical part of ureterolitholapaxy. In our patients no dilatation of the ureteral orifice was necessary as the instrument could be advanced to the stone passing the orifice with a torsion of the endoscope.

Laser stone fragmentation proved to be effective in all but five stones. Optimal conditions for stone disintegration with the Nd-YAG laser of 1064 nm wavelength were recorded with 8 ns pulse duration, 37–70 mJ single pulse energy, and 40–50 Hz repetition rate. Stone powder or particles created were so tiny (less than 0.5 mm) that they were flushed out of the ureter during the operation. Short contact of the fiber tip to the stone or the spray of fragments does not damage the fiber, while constant laser application with stone contact results in cracks of the fiber surface. The highly flexible quartz fiber, however, can be easily changed during the operation by removing the plug-formed end from the coupling device.

Optimization of all physical and clinical parameters lead to a laser system featuring the following properties:

1. No irritation of the eyes because of the use of infrared light
2. Tiny stone fragments
3. Easily interchangeable optical fibers
4. No stone contact necessary
5. Low cost and stable laser systems available
6. Insertion of the ureteroscope only once without frequent use of forceps for stone fragments ("one-step" procedure)
7. Small focussed pressure at the stone reduced incidence of flushing up stones in the ureter
8. No harm to the urothelium
9. No mutagenic effects

Just recently photofragmention with a flash-lamp pumped dye laser has been introduced (Watson et al. 1987). This laser works by absorption of laser energy directly in the calculus with 1 μsec pulse duration, up to 60 mJ single pulse energy, and 10 Hz repetition rate. Nanosecond laser pulses in our system act by cavitation and shock waves by inducing an LIB in a liquid and cavitation. Using the YAG laser, the liquid surrounding the stone acts in transforming the laser energy into mechanical energy. With the dye laser, the calculus itself is used as the energy converter, thus being dependent on the composition and color of the stone. The flexible quartz fibers used for LISL allow miniaturization of rigid instruments and application with small flexible probes. The laser action allows controlled fragmentation of the calculus, so that no additional measures such as removal of stone particles with forceps or basket are necessary.

Indications for LISL are ureteric calculi not suitable for ESWL or those which failed ESWL fragmentation, obstructing ureteric calculi with LISL as a primary therapy without percutaneous nephrostomy, "steinstrasse", and if there is no ESWL system operational.

Effective and secure stone disintegration with small flexible laser fibers has proved to be a prerequisite for application with flexible endoscopes, so far only used as diagnostic instruments. Flexible ureteroscopy in combination with laser stone disintegration implies the possibility of an atraumatic, one-step procedure for fragmentation of ureteral and kidney calculi without general anesthesia.

References

Begun FP, Jacobs SC, Lawson RK (1987) Shock wave lithotriptor pressure field analysis. Pres AUA Annual Meeting Anaheim, CA

Hofmann R, Schütz W (1984) Zerstörung von Harnsteinen durch Laserstrahlung. Urologe [Ausg A] 23:181–184

Hofmann R, Hartung R, Geissdörfer K, Ascherl R, Erhardt W, Schmidt-Kloiber H, Reichel E (1988) Laser induced shock wave lithotripsy-biologic effects of nanosecond pulses. J Urol 139: 1077–1079

Lingeman JE, Coury TA, Newman DM, Kahnoski RJ (1987) Comparison of results and morbidity of percutaneous nephrostolithotomy and extracorporeal shock wave lithotripsy. J Urol 138: 485–490

Riehle RA, Carter HB, Vaughn ED (1987) Quantitative and crystallographic analysis of stone fragments voided after extracorporeal shock wave lithotripsy. J Endourol 1:37–44

Schmidt-Kloiber H, Reichel E, Schöffmann H (1985) Laser induced shock wave lithotripsy (LISL). Biomed Technik 30:173–181

Watson G, Murray S, Dretler StP, Parrish JA (1987) The pulsed dye laser for fragmenting urinary calculi. J Urol 138:195–198

Subject Index

MIX
Papier aus verantwortungsvollen Quellen
Paper from responsible sources
FSC® C105338

If you have any concerns about our products,
you can contact us on
ProductSafety@springernature.com

In case Publisher is established outside the EU,
the EU authorized representative is:
Springer Nature Customer Service Center GmbH
Europaplatz 3, 69115 Heidelberg, Germany

Printed by Libri Plureos GmbH
in Hamburg, Germany